Auditory Brainstem Implants

Eric P. Wilkinson, MD, FACS
Surgeon and Associate
House Ear Clinic
House Institute
Los Angeles, California, USA

Marc S. Schwartz, MD
Clinical Professor of Neurosurgery
University of California San Diego
San Diego, California, USA

148 illustrations

Thieme
New York • Stuttgart • Delhi • Rio de Janeiro

Library of Congress Cataloging-in-Publication Data is available from the publisher.

Thieme Publishers New York
333 Seventh Avenue, New York, NY 10001, USA
+1-800-782-3488, customerservice@thieme.com

Georg Thieme Verlag KG,
Rüdigerstrasse 14, 70469 Stuttgart, Germany
+49 [0]711 8931 421, customerservice@thieme.de

Thieme Publishers Delhi
A-12, Second Floor, Sector-2, Noida-201301
Uttar Pradesh, India
+91 120 45 566 00, customerservice@thieme.in

Thieme Publishers Rio,
Thieme Publicações Ltda.
Edifício Rodolpho de Paoli, 25º andar
Av. Nilo Peçanha, 50 – Sala 2508
Rio de Janeiro 20020-906 Brasil
+55 21 3172 2297 / +55 21 3172 1896

Cover design: Thieme Publishing Group
Typesetting by TNQ Technologies, India

Printed in USA by King Printing Company, Inc.   5 4 3 2 1

ISBN 978-1-62623-826-8

Also available as e-book:
eISBN 978-1-62623-827-5

Important note: Medicine is an ever-changing science undergoing continual development. Research and clinical experience are continually expanding our knowledge, in particular our knowledge of proper treatment and drug therapy. Insofar as this book mentions any dosage or application, readers may rest assured that the authors, editors, and publishers have made every effort to ensure that such references are in accordance with **the state of knowledge at the time of production of the book**.

Nevertheless, this does not involve, imply, or express any guarantee or responsibility on the part of the publishers in respect to any dosage instructions and forms of applications stated in the book. **Every user is requested to examine carefully** the manufacturers' leaflets accompanying each drug and to check, if necessary in consultation with a physician or specialist, whether the dosage schedules mentioned therein or the contraindications stated by the manufacturers differ from the statements made in the present book. Such examination is particularly important with drugs that are either rarely used or have been newly released on the market. Every dosage schedule or every form of application used is entirely at the user's own risk and responsibility. The authors and publishers request every user to report to the publishers any discrepancies or inaccuracies noticed. If errors in this work are found after publication, errata will be posted at www.thieme.com on the product description page.

Some of the product names, patents, and registered designs referred to in this book are in fact registered trademarks or proprietary names even though specific reference to this fact is not always made in the text. Therefore, the appearance of a name without designation as proprietary is not to be construed as a representation by the publisher that it is in the public domain.

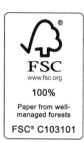

FSC
www.fsc.org
100%
Paper from well-managed forests
FSC® C103101

Contents

13 Programming, Rehabilitation, and Outcome Assessment for Adults: II 83
Cordula Matthies, Anja Kurz, and Wafaa Shehata-Dieler

14 Outcomes in Pediatric ABI: The Hacettepe University Experience 95
Levent Sennaroğlu, Gonca Sennaroğlu, Esra Yucel, and Burçak Bilginer

15 Auditory Brainstem Implantation in Tone Language Speakers 102
Michael C.F. Tong, John Ka Keung Sung, and Kathy Y.S. Lee

Preface

The auditory brainstem implant (ABI), through the course of its development, has brought together surgeons, audiologists, engineers, auditory physiologists, and researchers in psychoacoustics.

Although a very specialized and narrow topic, ABI development has involved clinicians and scientists working together. Those with interest in ABI are from a broad range of fields: audiologists, otolaryngologists, neurosurgeons, oncologists, speech therapists, neurophysiologists, social workers, educational specialists, engineers, and implant manufacturers. This textbook is designed to be suitable for all personnel working with the clinical and research application of ABI, both in adults and children. It is an effort to bring together materials and resources regarding ABI under one cover, with sensitivity to the fact that prospective readers may bring various levels of expertise in individual topics.

The ABI is a triumph of translational research. It was initially developed somewhat serendipitously: Surgeons recognized that the cochlear nucleus is directly in the surgical field during resection of neurofibromatosis type 2-associated acoustic tumors and it might respond to direct stimulation. After several iterations, today's devices capitalize on existing cochlear implant (CI) receiver-stimulator technology and apply it to the central auditory system. The ABI shows the benefit that can be derived from technology—the ability to convey auditory information electrically to the central nervous system—while also highlighting its limitations— a relatively small population of recipients who can understand open-set speech information. It shows how technology developed for one indication (neurofibromatosis

type 2) can fortuitously assist with other indications (nontumor adults and children with cochlear ossification, cochlear malformations, and cochlear nerve deficiency). The ABI can give insights into common, disabling conditions (e.g., tinnitus), and it can provide research insights into such areas as the central auditory pathways. The chapters in this textbook delve into these topics.

What does the future hold for ABI? In this textbook, the current state of ABI is explored, and future directions are mapped out. Questions regarding how we move forward are many: Should we completely reconsider how we are doing speech processing with ABI? Have conventional CI strategies been inadequate for the central auditory system? Can new electrode technologies (penetrating arrays, contoured paddles) help in creating a better interface between the device and the tissue? What new research areas, such as improved medical imaging and optical stimulation, might assist in improving outcomes? And, finally, how does the narrow topic of cochlear nucleus stimulation relate to the topic of neurostimulation in general?

Those of us in the ABI field continue to apply this technology for the benefit of our patients. We have been generally cautious in its expansion to wider populations, understanding that there are risks involved and that the measurement of benefits is an ongoing process. Although we are cautious, at the same time we understand that there may be preconceptions and assumptions that we need to move beyond.

Eric P. Wilkinson, MD, FACS
Marc S. Schwartz, MD

Contributors

Robert Behr, MD, PhD
Professor and Chairman
Department of Neurosurgery
University Medicine Marburg
Campus Fulda, Hessen, Germany

Ricardo F. Bento, MD, PhD
Chairman and Professor
Department of Otorhinolaryngology
University of São Paulo
São Paulo, Brazil

Burçak Bilginer, MD
Professor
Department of Neurosurgery
Hacettepe University
Ankara, Turkey

Derald E. Brackmann, MD
Surgeon and Associate
House Ear Clinic
House Institute
Los Angeles, California, USA

M. Christian Brown, PhD
Associate Professor
Harvard Medical School
Massachusetts Eye and Ear
Boston, Massachusetts, USA

Giacomo Colletti, MD
Maxillofacial Surgeon
Vascular Birthmarks Foundation
Latham, New York, USA;
Vascular Birthmarks Foundation
Milan, Italy

Liliana Colletti, PhD
Audiologist
ENT Department
University of Milan
Milan, Italy

Vittorio Colletti, MD
Professor
International Center for Performing and Teaching
   Auditory Brainstem Implantation in Children
Milan, Italy

Karl-Heinz Dyballa, PhD
Research Assistant
Department of Otorhinolaryngology
   Head and Neck Surgery
Hannover Medical School (MHH)
Hannover, Germany

Martin Han, PhD
Associate Professor
Biomedical Engineering Department
University of Connecticut
Storrs Mansfield, Connecticut, USA

Lawrence Kashat, MD, MSc
Resident (Otolaryngology)
School of Medicine
Division of Otolaryngology
University of Connecticut
Farmington, Connecticut, USA

Elliott D. Kozin, MD
Otologist/Neurotologist
Massachusetts Eye and Ear
Harvard Medical School
Boston, Massachusetts, USA

Anja Kurz, MA, PhD
Technical Director
Comprehensive Hearing Center (CHC)
Department of Otorhinolaryngology
Würzburg University Hospital
Bavaria, Germany

Daniel J. Lee, MD, FACS
Associate Professor
Harvard Medical School
Massachusetts Eye and Ear
Boston, Massachusetts, USA

Kathy Y.S. Lee, PhD
Associate Professor
Department of Otorhinolaryngology
   Head and Neck Surgery
Institute of Human Communicative Research
The Chinese University of Hong Kong
Shatin, Hong Kong

Gregory P. Lekovic, MD, PhD, FAANS
Chief
Division of Neurosurgery
House Institute
Los Angeles, California, USA

Thomas Lenarz, MD, PhD
Chairman, Professor, and Surgeon
Department of Otorhinolaryngology
    Head and Neck Surgery
Hannover Medical School (MHH)
Hannover, Germany

Hubert H. Lim, PhD
Associate Professor
Department of Biomedical Engineering
Department of Otolaryngology
    Head and Neck Surgery
Institute for Translational Neuroscience
University of Minnesota
Minneapolis, Minnesota, USA

Paula T. Lopes, MD
Assistant Physician
Department of Otorhinolaryngology
University of São Paulo
São Paulo, Brazil

Marco Mandalà, MD, PhD
Head of Department
Otolaryngology Department
University of Siena
Siena, Italy

Cordula Matthies, MD, PhD
Professor of Neurosurgery
Vice Clinic Director
Department of Neurosurgery
Director
Functional Neurosurgery
Würzburg University Hospital
Bavaria, Germany

Douglas B. McCreery, PhD
Scientist Emeritus
Neural Engineering Program
Huntington Medical Research Institutes
Pasadena, California, USA

Mia E. Miller, MD
Surgeon and Associate
House Ear Clinic
House Institute
Los Angeles, California, USA

Barry Nevison, DPhil
Clinical and Technical Support Manager
Cochlear Europe Ltd
Addlestone, Surrey, United Kingdom

Kathryn Y. Noonan, MD
Assistant Professor
Department of Otolaryngology
    Head and Neck Surgery
Tufts Medical Center
Boston, Massachusetts, USA

Steven R. Otto, MA
Audiologist Emeritus
House Ear Clinic
House Institute
Los Angeles, California, USA

Burce Ozgen, MD
Associate Professor of Radiology
Department of Radiology
University of Illinois at Chicago
Chicago, Illinois, USA

Kevin A. Peng, MD
Surgeon and Associate
House Ear Clinic
House Institute
Los Angeles, California, USA

Marek Polak, PhD
Head
Electrophysiology for Assessment/Research
    and Development
MED-EL Medical Electronics
Innsbruck, Austria

Daniel S. Roberts, MD, PhD
Assistant Professor
Division of Otolaryngology
School of Medicine
University of Connecticut
Farmington, Connecticut, USA;
Adjunct Faculty
House Institute
Los Angeles, California, USA

Jordan M. Rock, AuD
Audiologist
House Ear Clinic
House Institute
Los Angeles, California, USA

Steffen K. Rosahl, MD, PhD
Professor of Neurosurgery
Albert-Ludwigs-University
Freiburg, Germany;
Chairman
Helios Klinikum
Erfurt, Germany

Amir Samii, MD, PhD
Chairman, Professor, and Surgeon
Department of Neurosurgery
International Neuroscience Institute
Hannover, Germany

Marc S. Schwartz, MD
Clinical Professor of Neurosurgery
University of California San Diego
San Diego, California, USA

Gonca Sennaroğlu, PhD
Professor and Head
Department of Audiology
Hacettepe University
Ankara, Turkey

Levent Sennaroğlu, MD
Professor
Department of Otolaryngology
Hacettepe University
Ankara, Turkey

Wafaa Shehata-Dieler, MD, PhD
Professor (Otolaryngology)
Department of Otorhinolaryngology
  Head and Neck Surgery
and Plastic Aesthetic Surgery;
Medical Director
Audiology and Phoniatrics
Comprehensive Hearing Center (CHC)
Würzburg University Hospital
Bavaria, Germany

John Ka Keung Sung, MD
Clinical Associate Professor (Honorary)
Department of Otorhinolaryngology
  Head and Neck Surgery
Institute of Human Communicative Research
The Chinese University of Hong Kong
Shatin, Hong Kong

Osama Tarabichi, MD
Resident Physician
Department of Otolaryngology
University of Iowa
Iowa City, Iowa, USA

Michael C.F. Tong, MD
Professor and Chairman
Department of Otorhinolaryngology
  Head and Neck Surgery
Institute of Human Communicative Research
The Chinese University of Hong Kong
Shatin, Hong Kong

Eric P. Wilkinson, MD, FACS
Surgeon and Associate
House Ear Clinic
House Institute
Los Angeles, California, USA

Esra Yucel, PhD
Professor
Department of Audiology
Hacettepe University
Ankara, Turkey

1 The History and Development of Auditory Brainstem Implants

Kevin A. Peng and Derald E. Brackmann

Abstract

The auditory brainstem implant (ABI), which was conceived by William F. House at the House Ear Institute in Los Angeles, California in the 1970s, is a device that provides auditory sensation by directly stimulating the cochlear nucleus of the brainstem. By bypassing the cochlea and the cochlear nerve, it has become an invaluable resource for hearing rehabilitation in patients with neurofibromatosis type 2. Additional clinical advances have expanded the use of ABIs to pediatric patients, and additional research may establish other clinical applications.

Keywords: auditory brainstem implant, neurofibromatosis type 2

1.1 Early Work in Stimulation of the Brainstem

The first report of stimulation of the human brainstem was published in 1964. In this study, Simmons et al stimulated the inferior colliculus, but this yielded no sound perception or awareness.[1] Several years elapsed before any significant advances were made. At the House Ear Institute (HEI) in Los Angeles, California, William F. House had begun surgical placement of cochlear implants in the late 1960s. He realized that auditory rehabilitation in patients with no auditory nerves, such as patients with neurofibromatosis type 2, remained unaddressed.

House began to design a device to stimulate the cochlear nucleus of the brainstem directly. He enlisted the assistance of Jean Moore, a neuroanatomist at HEI. Moore mapped out the target area for brainstem implantation. Based on his prior experience with the development of the cochlear implant, House designed an initial device with a two-ball-electrode configuration. This communicated percutaneously with an external receiver.

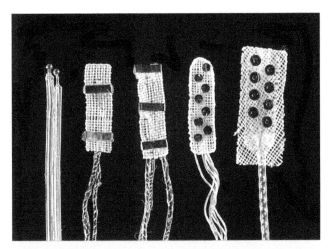

Fig. 1.1 Chronological design of early auditory brainstem implants. Earliest implant with two electrodes (*leftmost*) and prototype of modern multi-channel implant (*rightmost*).

On May 24, 1979, House and William E. Hitselberger operated on a 51-year-old female with a vestibular schwannoma in her only-hearing ear. Following tumor resection, they placed the first auditory brainstem implant (ABI) with the electrode residing next to the cochlear nucleus. This was percutaneously coupled with a modified body-worn Bosch hearing aid. This provided the patient with sound awareness, but by 1980, the patient developed a sensation of "twitching" in the ipsilateral leg. The electrode was deemed to have migrated. The patient continued to use the ABI and external processor until her death in her late 80s.

In conjunction with Douglas McCreery of the Huntington Medical Research Institute (HMRI), House designed a new electrode with a Dacron mesh backing, to which an increasing number of electrodes was later added (▶ Fig. 1.1). This mesh was designed to provide increased stability of the electrode after implantation. In 1981, the original subject underwent a second surgery. The prior electrode was removed, and the new Dacron mesh electrode was placed on the surface of the brainstem. This ABI allowed once again for auditory sensation, and was paired several years later with a House-Sigma single-channel cochlear implant processor. The patient continues to use the ABI and external processor to this day.[2] A seminal paper by Edgerton et al later summarized the preliminary efforts and physiology of direct stimulation of the cochlear nucleus.[3]

1.2 Auditory Brainstem Response and Advances in Device Manufacturing

In 1982, Michael D. Waring, an audiologist working with HEI, recorded the first electrically evoked auditory brainstem response from the first ABI recipient previously discussed. This provided additional encouragement, and HEI began to construct and evaluate electrode designs for future ABI devices. J. Phil Mobley and Franco Portillo, engineers with HEI, supervised the installation of fabrication facilities at HEI. In 1984, the first implantation of an ABI device fabricated at HEI was performed.

In 1985, three patients underwent ABI placement. Broken wires and electrode migration were both encountered, but nonetheless the implants showed promise. Technical details were described in a subsequent publication by McElveen et al, which confirmed the feasibility of using the ABI for auditory stimulation.[4] In 1986, HEI received investigational device exemption status from the Food and Drug Administration (FDA) to pursue the ABI program.

Another advance came in 1987, when Portillo suggested the use of braided wires rather than single-stranded wires. Braided wires were more flexible and less prone to breakage. Derald E. Brackmann, a neurotologist at HEI, worked with Portillo to improve the reliability and biocompatibility of the percutaneous plug. The same year, Eisenberg et al published the first audiological perspective on the ABI, confirming that ABI recipients experienced tone perception and significant auditory discrimination exceeding what is expected due to chance.[5]

1.3 Development of Modern Processors and Multi-electrode Arrays

House-Sigma cochlear implant processors were adapted for ABIs in 1984. Thereafter, a collaboration between 3M (Maplewood, Minnesota, USA) and HEI led to the development of the Alpha processor, again an improvement over the House-Sigma cochlear implant processors. In 1991, HEI and Cochlear (Sydney, Australia) began to collaborate on developing an eight-electrode array. This was completed in 1992.

Steve R. Otto, a clinical audiologist at HEI, began to provide and refine maps for ABI patients around this time, including performance testing. Meanwhile, the ABI program was clinically spearheaded by Derald E. Brackmann. Research on auditory performance at HEI was overseen by Robert V. Shannon. Clinical trials for the ABI were initiated in the United States in 1993, and the device later gained FDA approval in 2000. Array development had continued during this time, and by the time FDA approval was obtained, the new array contained 21 electrodes paired with Cochlear's nucleus speech processor.[6]

In parallel, MED-EL (Innsbruck, Austria) began to develop a multi-electrode array. Advanced Bionics (Valencia, California, USA) also began work on a proprietary ABI. In 1997, Robert Behr performed the first ABI in Europe at the University of Wurzburg, Germany. This device was a 12-electrode array developed by MED-EL with a speech processor based on the Combi 40 + cochlear implant processor.

1.4 The Penetrating Auditory Brainstem Implant

In the early 2000s, the HEI began work on development of a penetrating electrode for the ABI. This was conceived on the basis of the tonotopic organization of the cochlear nucleus, where low acoustic frequencies were located superficially and high frequencies were located more deeply. The pilot penetrating ABI (PABI) device included eight penetrating electrodes paired with a 12-electrode surface electrode array, and the first PABI was implanted in July 2003. A second-generation device, with two additional penetrating electrodes and a higher allowable charge limit, was first implanted in 2005.

By 2007, nine PABI patients had been implanted. The benefits of the PABI included a lower threshold for stimulation, increased frequency range, and high selectivity. Fewer than 25% of penetrating electrodes resulted in auditory stimulation, while more than 60% of surface electrodes were effective.

PABI patients were evaluated with three different maps: surface electrodes only, penetrating electrodes only, and a combination of the two. Patients with the PABI did not demonstrate improved speech recognition when compared to a cohort of patients implanted with surface electrode devices.[7] As the device was more complex to manufacture and implant than the surface-array-only ABI, further development of the PABI was deferred.

1.5 New Horizons for ABI

In 1999, Vittorio Colletti, of the University of Verona, implanted the first ABI in a pediatric patient with deficient cochlear nerves.[8] He proceeded to implant the ABI in several additional pediatric patients, and some achieved open-set recognition. Pediatric ABI is now being performed at select centers in the United States and elsewhere. Recently, Roberts et al once again described the phenomenon of tinnitus suppression in a subset of ABI patients, a topic that will require further research.[9]

Over the past four decades, the ABI has been established as an invaluable tool for hearing rehabilitation in NF2 patients. Additional research is planned to determine candidacy, identify predictive factors for performance, and expand clinical applications.

Acknowledgments

The authors wish to acknowledge Steve R. Otto, MA, and William M. Luxford, MD, for their invaluable assistance with elucidating the chronology of the development of the ABI.

References

[1] Simmons FB, Mongeon CJ, Lewis WR, Huntington DA. Electrical stimulation of acoustical nerve and inferior colliculus. Arch Otolaryngol. 1964; 79: 559–568

[2] Hitselberger WE, House WF, Edgerton BJ, Whitaker S. Cochlear nucleus implants. Otolaryngol Head Neck Surg. 1984; 92(1):52–54

[3] Edgerton BJ, House WF, Hitselberger W. Hearing by cochlear nucleus stimulation in humans. Ann Otol Rhinol Laryngol Suppl. 1982; 91(2 Pt 3):117–124

[4] McElveen JT, Jr, Hitselberger WE, House WF, Mobley JP, Terr LI. Electrical stimulation of cochlear nucleus in man. Am J Otol. 1985 Suppl:88–91

[5] Eisenberg LS, Maltan AA, Portillo F, Mobley JP, House WF. Electrical stimulation of the auditory brain stem structure in deafened adults. J Rehabil Res Dev. 1987; 24(3):9–22

[6] Shannon RV. Auditory implant research at the House Ear Institute 1989–2013. Hear Res. 2015; 322:57–66

[7] Otto SR, Shannon RV, Wilkinson EP, et al. Audiologic outcomes with the penetrating electrode auditory brainstem implant. Otol Neurotol. 2008; 29 (8):1147–1154

[8] Colletti V, Fiorino FG, Carner M, Miorelli V, Guida M, Colletti L. Auditory brainstem implant as a salvage treatment after unsuccessful cochlear implantation. Otol Neurotol. 2004; 25(4):485–496, discussion 496

[9] Roberts DS, Otto S, Chen B, et al. Tinnitus suppression after auditory brainstem implantation in patients with neurofibromatosis type-2. Otol Neurotol. 2017; 38(1):118–122

2 Neuroanatomy and Physiology Relevant to Auditory Brainstem Implants

Steffen K. Rosahl

Abstract

Placing an electrode for functional restoration of an injured auditory pathway at the base of the brain requires fundamental understanding of anatomical and physiological constraints. The auditory system has been extensively studied in the past. In fact, it is the single most researched human sensory modality. The following chapter attempts to deliver the massive collection of data on anatomy and physiology of the human auditory brainstem system in a comprehensive for anybody who approaches the topic of a neuroelectronic interface to the process and perceive sounds.

Basic aspects of each anatomical structure in and around the brain-stem auditory pathway, focusing on the cochlear nuclei, but also touching the cochlea, the cochlear nerve, and higher auditory nuclei will be discussed.

The chapter serves as a reference for the biological specifics just as much as an inspiration and guide to overcome obstacles in the development of most effective auditory brain-stem implants.

Keywords: auditory brainstem implant, retrosigmoid, semi-sitting position, vestibular schwannoma, neurofibromatosis type 2

2.1 Introduction

It stretches human imagination that in a profoundly deaf person speech perception can be partially re-established by a device implanted by a surgeon that activates fewer than 10 effective electrodes placed over a biological structure containing nearly 30,000 neurons. It is even more astonishing if we consider that these neurons are modulated by multiple other neurons, and that the target region cannot be visually distinguished from surrounding neural structures.

To understand why auditory brainstem implants (ABIs) function at all, we will focus on two major aspects here:
- Why do present ABI actually work?
- How can these neurotechnical interfaces be improved based on what is known about the microanatomy and physiology of the auditory system?

The neural processing of two of the basic physical properties of sound—volume and pitch levels—starts as far peripheral as the cochlea itself. Pitch is transferred from a specific frequency into a spatial location along the hair cells of the basilar membrane and their associated neurons.

The brain deciphers pitch by determining which fibers of the cochlear nerve are maximally active at a given point of time.

Volume or loudness is coded in the cochlea by the firing frequency of these primary sensory neurons. The brain interprets volume as a function of both the number of axons firing and their frequency.

The other function of sound perception, localization, requires bilateral input from both ears, and this function cannot be restored with any unilateral hearing prosthetic.

In this chapter, I will discuss the basic morphological and physiological aspects of each anatomical structure in the brainstem portion of the hearing pathway where the electrodes of current ABIs located as well as the adjacent sites of the hearing pathway (▶ Fig. 2.1). I will delineate opportunities and obstacles for the development of effective ABIs presented by these biological specifics.

2.2 The Cochlea and the Cochlear Nerve

While patients to be implanted with an ABI usually do not have a functional cochlear nerve, it remains important to consider this nerve in order to understand the concept of tonotopy. The cochlear nerve relates cochlear tonotopy to the brainstem. The fibers of the cochlear nerve originate from the nerve cell bodies of the spiral ganglion, in the modiolus of the cochlea. The neurons of the spiral ganglion are the first (of four) order neurons between the cochlea and the cerebrum.

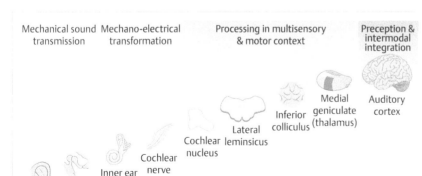

Mechanical sound transmission Mechano-electrical transformation Processing in multisensory & motor context Preception & intermodal integration

Medial geniculate (thalamus) Auditory cortex Inferior colliculus Lateral leminsicus Cochlear nucleus Cochlear nerve Inner ear (cochlea) Middle ear Outer ear

Fig. 2.1 Simplified depiction of the main waypoints of the human auditory system and their basic functional roles.

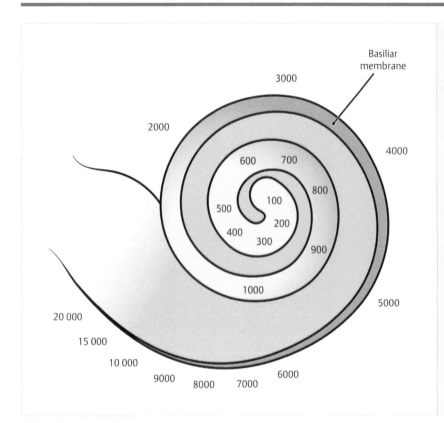

Basiliar membrane

3000

2000

600 700

800

100

500

200

400

300

900

1000

4000

5000

20 000

15 000

10 000

9000 8000 7000 6000

Fig. 2.2 Schematic tonotopic map of sound representation along the basilar membrane in the cochlea. High frequencies (in Hz) are represented at the base of the spiral and low frequencies at the top (= "apex").

The inner and outer hair cells in the spiral organ (of Corti[a]) are the sensory receptor cells for the mechanical impulses that are primarily generated when sounds hit the eardrum and are transmitted via the middle ear structures to the cochlea. A single inner hair cell is innervated by numerous myelinated nerve fibers, whereas a single—unmyelinated—nerve fiber innervates many outer hair cells. A particular region with a number of hair cells which supply input to a particular afferent nerve fiber is considered to be the "receptive field" of this fiber. High frequencies are represented at the base turn of the cochlea while low frequencies have their receptive field at its apex (▶ Fig. 2.2). This arrangement of neurons in the auditory system is "cochleotopic" or "tonotopic."

There are different types of hair cells corresponding to two different types of auditory nerve fibers: *Inner* hair cells convey their signals through type I fibers of the cochlear nerve. Type I fibers are myelinated, constitute 90 to 95% of the fibers in the auditory nerve, and are the primary afferent input to most of the cell types in the cochlear nucleus.[1,2]

Outer hair cells are innervated by type II fibers, which are unmyelinated and project to nonprincipal cell regions of the cochlear nucleus.[3,4] Responses to sound have not been recorded from type II fibers and it is not clear what role they play.[5] Outer hair cells appear to participate in the mechanical response of the basilar membrane; loss of outer hair cells leads to a loss of sensitivity to soft sounds and a decrease in the sharpness of tuning (i.e., the frequency selectivity) of the basilar membrane.

About 95% of the cochlear nerve fibers innervate the inner hair cells. The cochlear nerve trunk exits the modiolus to run into the internal auditory canal (IAC). The peripheral segment of the cochlear nerve joins the vestibular nerve to form the vestibulocochlear nerve (VIII cranial nerve) at the lateral part of the IAC. In cadaver studies, the two portions of the nerve have been found to have a distinct and quite constant spatial relationship: in the IAC the cochlear portion lies anterior to become located inferior to the vestibular nerve in the middle of the nerve and remain there until its entrance into the brainstem.[6] In a magnetic resonance (MR) study, the spatial relationship between the cochlear nerve and the superior portion of the vestibular nerve was more variable. In general, the prevailing—cadaver study based—textbook notion that the three nerves rotate around each other needs to be corrected. It is more accurate to describe the cochlear nerve and inferior vestibular nerve as coursing beneath the superior vestibular nerve in either the IAC or cerebellopontine cistern.[7]

Glial tissue surrounds the nerve in the inner ear canal. Close to its exit, the porus acousticus, the glia encasement changes into by Schwann[b] cells ("Obersteiner-Redlich zone"). It is here where most vestibular schwannomas originate.

The primary terminal of the cochlear nerve is the cochlear nucleus in the medulla oblongata. The length of the vestibulocochlear nerve, from the glial–Schwann junction to the brainstem, is 10 to 13 mm in human males and 7 to 10 mm in females.[8]

[a] Alfonso Giacomo Gaspare Corti, Italian anatomist, 1822–1876.

[b] Theodor Ambrose Hubert Schwann, German anatomist and physiologist, 1810–1882.

The pars cochlearis of the human cochlear nerve contains 32,000 to 41,000 fibers with a diameter of 2 to 3 μm, with nearly all myelinated for fast conduction.[9] The fibers reach the ventral cochlear nucleus (VCN) at its ventromedial surface. At the root entry zone, each axon splits into an ascending and a descending fiber.[10] Ascending fibers run dorsolaterally into the VCN, and descending fibers run caudal and dorsal straight through this portion and diverge into the dorsal cochlear nucleus (DCN). In contrast to other mammals, the human DCN is entirely penetrated by these descending fibers, forming a rather homogeneous plexus with the neurons.[10] Therefore, the DCN in humans does not have a laminar structure as in the cat.[11]

2.3 Cochlear Nuclei

2.3.1 Two Nuclei in One: The Ventral and Dorsal Cochlear Nucleus

Based on histomorphological criteria, one of the pupils of Cajal, Lorente de No, distinguished a compact ventral and a flatter, longer portion of the cochlear nucleus well before more detailed investigations.[12] On the cellular level, this subclassification has been confirmed.[13,14,15,16,17,18]

The intramedullary portion of the cochlear nerve runs through the VCN resulting in secondary, more macroanatomical descriptive division into a "nucleus cochlearis ventralis superior" (NCVS) and "nucleus cochlearis ventralisinferior" (NCVI).[16,19,20,21]

It is important that there are differences in nomenclature between animal and human research because of the spatial orientation of the brainstem: "anterior" in the animal refers to "superior" in the human. The same is true for the pairing of "inferior" and "posterior."

Another histological subdivision of the VCN in the animal into a "pars anteroventralis" and a "pars posteroventralis" is not recognizable in humans due to the curved course of the cochlear nucleus.[18]

2.3.2 Physiology

Animal Research

The cochlear nucleus contains the circuits through which information about sound is coupled to the brain. In the nucleus, fibers of the auditory nerve contact neurons that form multiple, parallel representations of the acoustic environment, each performing a different analysis of the auditory signal.[22] Calculations such as source localization and the identification of a particular sound are separated and performed in parallel as signals travel through the brainstem auditory nuclei.

The modern definitions of the cell types in the cochlear nucleus were developed by Kirsten Osen on the basis of cytoarchitecture in the cat.[23] Incoming auditory nerve fibers bifurcate in the central region of the VCN and send an ascending branch to the anterior division of the VCN and a descending branch to the posterior division of the VCN. The descending branch also curves back to innervate the DCN. To understand the neural ABI interface, it is important to note that the primary terminal of the auditory nerve fibers is the VCN. As we will see below, that is a reason why electrical stimulation with brainstem-penetrating electrodes evoke auditory responses at lower intensities than

stimulation with surface electrodes.[24] The innervation of the cochlear nucleus by auditory nerve fibers reflects the tonotopic organization of the cochlea.

The principal cells in the cochlear nucleus are arranged such that each type receives input from auditory nerve fibers over the whole tonotopic range, that is, each principal cell type carries a separate but complete representation of the sound coming to the ear on that side of the head. In projecting to different targets in the brainstem, the principal cell types form separate, parallel pathways.[5] Innervation by auditory nerve fibers both in the VCN and in the deep layer of the DCN is tonotopically organized. In the cat, low-frequency encoding fibers innervate bands ventrally and high-frequency encoding fibers innervate bands dorsally.

McCreery et al proved that it is possible to access the tonotopic gradient of the cochlear nucleus of the cat by electrical stimulation by measuring evoked potentials in different layers of the inferior colliculus (IC) higher up in the brainstem auditory pathway.[25] It is well known that the IC has a layered tonotopy. These researchers demonstrated the tonotopic order in the cochlear nucleus (CN) by stimulating at different sites along its ventro-dorsal axis. Stimulation at various depth in the CN resulted in electrical activity in specific frequency layers in the IC.[25] This finding was an important motivation to design penetrating electrodes for ABIs.

There are at least five primary cell types in the cochlear nucleus, and each has its own unique pattern of response to sound, consistent with the idea that each type is involved in a different aspect of the analysis of the information in the auditory nerve. The diversity of these patterns can be accounted for by three features that vary among the principal cell types: (1) the pattern of the innervation of the cell by auditory nerve fibers; (2) the electrical properties of the cells that shape synaptic inputs; and (3) the interneuronal circuitry associated with the cell.[5]

Auditory nerve fibers make synapses on most of the cell types in the cochlear nucleus. Their terminals range in size from small boutons to large endbulbs.[26] Release of neurotransmitters like glutamate activates miniature synaptic currents whose time constants of decay are shorter than 1 millisecond. These kinetics are fast for activation, deactivation, and desensitization; in fact, they match the most rapid that have been measured in any neural structures. Conductances of single glutamate receptors on VCN cells average 28 picoseconds. On average 40 to 50 receptors are activated in a miniature synaptic event.[27,28,29] In responding to sounds, mammalian auditory nerve fibers fire up to 300 action potentials/second in vivo.[30] Synaptic transmission in the cochlear nucleus is remarkable in showing little plasticity, a feature that is useful for transmitting ongoing acoustic information faithfully and with minimal distortion by preceding sounds.[5]

In addition to the frequency information, natural auditory stimuli also contain information on its temporal structure, which is especially important in speech perception. In experiments in which the information encoded in the frequency content of sound is removed, leaving only the temporal structure, much speech discrimination can still be made.[31] This is important since as with cochlear implants, ABIs convey much information via the temporal structure of stimulation.[32] Cochlear nucleus neurons are sensitive to temporal fluctuations and—compared to auditory nerve fibers—generally sharpen the representation of temporal information, to changes in stimulus amplitude.[33,34]

With different response patterns, these neurons act to separate specific pieces of information from sound stimuli. For example, "onset neurons" show the largest enhancement of the temporal sound structure. The representation of temporal and spectral information encoded in various types of neurons allows the identity of sounds to be determined, that is, one speech sound versus another.

The important aspect with respect to auditory implants is that aspects of the acoustic environment are separated out at the brainstem level, and that they are selectively processed and represented in the cochlear nuclei.

There are even more sophisticated mechanisms of feature detection in the mammalian DCN. Principal cells of the DCN integrate inputs from auditory nerve fibers and from parallel fibers that carry a mixture of auditory and nonauditory information. In contrast to the VCN, where effects of inhibition are relatively weak, DCN neurons in unanesthetized animals receive strong inhibition from both sets of inputs. Spectrally complex sounds evoke a summation of excitation and inhibition that enables neurons to detect spectral features, which are often the information-bearing elements of sounds.[35,36] DCN principal cells seem to signal "interesting" features in the stimulus spectrum, by being inhibited where such features lie near the best frequency.[5]

The second set of inputs to DCN principal cells conveys multimodal sensory information, from the somatosensory spinal nuclei. A number of researchers have suggested that the DCN is involved in coordinating motor and sensory information in sound localization and that it might be performing a role similar to one kind of cerebellar learning.[5]

All parallel ascending auditory pathways through the brainstem converge in the IC. Some fibers of the cochlear nerve send signals from the brainstem (olivary nucleus) back to the cochlea (efferent feedback) which reduce the sensitivity of the cochlea in the presence of loud sounds, reducing saturation.[37]

2.4 Human Research

Functional data about the auditory brainstem nuclei in humans are scarce. In the 1970s Dublin attempted to establish a "cochlear nucleogram" to chart tonotopy in the cochlear nuclei. He measured the loss of spheric cells in the VCN and of spiral ganglion hair cells in postmortem specimens and correlated these with the estimated audiogram in sensorineural hearing loss to determine a "best fit" frequency map ("audiohistogram"). His data revealed an intranuclear gradient with low frequencies represented ventral and high frequencies dorsal.[19,38,39] These and other findings basically matched the tonotopic map that was found in animal research.[11,18,40]

The next step in charting tonotopy in humans came with the advent of ABIs when pitch ranking became possible by selectively activating stimulating electrodes along the brainstem surface of the cochlear nucleus. Pitch ranking showed the lower frequencies to be represented more medial (deeper inside the so-called "lateral recess" of the fourth ventricle) and caudal, and higher frequencies more lateral and cranial.[41]

The significance of these data, however, is arguable since the inner (medial) electrodes primarily stimulate the DCN and electrodes located on the outer (lateral) portion of the carriers overlap and may stimulate primarily the VCN. Moreover, the location of the electrodes varies inter-individual and, as we will see, most of the VCN cannot be reached by surface implants at all. In addition, one must bear in mind that the distribution of the electric field around the electrodes is inconsistent, so that it is not easy to calculate at what depth neurons underlying specific electrodes would be excited or inhibited by the electric stimulation. Again, it is notable that threshold-distance measurements were similar in human and animal research.[42,43] When it comes to charting tonotopy, however, the possibility that perceived pitch will also be a function of depth penetration of the electrical field generated by surface electrodes, is detrimental.

The key point demonstrated by these studies is that axons conveying higher frequencies penetrate to terminals deep inside the VCN while axons representing lower frequencies terminate more superficial.[10,18,19,44] In the human DCN, fibers carrying higher frequencies terminate more ventral than fibers carrying lower frequencies.[10,18]

Another line of functional data on the human cochlear nucleus stems from degeneration studies. Axons in the cochlear nerve have a trophic function for the second-order neuron of the auditory pathway that originates in the cochlear nucleus. It has been shown that following destruction of the cochlea resulting in deafness, neurons in the DCN degenerate much less than those in the VCN.[11,45] This suggests that most of these neurons do not primarily receive their input from the cochlear nerve.

In a group of deaf patients suffering from sensorineural hearing loss, Jean Moore and colleagues found a 20 to 30% shrinkage of cells in the VCN in postmortem studies. They found the same effect in a deceased patient with a cochlear implant, suggesting that electrical stimulation alone cannot substitute for the trophic function of afferent nerve fibers.[46]

Interestingly, the authors saw the same cell shrinkage in higher centers of the auditory pathway, namely the olive and the IC. The necessity of trophic input from the cochlear nerve, however, is limited, since 70% of the cochlear nucleus cells do not show signs of degeneration even a long as 10 years after the onset of deafness. Again, data from human and mammalian animal research overlap considerably.[47] Still, data from both sources are of limited use for the surgeon tasked to place an implant as close to the auditory brainstem nuclei as possible.

2.5 Anatomy and Surgical Approach

2.5.1 Extrinsic Anatomy of the Cochlear Nuclei

In contrast to the favorite auditory research animal, the cat, only a small portion of the ventral human cochlear nucleus lies superficial.[42] The cochlear nucleus itself is not visible on the surface of the human brainstem. However, there are some structural patterns that are helpful in guiding surgeons during ABI implantation. Neurosurgeons have become more acquainted with the surface anatomy of this particular brainstem area, with attempts made to

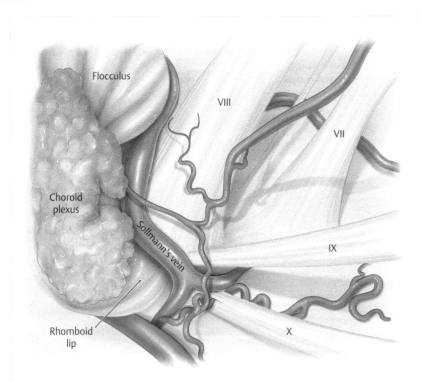

Fig. 2.3 Extrinsic anatomy of the brainstem region around the entrance to the lateral recess (foramen of Luschka): CN VIII vestibulocochlear nerve; CN VII facial nerve; CN IX glossopharyngeal nerve; CN X vagus nerve.

correlate intrinsic anatomy to outer landmarks such as the "torus" and the "auditory tubercle."[c,48,49,50]

In the 1980s, researchers of the House Ear Institute (HEI) in Los Angeles reported that part of the wall of the lateral recess of the fourth ventricle is formed by the cochlear nuclei, and that the dorsal surface of the DCN—with the exception of a tiny caudal portion—is almost entirely accessible from the surface of this region of the brainstem.[20,21,51] Jacob et al measured this accessible area inside the lateral recess to be 7.5 × 2.5 mm.[52]

Anatomically, a 0.5-mm-thin cell layer of the so-called pontobulbar body, a relay station between the brainstem and the cerebellum, can overlap the dorsal aspect of the DCN.[42] More recently, Abe et al revisited this anatomical region and showed that the DCN, which lies back to back with the cerebellar peduncle, forms a slight elevation on the surface of the brainstem—the "auditory tubercle."[53] This elevation, however, is probably only partially formed by the DCN; the pontobulbar body, the vestibular nucleus, and the ependymal lining of the fourth ventricle may be responsible for another portion.[55,56] Therefore, and because it is not even present in each case,[49] the auditory tubercle is not a reliable surgical landmark, even with normal anatomy.

The "visible area of the cochlear nucleus" on the surface of the brainstem has been reported to be 11.7 ± 2.7 × 3.1 ± 0.7 mm.[23] Moreover, the mean distance between the auditory tubercle and another visible structure on the surface in this area of the brainstem, the median sulcus, has been measured to be 6.5 to 6.9 mm,[49] while the mean distance between the DCN and the median sulcus is about 10 mm. As such the auditory tubercle is longer than and lies medial to the DCN.[54]

"Nuclear torus" is a term that is used for a more extended eminence on the surface of the medulla oblongata that is supposed to be created by the DCN, the lower part of the VCN, and the root entry zone of the vestibulocochlear nerve. This makes it a structure that curves around the posterior lateral border of the brainstem.[52] Both the auditory tubercle and the torus have been measured by these researchers. The mean length of the torus was 12.8 mm. The length range of the tubercle was reported to be 3.5 to 9 mm and its height (rostrocaudal extension) 1.2 to 3 mm.

The most striking result of these definitions and measurements is their vagueness and variability. This holds true for the cochlear nucleus itself, too. Abe et al note that the VCN may reach the entrance of the lateral recess of the fourth ventricle (foramen of Luschka). However, since most of the VCN is located deep inside the brainstem, it is unlikely that this structure causes much of an outer landmark on the surface. Moreover, it is difficult to define a clear border between DCN and VCN even in histological section.

More interesting may be the distance from the apparent origin of the borders of the VCN to the facial nerve, because this nerve usually is, even in cases of neurofibromatosis, often well visible during surgery in this area. While the DCN is located below the facial nerve exit zone in most cases, the more deeply located VCN stretches right across the apparent origin of this nerve from the brainstem. This would make access to the VCN from the outer surface of the brainstem problematic. Notably, the cochlear nerve enters the middle portion of the VCN at its root entry zone (▶ Fig. 2.4).[56]

The classical landmark for the surgical introduction of a surface electrode into the lateral recess is the foramen of Luschka. Komune et al have precisely described the anatomy around this entrance into the lateral recess (▶ Fig. 2.3). They used the term

c "Tuberculum auditivum."

"rhomboid lip" for the ventral border of the foramen, a structure that is probably consistent with the lateral part of the taenia of the choroid plexus.[48,49,57] At the HEI, Terr and Edgerton created three-dimensional models of the cochlear nucleus based on light microscopy analysis in cadaveric specimens to determine the optimal surgical approach to the cochlear nucleus complex (CNC).[20,58] They showed that the terminal part of the cochlear nerve approximately coincides with the line of attachment of the taenia of the choroid plexus (= inferior medullary velum of the fourth ventricle).

The glossopharyngeal nerve guides the approach to the foramen of Luschka and it also serves as an estimate of the trajectory for the implantation of a surface ABI electrode array. Klose and Sollmann noted that in two-thirds of cases, a branch of the lateral pontine vein runs over the entrance of the lateral recess (Sollmann's vein, ▶ Fig. 2.3).[48] In formalin-fixed specimens, the foramen of Luschka has a size of about 3.5 × 2 mm.[48,49]

2.6 Intrinsic Anatomy of the Cochlear Nuclei

It has been suggested that the volume of the cochlear nucleus almost triples over the first five decades of life, and then decreases again by about one-third until toward the end of life.[59] Seldon and Clark found a larger volume of the human cochlear nucleus on the right side.[45] This may be attributed to a preference of the right ear in right-handed people.[60,61,62] The fact that neurons in the hearing cortex of the dominant left hemisphere have been found to be larger than on the right side would be well in line with this finding since a majority of fibers of the auditory pathway cross over to the contralateral side.[63]

The inferior cerebellar peduncle, a large neural fiber connection between the pons and the cerebellum, borders on and partially overlaps the most ventral portion of the cochlear nucleus

(▶ Fig. 2.4).[10,11,18] The floccular peduncle, which originates from the cerebellar flocculus, forms part of the lateral border of the VCN. From the caudolateral portion to its ventrolateral aspect, the VCN is crossed by myelinated fibers ("peripheral astrocytic border") of the pontobulbar body. This nucleus is a neuronal relay site with connections to visual and auditory regions of the cerebellum, the trigeminal system, and to the spinal cord.[18,64,65]

For several reasons, the real dimensions of the human cochlear nucleus are difficult to assess. In histological sections, the borders of the VCN and DCN are not clearly delineated. Also, histological fixation ultimately leads to shrinkage of specimen in the range of 10 to 17%, more pronounced in longitudinal than in transversal direction, so that measurements need to be multiplied by a correction factor.[46,54,59,66] Until recently, the intrinsic morphological dimensions of the cochlear nucleus in the human brainstem and measurements of protruding structures have only been examined in case studies.[18,21,49,53,67] On magnetic resonance imaging (MRI) the nucleus is hardly detectable, but its length and width on a horizontal plane have been estimated to be 8 × 3 mm.[68]

Previous attempts to determine the dimensions of the cochlear nucleus have resulted in varying results. Measured rostrocaudal dimensions have ranged from 2.3 to 4.5 mm.[13,17,45,52,69] Moore and Osen were the first to investigate the shape and the spatial orientation of the human CNC.[18] They noted that its rostrocaudal ("up to down") axis is tilted to the brainstem axis by an angle of 30 to 35 degrees. Other authors attempting to better refine this have come up with sometimes paradoxical results.[70,71,72] Other attempts were made to measure the distance of the nucleus from the surface of the brain over its length.[20] Needless to say, measurement of this complex structure is far from a simple issue.

In order to attempt to synthesize the complex issue of dimension, spatial orientation, and depth of the cochlear nucleus, we undertook a three-dimensional study of 20 brainstem specimens (33 nuclei).[54] The most striking finding in this analysis

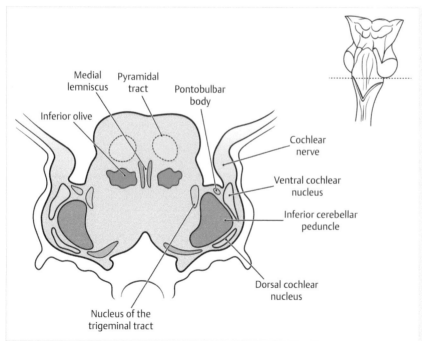

Medial lemniscus
Pyramidal tract
Pontobulbar body
Inferior olive
Cochlear nerve
Ventral cochlear nucleus
Inferior cerebellar peduncle
Dorsal cochlear nucleus
Nucleus of the trigeminal tract

Fig. 2.4 Schematic axial section through the brainstem at the level of the entry zone of the cochlear nerve.

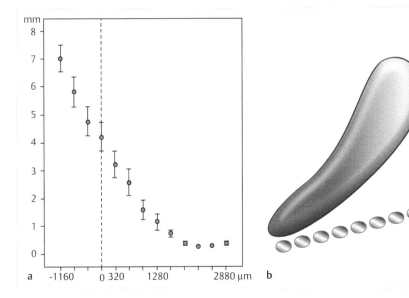

Fig. 2.5 Distance of the ventral cochlear nucleus (VCN) to the surface of the brainstem. **(a)** Minimal surface depth (mean ± standard error) of the VCN. The broken line represents the first histological section of the facial nerve. **(b)** Three-dimensional rendering of the cochlear nucleus complex (CNC) on the right side (view from above) in relation to an auditory brainstem implant (ABI) surface electrode. Note the distance of the rostral part of the VCN from a surface electrode placed in the lateral recess of the fourth ventricle (*dashed arrow*).

Table 2.1 Means and standard deviations of the maximum dimensions measured in each histological slice of the human cochlear nuclei (mm). The variables were assessed in along the intrinsic axis of the cochlear nuclei

	Length	Width	Height
DCN	3.42 ± 1.21	0.68 ± 0.20	1.90 ± 0.66
VCN	4.59 ± 0.89	1.53 ± 0.64	3.18 ± 0.69
CNC	8.02 ± 1.05	1.53 ± 0.64	3.76 ± 0.89

Abbreviations: CNC, cochlear nucleus complex; DCN, dorsal cochlear nucleus; VCN, ventral cochlear nucleus.

was that the inward rotation of the VCN to the longitudinal axis of the brainstem is so pronounced that the rostral half of the VCN has a distance of several millimeters to the surface of the brainstem (▶ Fig. 2.5).

The overall extension of the CNC as a whole was 8.01 × 1.53 × 3.76 mm (length × width × height) with respect to the intrinsic axis of the complex, with standard deviations between 0.2 and 1.21 mm (▶ Table 2.1). The VCN becomes wider in more rostral (upper) slices of the brainstem and its longitudinal axis (length) was longer in more caudal (lower) sections.

Individual variability of the dimensions of the cochlear nucleus is high. In this study, the smallest and largest values for maximum dimensions and maximum surface depths varied by factor of 3 (▶ Table 2.2). Of note, there was no single CNC that was smallest or largest in all three dimensions.

In each CNC, width and length of the VCN and DCN correlated with each other, that is, if the DCN was smaller in these dimensions, the VCN was too. Interestingly, the height of the DCN correlated inversely with the length of the VCN and that of the whole CNC.

In this particular study, there were no significant side differences with respect to length and height of the cochlear nucleus. On the contrary, most data regarding these variables and the surface depth of the nuclei on either side of the brainstem correlated linearly with each other. The only exception was the mean length of the DCN in the sagittal plane: it was greater on the left side than on the right. With advancing age, the height of

the CNC was reduced, a finding that correlates to the pattern of degenerative shrinkage without reduction in the number of cells described in the literature.[47,56]

There are few data on three-dimensional shape of the human cochlear nuclei. At the HEI, Terr and Sinha have produced two models, one demonstrating the CN in relation to the brainstem and the other showing the CN completely dissected out of the brainstem (▶ Fig. 2.6).[65] Of course, measures of variance are unobtainable with this method, but still the models helped to design the first ABIs. In our molded three-dimensional renderings of the CNC, it has a distorted X-like or bootlike shape viewed from the side and looks like a wedge from above (▶ Fig. 2.7).[54,55,73]

2.7 The Cochlear Nucleus as an Anatomic Interface for Auditory Brainstem Implants

Despite a presumed point-to-point connection between the origins of auditory nerve fibers at the cochlea and neurons located in the cochlear nucleus of the brainstem, these implants are not nearly as effective as cochlear implants.

In view of what we learned about the surgical and functional anatomy of the cochlear nucleus (▶ Fig. 2.8), there are five main difficulties for interfacing it with a neuroprosthetic implant:

- First, there are very few landmarks helping to guide a surgeon to the cochlear nucleus.
- Second, the cochlear nucleus, especially its ventral portion, has a very complex shape that cannot be properly anticipated by one or two external landmarks.
- Third, the size and spatial orientation of the nucleus inside the brainstem vary individually.
- Fourth, most of the primary terminals of afferent cochlear nerve fibers are located at a depth of several millimeters whereby only penetrating electrodes can contact them directly. What is more, they are partially hidden behind the intrinsic course of the facial nerve so that penetrating electrodes have a risk to damage facial nerve fibers.

Table 2.2 Means and standard deviations of the smallest and largest maximum dimensions of the human cochlear nuclei as measured in about 825 histological slices. Because measurements were performed in axial sections, height was calculated by multiplying slice thickness (320 μm) by number of sections on which the nuclei were visible. Therefore, standard deviations are not given for this variable

	Length		Width		Height	
	Smallest	Largest	Smallest	Largest	Smallest	Largest
DCN	1.46 ± 1.00	4.24 ± 1.67	0.29 ± 0.19	0.81 ± 0.19	0.77	3.10
VCN	1.92 ± 1.11	5.42 ± 1.75	0.780 ±.31	2.10 ± 0.91	2.32	4.26
CNC	3.38 ± 1.05	9.66 ± 3.42	0.78 ± 0.31	2.10 ± 0.91	2.32	7.36

Abbreviations: CNC, cochlear nucleus complex; DCN, dorsal cochlear nucleus; VCN, ventral cochlear nucleus.

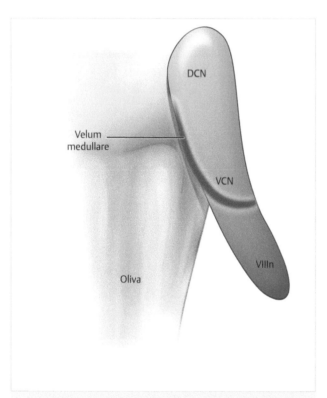

Fig. 2.6 Lateral view of a three-dimensional model of the brainstem at the level of the cochlear nucleus. The arrows point to the velum medullare (i.e., the taenia of the choroid plexus; white line). DCN, dorsal cochlear nucleus; ol, oliva; VCN, ventral cochlear nucleus; VIIIn, vestibulocochlear nerve.

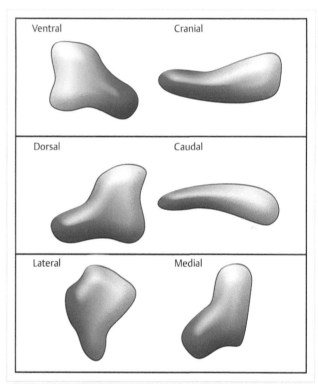

Fig. 2.7 Aspects of a three-dimensional, true-to-scale model based on the measurements in about one thousand histological sections. The model was molded from plasticine, photographed from several angles and uploaded onto a graphic computer for smoothing of the surfaces and re-coloring. Views are spatially rotated according to the axes of the brainstem.

- Fifth, large neoplasms may compromise the cochlear nuclei or permanently displace them. This assumption is sustained by the fact that the best results with ABIs are often obtained in deaf patients with nontumor pathologies, albeit with a wide variation in speech recognition from 10 to 100%.[74,75]

Current ABI surface electrodes reach the cochlear nucleus at its caudal end, which is about 0.8 mm thin and about 0.5 mm deep to the surface. These electrodes overlap by about two-thirds on the area of the nucleus that projects itself to the lateral brainstem border. They preferably stimulate the DCN and about one-third of the length of the VCN. These superficially lying parts of the CNC do not include all the primary terminals of the cochlear nerve fibers. They constitute a maximal area of about 3.4 mm + (one-third of 4.6 mm) × 3.8 mm or 4.9 mm × 3.8 mm.

Electrodes outside and deep to this area cannot really be expected to stimulate the cochlear nucleus at reasonable charge densities.

While the glossopharyngeal nerve, the lateral recess with its choroid plexus, and Sollmann's vein are sufficient guiding structures for surface electrodes, clear landmarks and trajectories for penetrating implants are lacking and will generally be hard to obtain on an individual basis for the VCN that is slanted inside the brainstem. Most of the ventral portion of the CN is still out of reach. If a new attempt is undertaken to reach this target with penetrating electrodes the entry point will have to be cranial to the lateral recess at the level of the pontocerebellar junction and at the lateral vertex of the brainstem, a site that roughly correlates with the middle portion of the VCN. The trajectory of the electrodes would be running obliquely upwards (from caudal to rostral), avoiding the exit zone and the

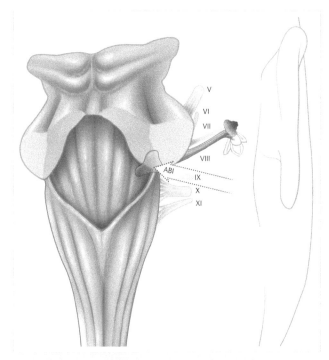

Fig. 2.8 Surgical and functional anatomy of the brainstem, vestibulo-cochlear structures in the petrous bone and the cranial nerves in the cerebellopontine angle. View from a retrosigmoid perspective. Tonotopy in the cochlea, the cochlear nerve, and the cochlear nucleus is approximated by the blue gradient from high frequencies (*light blue*) to low frequencies (*dark blue*).

intra-axial course of the facial nerve. Because of the close spatial relationship to the rubrospinal tract medially, the tectospinal tract ventrally, the pontobulbar body, the trigeminal tract, the second motor neuron of the long sensory tracts, the middle and inferior cerebellar peduncle, the vestibular nucleus, and the glossopharyngeal nerve caudally, side effects caused by the electrical stimulation with both superficial and in-depth electrodes are always possible.[76,77,78,79]

An individual approach would be desirable in any case, but this will depend on further improvement of MRI of the CNC.

2.8 Higher Up in the Auditory Pathway

Apart from the cochlear nucleus, the only other site that has clinically been implanted with electrodes for restoration of hearing is the IC in a very limited number of patients.

Therefore, the auditory pathway above the cochlear nuclei will only be briefly described here.

The cochlear nuclei contain second-order neurons. Thereafter, the auditory pathway crosses and runs bilaterally with a multitude of interneurons and synapses. More fibers decussate at the level of the trapezoid body than remain ipsilateral; then the pathway ascends in the lateral lemniscus and the brachium of the caudal colliculus. Next, the pathway synapses in the medial geniculate body. From there, neurons send their axons through the internal capsule to the portion of cerebral cortex

that surrounds the Sylvian sulcus, that is, the primary auditory cortex.

2.8.1 Dorsal Nucleus of Trapezoid Body

Via the cochlear nuclei, each trapezoid body receives input from right and left ears. The nucleus functions in sound localization, that is, detecting phase and intensity differences between the two ears.

Interestingly, this nucleus also sends output to the trigeminal and facial nerves for reflex contraction of tensor tympani and stapedius muscles, which dampen loud sounds. It is also the source of efferent axons to outer hair cells in the cochlea, which selectively "tune" the spiral organ for frequency discrimination.

2.8.2 Inferior Colliculus

The IC receives input via the lateral lemniscus and connects the auditory brainstem to sensory, motor, and limbic systems. It is also a significant midbrain site for auditory processing.[80]

The colliculus contains neurons that are sensitive to phase and intensity differences between the ears.[81] IC neurons projecting to the medial geniculate are part of a conscious auditory pathway. Via the tectospinal and tectobulbar tracts, output from the IC produces reflex turning of the head, ears, and eyes toward a sudden sound stimulus. Collateral branches of auditory pathway axons go to the reticular formation to alert the whole brain to a loud sound stimulation.

In general, the further a neuron is located up in the auditory pathway, the more complex the stimulation patterns will have to be to activate these neurons in a meaningful way.[82] Many neurons in the auditory pathway far away from the cochlea do not react to pure tones.

In the IC, some cell types can only be activated by frequency-modulated tones of a particular direction or degree. Other neurons still react to a pure tone, but only if it is frequency-modulated.[81] Whether midbrain auditory implants as an alternative to ABIs will improve speech perception in the future is yet to be determined.[83,84,85]

2.8.3 Medial Geniculate

This anatomical structure in the "conscious" auditory pathway receives input via the brachium of the IC. Imprecise sound consciousness takes place at this level.

The axons of the geniculate neurons project through the internal capsule to the primary auditory cortex. The geniculate body functions for sound like the thalamus functions for tactile sense.[22]

2.8.4 Primary Auditory Cortex

The primary endpoint of the auditory pathway is located around the Sylvian sulcus. This cortex is necessary for recognizing temporal patterns of sound and direction of pitch change. Melodies and speech are represented at this site. The primary auditory cortex has tonotopic maps, but they are separated for detecting pitch and direction of sound since both modalities are relayed to the cortex by separate pathways.

2.8.5 Auditory Association Cortex

This cortex surrounds the primary auditory cortex from which it receives input. The association cortex extracts meanings of sound patterns and associates with learned significance stored in memory with a particular sound pattern.

References

[1] Kiang NY, Rho JM, Northrop CC, Liberman MC, Ryugo DK. Hair-cell innervation by spiral ganglion cells in adult cats. Science. 1982; 217(4555):175–177

[2] Spoendlin H, Brun JP. Relation of structural damage to exposure time and intensity in acoustic trauma. Acta Otolaryngol. 1973; 75(2):220–226

[3] Brown MC, Berglund AM, Kiang NY, Ryugo DK. Central trajectories of type II spiral ganglion neurons. J Comp Neurol. 1988; 278(4):581–590

[4] Brown MC, Ledwith JV, III. Projections of thin (type-II) and thick (type-I) auditory-nerve fibers into the cochlear nucleus of the mouse. Hear Res. 1990; 49(1–3):105–118

[5] Young, E. D., & Oertel, D. (2003). Cochlear nucleus. In G. M. Shepherd (Ed.), The synaptic organization of the brain (5th ed., ch. 4, pp.125–163). Oxford, England: Oxford University Press.

[6] Kunel'skaya NL, Yatskovsky AN, Mishchenko VV. [Microanatomy of the cranial segment of the vestibulocochlear nerve: possible correlations with the symptoms of neurovascular compression syndrome]. Vestn Otorinolaringol. 2016; 81(1):25–28

[7] Ryu H, Tanaka T, Yamamoto S, Uemura K, Takehara Y, Isoda H. Magnetic resonance cisternography used to determine precise topography of the facial nerve and three components of the eighth cranial nerve in the internal auditory canal and cerebellopontine cistern. J Neurosurg. 1999; 90(4):624–634

[8] Lang J. Skull Base and Related Structures: Atlas of Clinical Anatomy. 2nd ed. Stuttgart:Schattauer Verlag; 2001

[9] Spoendlin H, Schrott A. Analysis of the human auditory nerve. Hear Res. 1989; 43(1):25–38

[10] Moore JK. Cochlear nuclei: relationship to the auditory nerve. In: Altschuler RA, Hoffmann DW, Bobbin RP, eds. Neurobiology of Hearing: The Cochlea. New York: Raven Press; 1986:283–301

[11] Moore JK. The human auditory brain stem: a comparative view. Hear Res. 1987; 29(1):1–32

[12] Lorente de No R. Anatomy of the eighth nerve. III. General plan of structure of the primary cochlear nuclei. Laryngoscope. 1933; 43:327–350

[13] Bacsik RD, Strominger NL. The cytoarchitecture of the human anteroventral cochlear nucleus. J Comp Neurol. 1973; 147(2):281–289

[14] Brawer JR, Morest DK, Kane EC. The neuronal architecture of the cochlear nucleus of the cat. J Comp Neurol. 1974; 155(3):251–300

[15] Gandolfi A, Horoupian DS, De Teresa RM. Quantitative and cytometric analysis of the ventral cochlear nucleus in man. J Neurol Sci. 1981; 50(3):443–455

[16] Luxon LM. The anatomy and pathology of the central auditory pathways. Br J Audiol. 1981; 15(1):31–40

[17] Mobley JP, Huang J, Moore JK, McCreery DB. Three-dimensional modeling of human brain stem structures for an auditory brain stem implant. Ann Otol Rhinol Laryngol Suppl. 1995; 166:30–31

[18] Moore JK, Osen KK. The cochlear nuclei in man. Am J Anat. 1979; 154(3):393–418

[19] Dublin WB. The cochlear nuclei revisited. Otolaryngol Head Neck Surg. 1982; 90(6):744–760

[20] Terr LI, Edgerton BJ. Surface topography of the cochlear nuclei in humans: two- and three-dimensional analysis. Hear Res. 1985; 17(1):51–59

[21] Terr LI, Sinha UK, House WF. Anatomical relationships of the cochlear nuclei and the pontobulbar body: possible significance for neuroprosthesis placement. Laryngoscope. 1987; 97(9):1009–1011

[22] Young ED, Oertel D: Cochlear Nucleus, in Shepherd GM (ed): The synaptic organization of the brain. New York: Oxford University Press, 2003, pp 125-163

[23] Osen KK. Cytoarchitecture of the cochlear nuclei in the cat. J Comp Neurol. 1969; 136(4):453–484

[24] Rosahl SK, Mark G, Herzog M, et al. Far-field responses to stimulation of the cochlear nucleus by microsurgically placed penetrating and surface electrodes in the cat. J Neurosurg. 2001; 95(5):845–852

[25] McCreery DB, Shannon RV, Moore JK, Chatterjee M. Accessing the tonotopic organization of the ventral cochlear nucleus by intranuclear microstimulation. IEEE Trans Rehabil Eng. 1998; 6(4):391–399

[26] Rouiller EM, Cronin-Schreiber R, Fekete DM, Ryugo DK. The central projections of intracellularly labeled auditory nerve fibers in cats: an analysis of terminal morphology. J Comp Neurol. 1986; 249(2):261–278

[27] Golding NL, Robertson D, Oertel D. Recordings from slices indicate that octopus cells of the cochlear nucleus detect coincident firing of auditory nerve fibers with temporal precision. J Neurosci. 1995; 15(4):3138–3153

[28] Manis PB, Marx SO. Outward currents in isolated ventral cochlear nucleus neurons. J Neurosci. 1991; 11(9):2865–2880

[29] Oertel D. Synaptic responses and electrical properties of cells in brain slices of the mouse anteroventral cochlear nucleus. J Neurosci. 1983; 3(10):2043–2053

[30] Sachs MB, Abbas PJ. Rate versus level functions for auditory-nerve fibers in cats: tone-burst stimuli. J Acoust Soc Am. 1974; 56(6):1835–1847

[31] Van Tasell DJ, Soli SD, Kirby VM, Widin GP. Speech waveform envelope cues for consonant recognition. J Acoust Soc Am. 1987; 82(4):1152–1161

[32] Shannon RV, Zeng FG, Kamath V, Wygonski J, Ekelid M. Speech recognition with primarily temporal cues. Science. 1995; 270(5234):303–304

[33] Frisina RD. Subcortical neural coding mechanisms for auditory temporal processing. Hear Res. 2001; 158(1–2):1–27

[34] Wang X, Sachs MB. Neural encoding of single-formant stimuli in the cat. II. Responses of anteroventral cochlear nucleus units. J Neurophysiol. 1994; 71(1):59–78

[35] Nelken I, Young ED. Why do cats need a dorsal cochlear nucleus? J Basic Clin Physiol Pharmacol. 1996; 7(3):199–220

[36] Parsons JE, Lim E, Voigt HF. Type III units in the gerbil dorsal cochlear nucleus may be spectral notch detectors. Ann Biomed Eng. 2001; 29(10):887–896

[37] Guinan JJ, Jr, St, ankovic KM. Medial efferent inhibition produces the largest equivalent attenuations at moderate to high sound levels in cat auditory-nerve fibers. J Acoust Soc Am. 1996; 100(3):1680–1690

[38] Dublin WB. The combined correlated audiohistogram. Incorporation of the superior ventral cochlear nucleus. Ann Otol Rhinol Laryngol. 1976; 85(6 PT. 1):813–819

[39] Dublin WB. Cytoarchitecture of the cochlear nuclei:report of an illustrative case of erythroblastosis. Arch Otolaryngol. 1974; 100(5):355–359

[40] Irvine DRF. The Auditory Brainstem. Vol. 7. Berlin, Heidelberg, Tokyo: Springer; 1986

[41] Marangos N, Stecker M, Sollmann WP, Laszig R. Stimulation of the cochlear nucleus with multichannel auditory brainstem implants and long-term results: Freiburg patients. J Laryngol Otol Suppl. 2000(27):27–31

[42] Ranck JB, Jr. Which elements are excited in electrical stimulation of mammalian central nervous system: a review. Brain Res. 1975; 98(3):417–440

[43] Shannon RV, Moore JK, McCreery DB, Portillo F. Threshold-distance measures from electrical stimulation of human brainstem. IEEE Trans Rehabil Eng. 1997; 5(1):70–74

[44] Kelly JP. Hearing. In: Kandel EC, Schwartz JH, Jessell TM, eds. Principles of Neural Science. 3rd ed. New York, Amsterdam, London, Tokyo: Elsevier; 1991:481–498

[45] Seldon HL, Clark GM. Human cochlear nucleus: comparison of Nissl-stained neurons from deaf and hearing patients. Brain Res. 1991; 551(1–2):185–194

[46] Moore JK, Niparko JK, Perazzo LM, Miller MR, Linthicum FH. Effect of adult-onset deafness on the human central auditory system. Ann Otol Rhinol Laryngol. 1997; 106(5):385–390

[47] Shepherd RK, Hardie NA. Deafness-induced changes in the auditory pathway: implications for cochlear implants. Audiol Neurotol. 2001; 6(6):305–318

[48] Klose AK, Sollmann WP. Anatomical variations of landmarks for implantation at the cochlear nucleus. J Laryngol Otol Suppl. 2000(27):8–10

[49] Quester R, Schröder R. Topographic anatomy of the cochlear nuclear region at the floor of the fourth ventricle in humans. J Neurosurg. 1999; 91(3):466–476

[50] Schwalbe G. Lehrbuch der Neurologie. Jena: Gustav Fischer; 1881

[51] McElveen JT, Jr, Hitselberger WE, House WF. Surgical accessibility of the cochlear nuclear complex in man: surgical landmarks. Otolaryngol Head Neck Surg. 1987; 96(2):135–140

[52] Jacob U, Mrosack B, Gerhardt HJ, Staudt J. [The surgical approach to the cochlear nucleus area]. Anat Anz. 1991; 173(2):93–100

[53] Abe H, Rhoton AL, Jr. Microsurgical anatomy of the cochlear nuclei. Neurosurgery. 2006; 58(4):728–739, discussion 728–739

[54] Rosahl SK, Rosahl S. No easy target: anatomic constraints of electrodes interfacing the human cochlear nucleus. Neurosurgery. 2013; 72(1) Suppl Operative:58–64, discussion 65

[55] Rosahl SK, Rosahl S, Walter GF, Hussein S, Matthies C, Samii M. Cochlear region of the brainstem. J Neurosurg. 2000; 93(4):724–729

[56] Rosahl S: Ausdehnung, Lage und Form des menschlichen Nucleus cochlearis, Dissertation. Albert-Ludwigs-Universität Freiburg, Germany, 2008

[57] Komune N, Yagmurlu K, Matsuo S, Miki K, Abe H, Rhoton AL, Jr. Auditory brainstem implantation: anatomy and approaches. Neurosurgery. 2015; 11 Suppl 2:306–320, discussion 320–321

[58] Terr LI, Edgerton BJ. Three-dimensional reconstruction of the cochlear nuclear complex in humans. Arch Otolaryngol. 1985; 111(8):495–501

[59] Konigsmark BW, Murphy EA. Volume of the ventral cochlear nucleus in man: its relationship to neuronal population and age. J Neuropathol Exp Neurol. 1972; 31(2):304–316

[60] Geffen G. The development of the right ear advantage in dichotic listening with focused attention. Cortex. 1978; 14(2):169–177

[61] Kimura D. Functional asymmetry of the brain in dichotic listening. Cortex. 1967; 3:163–178

[62] Sidtis JJ. Predicting brain organization from dichotic listening performance: cortical and subcortical functional asymmetries contribute to perceptual asymmetries. Brain Lang. 1982; 17(2):287–300

[63] Seldon HL. The anatomy of speech perception: human auditory cortex. In: Peters A, Jones EG, eds. Cerebral Cortex. Vol. 4. New York: Plenum; 1985:73–324

[64] Terr LI, House WF. Neurons of the inferior medullary velum in the cerebello-pontine angle. Ann Otol Rhinol Laryngol. 1988; 97(1):52–54

[65] Terr LI, Sinha UK. Three-dimensional computer-aided reconstruction of the pontobulbar body. Am J Otol. 1987; 8(5):432–435

[66] Quester R, Schröder R. The shrinkage of the human brain stem during formalin fixation and embedding in paraffin. J Neurosci Methods. 1997; 75(1):81–89

[67] Musiek FE, Baran JA. Neuroanatomy, neurophysiology, and central auditory assessment. Part I: Brain stem. Ear Hear. 1986; 7(4):207–219

[68] Gebarski SS, Tucci DL, Telian SA. The cochlear nuclear complex: MR location and abnormalities. AJNR Am J Neuroradiol. 1993; 14(6):1311–1318

[69] Paxinos G, Huang X. Atlas of the Human Brainstem. San Diego: Academic Press; 1995

[70] Nevison B, Laszig R, Sollmann WP, et al. Results from a European clinical investigation of the nucleus multichannel auditory brainstem implant. Ear Hear. 2002; 23(3):170–183

[71] Rauschecker JP, Shannon RV. Sending sound to the brain. Science. 2002; 295 (5557):1025–1029

[72] Rosahl SK, Lenarz T, Matthies C, Samii M, Sollmann WP, Laszig R. Hirnstammimplantate zur Wiederherstellung des Hörvermögens. Dt. Aerzteblatt. 2004; 101: 180–188

[73] Rosahl SK, Rosahl S. Letter: anatomy and auditory brainstem implants. Neurosurgery. 2016; 78(4):E601–E602

[74] Choi JY, Song MH, Jeon JH, Lee WS, Chang JW. Early surgical results of auditory brainstem implantation in nontumor patients. Laryngoscope. 2011; 121 (12):2610–2618

[75] Colletti V, Shannon R, Carner M, Veronese S, Colletti L. Outcomes in nontumor adults fitted with the auditory brainstem implant: 10 years' experience. Otol Neurotol. 2009; 30(5):614–618

[76] Edgerton BJ, House WF, Hitselberger W. Hearing by cochlear nucleus stimulation in humans. Ann Otol Rhinol Laryngol Suppl. 1982; 91(2 Pt 3):117–124

[77] Matthies C, Thomas S, Moshrefi M, et al. Auditory brainstem implants: current neurosurgical experiences and perspective. J Laryngol Otol Suppl. 2000; 114 (27):32–36

[78] Shannon RV, Fayad J, Moore J, et al. Auditory brainstem implant: II. Postsurgical issues and performance. Otolaryngol Head Neck Surg. 1993; 108(6):634–642

[79] Sollmann WP, Laszig R, Marangos N. Surgical experiences in 58 cases using the Nucleus 22 multichannel auditory brainstem implant. J Laryngol Otol Suppl. 2000(27):23–26

[80] Winer JAS, C.E.: The central auditory system: a functional analysis, in Winer JAS, C.E. (ed): The Inferior Colliculus. New York: Springer Science and Business Media, 2005, pp 1–68

[81] Litovsky RY, Fligor BJ, Tramo MJ. Functional role of the human inferior colliculus in binaural hearing. Hear Res. 2002; 165(1–2):177–188

[82] Pickles JO. An Introduction to the Physiology of Hearing, 2nd ed. London: Academic Press; 1988

[83] Lenarz T, Lim HH, Reuter G, Patrick JF, Lenarz M. The auditory midbrain implant: a new auditory prosthesis for neural deafness—concept and device description. Otol Neurotol. 2006; 27(6):838–843

[84] Lim HH, Lenarz M, Lenarz T. Auditory midbrain implant: a review. Trends Amplif. 2009; 13(3):149–180

[85] Schierholz I, Finke M, Kral A, et al. Auditory and audio-visual processing in patients with cochlear, auditory brainstem, and auditory midbrain implants: an EEG study. Hum Brain Mapp. 2017; 38(4):2206–2225

3 Imaging of the Cochlea, Cochlear Nerve, Brainstem, and Auditory System

Burce Ozgen

Abstract

Imaging of the cochlea, cochlear nerve, brainstem, and auditory system is central to proper candidate selection and surgical planning in the setting of an auditory brainstem implantation. For the preoperative imaging of an auditory brainstem implant (ABI) candidate high-resolution computed tomography (CT) and magnetic resonance (MR) imaging provide complementary information. The imaging of an ABI candidate will not only help to fulfill the indication criteria but also help to assess the integrity of the auditory pathway from the brainstem up to the temporal cortex. Similarly imaging following implantation is again critical to confirm the appropriate electrode placement and, when needed, to evaluate possible complications.

Keywords: auditory brainstem implant, computed tomography, MR imaging, cochlear nerve, auditory pathway

3.1 Introduction

Imaging plays an important and indispensable role in the preoperative and postoperative assessment of cochlear and auditory brainstem implant (ABI) patients. The evaluation of the cochlea and cochlear nerve determines the eligibility of the patient for the cochlear versus auditory brainstem implantation. Additionally, the imaging of the posterior fossa as well as supratentorial structures is crucial for appropriate preoperative assessment of an ABI candidate. Following implantation, imaging is again required to confirm correct electrode placement as well as to evaluate possible complications; however, the implant itself becomes a source for artifact and potential hazard in a magnetic field. This chapter begins with a discussion of the radiological anatomy of the auditory pathway and will then address the important concepts related to preoperative and postoperative imaging of the ABIs.

3.2 Imaging Anatomy of the Inner Ear and Auditory Pathway

3.2.1 Cochlea

In modern-day practice the inner ear structures are evaluated with sectional imaging using computed tomography (CT) and magnetic resonance imaging (MRI). With either imaging technique, the cochlea appears as a spiral-shaped structure with 2.5 turns and a normal measured height of 5.1 mm (with a range of 4.4 to 5.9 mm).[1] The cochlear turns (basal, middle, and apical) are separated by interscalar septae, a bony plate radiating from the modiolus that forms the base of the cochlea (▶ Fig. 3.1). The spiral lamina that also projects from the modiolus is a micro-anatomical osseous structure that separates the spiral of the cochlea into scala tympani (inferiorly), scala media, and scala vestibuli (superiorly). The spiral lamina can be seen with

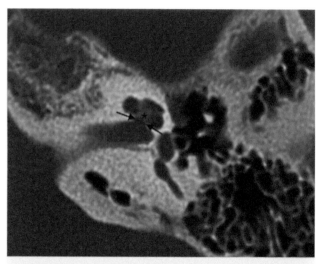

Fig. 3.1 Computed tomography (CT) anatomy of the cochlea. Axial temporal bone CT image demonstrates normal appearance of the cochlear aperture (*delineated by the arrows*). Note the normal appearance of the modiolus (*star*) at the base of the cochlea.

difficulty with conventional CT; however, it is easily appreciable with thin section MRI[2] (▶ Fig. 3.2a). The scala tympani and scala vestibuli that are filled with fluid can be separated with high-resolution clinical 1.5 and 3 Tesla MRI; however, the scala media can only be visualized with high Tesla imaging.[3,4] The cochlear nerve passes from the internal auditory canal (IAC) to the modiolus through a bony canal called the cochlear aperture (or bony cochlear nerve canal) (▶ Fig. 3.1). This "neck of the cochlea" has a normal measurable width of 1.9 mm (±0.24 mm).[2,5]

3.2.2 IAC and the Vestibulocochlear Nerve

The size of IAC varies but the mean canal diameter is 4.21 ± 0.79 mm (with a range of 2–8 mm), and the two ears have almost symmetric size with a difference of up to 2 mm.[6,7] The vestibulocochlear and the facial nerve can only be well appreciated with high-resolution, high T2-weighted imaging (▶ Fig. 3.2a). Although the axial slices can demonstrate the size of the IAC and help to evaluate the course of the vestibulocochlear nerve (VCN), the sagittal oblique images obtained perpendicular to the long axis of the IAC are best to distinguish each of the individual components of the VCN as the nerves are visualized in cross-section.[8] At the medial aspect of the IAC the VCN is seen as a crescent-shaped structure (▶ Fig. 3.2b); however, more laterally, in the fundus, the three components of the VCN can be seen separately and the cochlear nerve lies in the anteroinferior aspect (▶ Fig. 3.2c).[9] The normal size of the cochlear nerve on MRI measures 1.8 ± 0.2 mm at the porus acousticus and 1.2 ± 0.2 mm in the mid to distal IAC.[10] In the majority of cases, the cochlear nerve is larger than

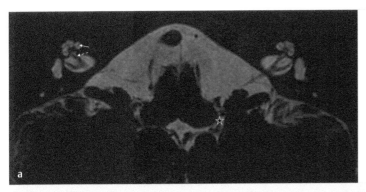
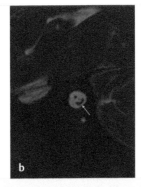
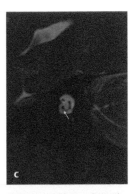

Fig. 3.2 Anatomy of the cochlea and cochlear nerve by high-resolution magnetic resonance imaging (MRI). Heavy T2-weighted driven equilibrium (DRIVE) images in axial (**a**) and sagittal oblique planes (**b, c**). The cochlear turns with internal spiral lamina (*arrow*) is visible with this high T2-weighted axial image in figure (**a**). The cochlear nerve (*dotted arrow*) is seen at the fundus of the internal auditory canal (IAC). With sagittal oblique imaging, the vestibulocochlear nerve (*arrow*) is seen as a crescenteric structure at the medial aspect of the IAC in figure (**b**); however, more laterally, the cochlear nerve (*arrow*) can be seen separately from the inferior and superior vestibular nerves in figure (**c**). Note is made of nice visualization the lateral recess (*empty star*) on the left.

both the superior or inferior vestibular nerves.[11] The cochlear nerve is of similar size or larger than the facial nerve in more than half of the cases.[9]

3.2.3 Cochlear Nucleus

MRI is better in delineating details of the brain anatomy but it is somewhat limited in the brainstem.[12] The difficulties in assessing the brainstem by using MRI arises not only from the small size of various brainstem structures, but also from the fact that those anatomical components do not exhibit enough contrast to enable their individual identification.[13] Therefore, when relaxation-based MR image contrast is used, despite high resolution, conspicuity of those structures such as cranial nerve nuclei cannot be achieved in clinical field strengths.[14] Nevertheless, the bulge of the medulla into the lateral recess of the fourth ventricle and to the foramen of Luschka caused by the cochlear nuclear complex can be easily identified by MRI (▶ Fig. 3.2a).[15]

3.2.4 Auditory Pathway

Morphologic Imaging Anatomy

Similar to the cochlear nuclear complex, the ascending fibers of the auditory pathway are not visible with normal visual inspection of routine MR sequences. The auditory radiation can only be demonstrated with dedicated fiber tracking obtained from the diffusion tensor imaging.[16] Functional MRI (fMRI) studies that allow noninvasive assessment of brain function can localize the auditory cortex (▶ Fig. 3.3).

3.3 Preoperative Imaging of the Auditory Brainstem Implants

3.3.1 Imaging Techniques

For the preoperative imaging of ABI candidates, high-resolution CT and MRI provide complementary information.

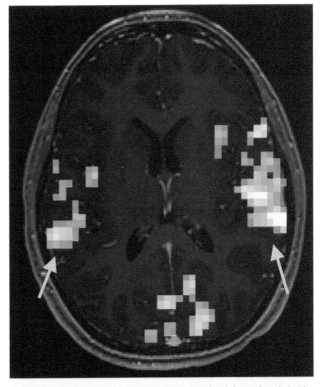

Fig. 3.3 Axial image from a blood oxygenation level dependent (BOLD) functional magnetic resonance imaging (fMRI) study demonstrating bilateral activation of the auditory cortex (*arrows*). (Courtesy of Dr. Keith Thulborn.)

CT

CT remains the preferred examination for the initial evaluation of congenital sensorineural hearing loss (SNHL). CT of the temporal bone is able to delineate the detailed anatomy of the inner ear; but more importantly it can also help to evaluate the dimensions of the IAC and cochlear aperture to subsequently refer the patient for possible ABI placement. The two currently available and recommended CT scanners for the imaging of the temporal bone are multi-detector CT (MDCT) and cone-beam CT (CBCT).

MDCT

MDCT has been and still is in most centers in the world the standard method to evaluate the temporal bone with CT. The image acquisition is performed in the axial plane; however, isotropic voxels allow reformatted images with high resolution in any additional plane. The imaging parameters are scanner specific but the collimation is usually 0.5 to 0.625 mm and has to be less than 1 mm. Images should always be processed with a bone algorithm and viewed with a window width of 4,000 HU and a window level of 200 to 500 HU.[17]

CBCT

Although MDCT is used worldwide, CBCT using flat panel detector technology is slowly taking over for detailed evaluation of the small temporal bone structures.[17] The CBCT uses a rotating gantry and a cone-shaped X-ray beam that generates three-dimensional volumetric dataset.[17] It results in higher resolution (0.15 mm thickness) with a lower dose. Additionally, it is less sensitive to metallic and beam hardening artifacts. It is however more sensitive to motion as the acquisition usually lasts for 40 seconds and anesthesia may be required for small children.

MRI

MRI is crucial in order to assess the cochlear nerve, the brain stem, and the integrity of the auditory pathways up to the temporal cortex. Again, the patient's cooperation in limiting the motion is paramount and anesthesia is required for small children. The MRI should be performed with a 3.0 Tesla scanner whenever possible as higher field strength improves the signal to noise ratio (SNR) and increases the spatial resolution.[18] The MRI for the evaluation of an implant candidate should include high-resolution heavily T2-weighted sequence for a detailed evaluation of the membranous labyrinth, and especially for the assessment of the cochlear nerve. These sequences can be achieved with both gradient-echo (GRE) and fast spin-echo (FSE) T2-weighted techniques but the choice of which sequence to prefer is a heavily debated and published topic.[19] The most commonly used and widely available sequences include: constructive interference into steady state (CISS), fast imaging employing steady-state acquisition (FIESTA), driven equilibrium radio frequency reset pulse (DRIVE), 3D true-fast imaging with steady-state precession (FISP), and 3D T2 FSE or 3D T2 FSE with fast recovery (FRFSE) depending on the scanner vendor. The resolution of these heavily T2-weighted sequence should be increased with a slice thickness less than or equal to 1 mm. Although sagittal oblique reformatted images can be obtained from the axial dataset, bilateral direct sagittal oblique images, perpendicular to the IACs, with the same heavily T2-weighted sequence should always be acquired as the direct sagittal oblique images have a better resolution than the reformatted images.[8] The T2-weighted imaging of the entire brain is also required to assess the auditory pathway.[20,21] For neurofibromatosis type 2 (NF2) patients, postcontrast imaging of the entire brain is also required to look for additional intracranial extra-axial tumors.

3.3.2 Radiological Evaluation of the Auditory Brainstem Implant Candidates

Evaluation of Eligibility Criteria for Implantation in Congenital SNHL

The initial radiological assessment of an ABI candidate with congenital SNHL is indeed one of a cochlear implant (CI) candidate with ineligibility for the latter determining indication for the former.[22,23] The selected congenital inner ear anomalies that result in an ABI candidacy will be discussed in detail in another chapter, but from an imaging point of view not only the specific anomaly has to be detected and correctly labeled but also the size of the cochlear aperture and the presence of the cochlear nerve and its size should be evaluated. The structures that need to be carefully evaluated in a pre-implant imaging study are the following.

Cochlea

Cochlear hypoplasia represents a group of cochlear malformations which have dimensions less than normal cochlea with decreased number or height of the cochlear turns.[24,25] When the cochlea is hypoplastic the nerve may be also be hypoplastic or aplastic and needs to be assessed with MRI.[26] Similarly, common cavity anomaly, and type 1 and 2 incomplete partition anomalies have also been reported to have accompanying cochlear deficiencies including aplasia and need to be evaluated with MRI.[7,27,28]

Cochlear Aperture

Atresia of the cochlear aperture is a strong indicator of underlying cochlear nerve anomaly.[7,29] Tahir et al reported that all 21 cases with cochlear aperture atresia in their series had accompanying cochlear nerve deficiency (either aplasia or hypoplasia).[7] The dimension of a patient's cochlear aperture also needs to be assessed, as its diameter is a marker of the cochlear nerve status.[7,30] The cochlear aperture is considered stenotic when it is narrower than 1.4 mm (▶ Fig. 3.4a).[5,31,32,33,34] In the series reported by Tahir et al, most of the stenotic cochlear aperture cases had accompanying hypoplasia/aplasia of the cochlear nerve with a normal size nerve in only 15% of the cases.[7] It is critical to realize that the aperture can be stenotic in the presence of a normal appearing and normal size cochlea; thus, a normal cochlear shape does not always indicate normal cochlear nerve structure and further imaging with MRI is required to assess the cochlear nerve status.[7]

Internal Auditory Canal

The IAC is considered stenotic when the diameter at its midpoint is smaller than 2 mm.[35] The IAC stenosis or atresia may be easily demonstrated by CT. Although the exact measurement of the IAC diameter is more difficult with MRI, the high-resolution T2-weighted images can still demonstrate IAC hypoplasia or atresia with deceased or absence of high T2 signal of cerebrospinal fluid (CSF) within the IAC. Again the finding of a narrow or aplastic IAC raises concern for a deficiency of the cochlear nerve.[29,36] However, the IAC morphology is an unreliable surrogate marker of cochlear nerve integrity and as reported by

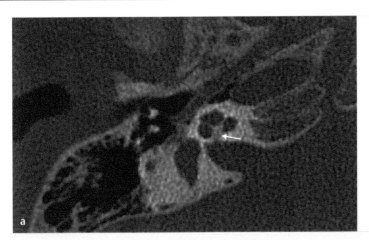 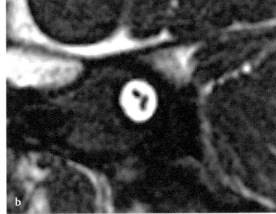

Fig. 3.4 **(a)** Axial temporal bone computed tomography (CT) **(b)** and sagittal oblique three-dimensional driven equilibrium (DRIVE) image of a patient with bilateral congenital severe sensorineural hearing loss (SNHL). The CT image of the right ear reveals atresia of the right cochlear aperture (*arrow*) with aplasia of the cochlear nerve on the corresponding magnetic resonance (MR) image in figure **(b)**.

Adunka et al, a normal IAC diameter can be seen in up to half of cochlear nerve aplasia patients.[7,37]

Cochlear Nerve

The evaluation of the VCN and especially its cochlear branch is of extreme importance prior to cochlear implantation. In a normal-sized IAC the diagnosis of cochlear nerve aplasia is relatively straightforward with dedicated sagittal oblique high-resolution images (▶ Fig. 3.4b).[38] However, in a very stenotic IAC, the diagnosis may be difficult because of the inability to separate the nerves.[35,37] Again the visualized inner ear may be normal or have subtle abnormality despite severe deficiency of the cochlear nerve.[38,39] Differentiation between hypoplasia and a normal size of the cochlear branch can also be challenging and require the highest possible resolution.[39] There isn't a well-defined consensus regarding the definition cochlear nerve hypoplasia. Li et al defined the cochlear nerve hypoplasia as a cochlear nerve with a diameter smaller than that of the facial nerve, seen on the oblique sagittal images.[29] Similarly, Glastonbury et al designated the cochlear nerve as small when it appeared decreased in size compared with the other nerves of the IAC.[39] It is critical to recognize that there might be occasional discrepancy between the imaging and audiological findings regarding the presence/functionality of the cochlear nerve.[40,41] Several studies have shown that subsets of patients with cochlear nerve aplasia have positive audiological responses and might derive benefit from cochlear implantation.[40,41,42] Anatomical connections between the cochlear nerve and other branches of the vestibulocochlear complex that are below the resolution of the current MRI might be responsible for this radiological–audiological inconsistency.[43] Imaging with ultra-high field magnets with diffusion tensor imaging (DTI) fiber tractography might solve this problem in the future.[3,44]

Brainstem and Supratentorial Brain

In every patient who is a candidate for an ABI placement, the imaging of the brainstem and supratentorial brain structures with MRI is crucial not only to verify the integrity of the auditory pathways up to the temporal cortex but also to determine

possible underlying congenital or acquired malformations that might hinder post implant rehabilitation.[22,45] There is significant variability of the anatomy of the lateral recess in children with congenital deafness due to abnormalities of embryonic and fetal development.[46] It has been previously reported that congenital developmental abnormalities of the brain are more common in patients with auditory neuropathy spectrum disorder.[21,46,47] In patients with bilateral cochlear nerve deficiency, hindbrain anomalies such as pontine hypoplasia were reported to be the most common abnormal intracranial finding.[46] Additionally, there might be evidence of central pathologies such as chronic changes of hypoxic-ischemic injury, kernicterus, and chronic changes of congenital central nervous system (CNS) infections.[48,49] White matter lesions are also common findings in the preimplant imaging of the CI/ABI candidates.[21,50] These lesions are nonspecific, and more diffuse and prominent parenchymal changes were found to represent negative prognostic factors for speech and language development.[20,49,50] It is therefore critical to make a comprehensive evaluation of the brainstem and cerebrum in each ABI candidate. Additionally, with new developing technologies, MRI also has the potential to study the anatomical and functional organization of the auditory cortex through voxel-based morphometry and fMRI.[51] DTI metrics, such as fractional anisotropy, may prove important in selecting patients and predicting outcomes after the implantation.[52]

Evaluation of Eligibility Criteria for Implantation in Acquired SNHL

The radiological evaluation of an ABI candidate with acquired SNHL is different from the cases with congenital SNHL as the imaging is more focused on the detection of possible surgical challenges and the following structures should be individually assessed.

The Brainstem

The posterolateral medulla where the cochlear nuclear complex is located should have no appreciable signal changes. Post-traumatic or postoperative encephalomalacic changes as well as potential injury from prior radiation therapy are important considerations for this location.[53,54] Similarly, ischemic changes involving the brainstem and especially posterolateral medulla should be absent.[55] Although currently T2-weighted imaging is the recommended method of assessment for pontomedullary junction, in the future DTI may enable depiction of more subtle anomalies such as early detection of radiation-induced changes on auditory pathways in patients with vestibular schwannomas and might predict the success of the implantation preoperatively.[44,56]

The Lateral Recess

The site of electrode placement should be normal in size without asymmetric widening as an enlargement at this location might contribute to the migration or rotation of the electrode array (▶ Fig. 3.5).[57] Additionally, in NF2 patients, the presence or previous resection of tumors may result in distortion of the brainstem and the lateral recess may be difficult to identify.[58] In the setting of scar tissue from previous surgery, visible as obliteration of normal CSF signal, accompanying enhancement might be seen at the site of contemplated implantation and may result in distortion of the normal anatomy.

Basal Cisterns

Anomalous lower cranial nerves and vascular anomalies around the lateral recess are potential variations that need to be looked for as those findings might prevent successful ABI placement or might cause unexpected surgical difficulties.[59] This assessment is best done with high-resolution heavily T2-weighted sequences. It has also been reported that previous meningitis might lead to excessive bleeding and increased surgical difficulties. It is thus

important to evaluate postcontrast T1-weighted images for possible increased leptomeningeal enhancement.[60]

Supratentorial Brain

In NF2 patients additional supratentorial masses such as meningiomas or meningiomatosis as well as parenchymal signal abnormalities should beinvestigated.[61] Similarly, possible accompanying traumatic encephalomalacia of the auditory cortex or sequel of shearing injury should be looked for in the setting of an ABI candidate with bilateral post-traumatic deafness.[60,62]

3.4 Postoperative Imaging of the Implanted Patient

3.4.1 Imaging Issues after ABI

Following implantation, imaging is usually performed to determine the location of the electrode array to check for appropriate electrode array placement.[63] Additionally, a brain imaging might be required to investigate immediate postoperative complications or for the follow-up of an NF2 patient.[64]

Radiographic Evaluation

Plain X-ray films in anteroposterior (AP) and modified Stenvers' views are the standard methods of imaging following ABI surgery and are sufficient in a majority of patients to depict the integrity and positioning of electrode array and to detect electrode kinking (▶ Fig. 3.6). The evaluation on those plain films were standardized by Cerini et al on lateral and AP views, where angles rather than distances from specific landmarks

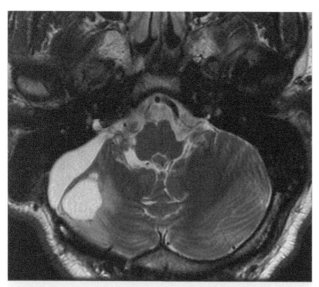

Fig. 3.5 The magnetic resonance imaging (MRI) of the ear of a patient with NF2 and prior resection of right-sided vestibular schwannomas. The axial T2-weighted image demonstrates marked asymmetric widening of the lateral recess on the right.

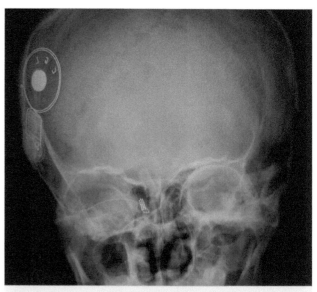

Fig. 3.6 Post implant anteroposterior (AP) plain film of a 31-year-old NF2 patient demonstrating the auditory brainstem implant (ABI) electrode array in place.

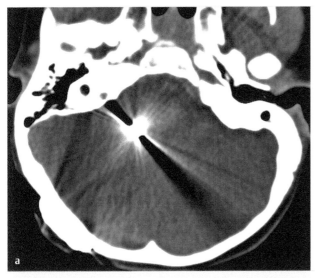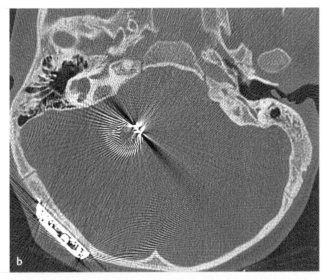

Fig. 3.7 Computed tomography (CT) of head of a child with auditory brainstem implant (ABI) performed for bilateral cochlear aplasia in **(a)** soft tissue and **(b)** bone windows. Although severely limited due to the artifact of the implant, the structures of the posterior fossa are visible on the soft-tissue window **(a)**. The bone window demonstrates the receiver-stimulator embedded within the temporal bone as well as the electrode array; however, the exact location of the implant is difficult to assess due to invisibility of the soft-tissue structures on this window **(b)**.

were used to establish correct electrode positioning.[65] However, only limited information concerning the exact positioning of the electrode array can be extrapolated from plain films due to the innate planar representation.[66]

CT Imaging

CT evaluation is especially useful when postoperative radiographs fail to properly demonstrate the location of the electrode array or if a postoperative complication is suspected.[65] CT is suitable to assess the integrity of the device. Although the soft-tissue algorithm adequately demonstrates brainstem structures, it fails to distinguish the metallic electrodes and wires (▶ Fig. 3.7a). Correspondingly, the bone algorithm delineates the electrodes well, but accompanying streak artifact limits the determination of the implant positioning with respect to surrounding soft tissues (▶ Fig. 3.7b).[65] To overcome this limitation Lo et al suggested a superposition technique with inverted bone windows that were superimposed onto soft-tissue windows to better delineate the electrodes in relation to surrounding soft-tissue structures.[67] Advanced techniques such as View Angle Tilting (VAT) and Slice-Encoding for Metal Artefact Reduction (SEMAC) are also being developed to address the device artifacts with promising results.[66] CT is usually the adequate and the recommended imaging for the evaluation of potential early postoperative complications such as hemorrhage or CSF leak.[22]

MRI Safety

Currently MRI is not used for standard postoperative imaging due to artifacts and poor resolution in the presence of the implant. However, as the majority of ABI candidates are NF2 patients who require continued follow-up imaging, the issue of

MRI safety for the ABI devices is an important consideration.[68] The original ABIs were magnetic and incompatible with MRI, but most of the current models are reported to be nonmagnetic and MRI-compatible for 1.5 Tesla.[69] The major issue with respect to MRI safety of ABIs relates to the internal magnet.[66] The magnetic field force may rotate the internal magnet with resultant pain and dislodgement during scan, with the greatest risk of deflection in young children (due to thin recipient bone) and with head MRI studies. For the dislocation risk, magnet removal using local anesthetic has been advised; however, this is costly, invasive and with a risk of skin flap infection (▶ Fig. 3.8a, b).[66] Another suggested solution is head bandaging with successful results even with 3 Tesla.[70,71] The magnet technology is advancing and has also led to the development of a freely rotating magnet that can be used without magnet removal or even a pressure dressing, with no reported risk of dislocation or demagnetization.[72]

The artifacts generated by the magnet of the implant might cause blooming artifact and distortion of the adjacent regions. However, it has been reported that the ipsilateral posterior fossa is rarely completely obscured. Thus, follow-up imaging for residual/recurrent vestibular schwannomas can be performed (▶ Fig. 3.8c).[71]

The present preoperative imaging for ABI is central to proper candidate selection and surgical planning but postoperative imaging is still limited due to artifacts from the electrode and magnet but especially due to inability of the current imaging to delineate the cochlear nuclear complex. Nevertheless, higher Tesla imaging with new sequence designs and postprocessing software technologies are likely to improve our imaging capabilities in the future with possibly better evaluation of microstructural changes of the higher auditory pathways that will allow better prognostic evaluation of the implant candidate.

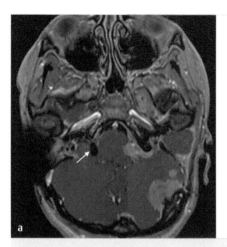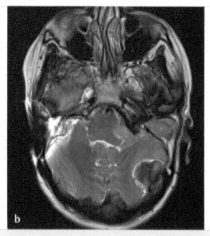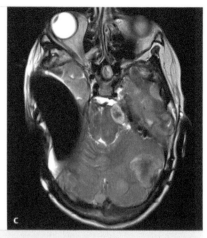

Fig. 3.8 Postimplant magnetic resonance (MR) study of a NF2 patient with prior resection of schwannoma on the right with auditory brainstem implant (ABI) placement. **(a)** The postcontrast T1-weighted and **(b)** T2-weighted images performed after removal of the magnet reveal the postoperative changes from prior posterior fossa surgery. The electrode array (*arrow*) is only visible on the T1-weighted image **(a)**. Note the residual vestibular schwannoma on the left with multiple accompanying meningiomas in the posterior fossa. **(c)** T2-weighted image from another MR study of the same patient obtained a year later with the magnet in place demonstrating a more prominent artifact of the magnet in place. (Courtesy of Dr. Bert De Foer.)

References

[1] Purcell DD, Fischbein N, Lalwani AK. Identification of previously "undetectable" abnormalities of the bony labyrinth with computed tomography measurement. Laryngoscope. 2003; 113(11):1908–1911

[2] Fatterpekar GM, Doshi AH, Dugar M, Delman BN, Naidich TP, Som PM. Role of 3D CT in the evaluation of the temporal bone. Radiographics. 2006; 26 Suppl 1:S117–S132

[3] Thylur DS, Jacobs RE, Go JL, Toga AW, Niparko JK. Ultra-high-field magnetic resonance imaging of the human inner ear at 11.7 Tesla. Otol Neurotol. 2017; 38(1):133–138

[4] van der Jagt MA, Brink WM, Versluis MJ, et al. Visualization of human inner ear anatomy with high-resolution MR imaging at 7T: initial clinical assessment. AJNR Am j Neuroradiol. 2015; 36(2):378–383

[5] Stjernholm C, Muren C. Dimensions of the cochlear nerve canal: a radioanatomic investigation. Acta Otolaryngol. 2002; 122(1):43–48

[6] Valvassori G, Palacios E. The abnormal internal acoustic canal. Ear Nose Throat J. 1998; 77(4):260–262

[7] Tahir E, Bajin MD, Atay G, Mocan BO, Sennaroğlu L. Bony cochlear nerve canal and internal auditory canal measures predict cochlear nerve status. J Laryngol Otol. 2017; 131(8):676–683

[8] Noij KS, Remenschneider AK, Kozin ED, et al. Direct parasagittal magnetic resonance imaging of the internal auditory canal to determine cochlear or auditory brainstem implant candidacy in children. Laryngoscope. 2015; 125 (10):2382–2385

[9] Rubinstein D, Sandberg EJ, Cajade-Law AG. Anatomy of the facial and vestibulocochlear nerves in the internal auditory canal. AJNR Am J Neuroradiol. 1996; 17(6):1099–1105

[10] Nadol JB, Jr, Xu WZ. Diameter of the cochlear nerve in deaf humans: implications for cochlear implantation. Ann Otol Rhinol Laryngol. 1992; 101(12): 988–993

[11] Lou J, Gong WX, Wang GB. Cochlear nerve diameters on multipoint measurements and effects of aging in normal-hearing children using 3.0-T magnetic resonance imaging. Int J Pediatr Otorhinolaryngol. 2015; 79(7):1077–1080

[12] Sclocco R, Beissner F, Bianciardi M, Polimeni JR, Napadow V. Challenges and opportunities for brainstem neuroimaging with ultrahigh field MRI. Neuroimage. 2018;168:412–426

[13] Beissner F. Functional MRI of the brainstem: common problems and their solutions. Clin Neuroradiol. 2015; 25 Suppl 2:251–257

[14] Lambert C, Lutti A, Helms G, Frackowiak R, Ashburner J. Multiparametric brainstem segmentation using a modified multivariate mixture of Gaussians. Neuroimage Clin. 2013; 2:684–694

[15] Gebarski SS, Tucci DL, Telian SA. The cochlear nuclear complex: MR location and abnormalities. AJNR Am J Neuroradiol. 1993; 14(6):1311–1318

[16] Javad F, Warren JD, Micallef C, et al. Auditory tracts identified with combined fMRI and diffusion tractography. Neuroimage. 2014; 84:562–574

[17] Lemmerling M, de De Foer B. Temporal Bone Imaging. Berlin Heidelberg: Springer; 2014

[18] Schulze M, Reimann K, Seeger A, Klose U, Ernemann U, Hauser TK. Improvement in imaging common temporal bone pathologies at 3 T MRI: small structures benefit from a small field of view. Clin Radiol. 2017; 72(3): 267.e1–267.e12

[19] Glastonbury C. The vestibulocochlear nerve, with an emphasis on the normal and diseased internal auditory canal and cerebellopontine angle. In: Swartz JD, Loevner LA, eds. Imaging of the Temporal Bone. New York, NY: Thieme Medical Publishers; 2009:480–558

[20] Moon IJ, Kim EY, Park GY, et al. The clinical significance of preoperative brain magnetic resonance imaging in pediatric cochlear implant recipients. Audiol Neurotol. 2012; 17(6):373–380

[21] Lapointe A, Viamonte C, Morriss MC, Manolidis S. Central nervous system findings by magnetic resonance in children with profound sensorineural hearing loss. Int J Pediatr Otorhinolaryngol. 2006; 70(5):863–868

[22] Sennaroglu L, Ziyal I. Auditory brainstem implantation. Auris Nasus Larynx. 2012; 39(5):439–450

[23] Sennaroğlu L, Colletti V, Lenarz T, et al. Consensus statement: long-term results of ABI in children with complex inner ear malformations and decision making between CI and ABI. Cochlear Implants Int. 2016; 17(4):163–171

[24] Giesemann AM, Goetz F, Neuburger J, Lenarz T, Lanfermann H. Appearance of hypoplastic cochleae in CT and MRI: a new subclassification. Neuroradiology. 2011; 53(1):49–61

[25] Shim HJ, Shin JE, Chung JW, Lee KS. Inner ear anomalies in cochlear implantees: importance of radiologic measurements in the classification. Otol Neurotol. 2006; 27(6):831–837

[26] Cinar BC, Batuk MO, Tahir E, Sennaroglu G, Sennaroglu L. Audiologic and radiologic findings in cochlear hypoplasia. Auris Nasus Larynx. 2017; 44(6): 655–663

[27] Özbal Batuk M, Çınar BC, Özgen B, Sennaroğlu G, Sennaroğlu L. Audiological and radiological characteristics in incomplete partition malformations. J Int Adv Otol. 2017; 13(2):233–238

[28] Giesemann AM, Kontorinis G, Jan Z, Lenarz T, Lanfermann H, Goetz F. The vestibulocochlear nerve: aplasia and hypoplasia in combination with inner ear malformations. Eur Radiol. 2012; 22(3):519–524

[29] Li Y, Yang J, Liu J, Wu H. Restudy of malformations of the internal auditory meatus, cochlear nerve canal and cochlear nerve. Eur Arch Otorhinolaryngol. 2015; 272(7):1587–1596

[30] Fatterpekar GM, Mukherji SK, Alley J, Lin Y, Castillo M. Hypoplasia of the bony canal for the cochlear nerve in patients with congenital sensorineural hearing loss: initial observations. Radiology. 2000; 215(1):243–246

[31] D'Arco F, Talenti G, Lakshmanan R, Stephenson K, Siddiqui A, Carney O. Do measurements of inner ear structures help in the diagnosis of inner ear malformations? A review of literature. Otol Neurotol. 2017; 38(10):e384–e392

[32] Lan M-Y, Shiao J-Y, Ho C-Y, Hung H-C. Measurements of normal inner ear on computed tomography in children with congenital sensorineural hearing loss. Eur Arch Otorhinolaryngol. 2009; 266(9):1361–1364

[33] Miyasaka M, Nosaka S, Morimoto N, Taiji H, Masaki H. CT and MR imaging for pediatric cochlear implantation: emphasis on the relationship between the cochlear nerve canal and the cochlear nerve. Pediatr Radiol. 2010; 40(9): 1509–1516

[34] Yi JS, Lim HW, Kang BC, Park S-Y, Park HJ, Lee K-S. Proportion of bony cochlear nerve canal anomalies in unilateral sensorineural hearing loss in children. Int J Pediatr Otorhinolaryngol. 2013; 77(4):530–533

[35] Romo LV, Casselman JW, Robson CD. Temporal bone: congenital anomalies. In: Som PM, Curtin HD, eds. Head and Neck Imaging. 5th ed. St. Louis, Missouri: Elsevier Health Sciences; 2011:1097–1165

[36] Shelton C, Luxford WM, Tonokawa LL, Lo WW, House WF. The narrow internal auditory canal in children: a contraindication to cochlear implants. Otolaryngol Head Neck Surg. 1989; 100(3):227–231

[37] Adunka OF, Roush PA, Teagle HFB, et al. Internal auditory canal morphology in children with cochlear nerve deficiency. Otol Neurotol. 2006; 27(6):793–801

[38] Casselman JW, Offeciers FE, Govaerts PJ, et al. Aplasia and hypoplasia of the vestibulocochlear nerve: diagnosis with MR imaging. Radiology. 1997; 202 (3):773–781

[39] Glastonbury CM, Davidson HC, Harnsberger HR, Butler J, Kertesz TR, Shelton C. Imaging findings of cochlear nerve deficiency. AJNR Am J Neuroradiol. 2002; 23(4):635–643

[40] Peng KA, Kuan EC, Hagan S, Wilkinson EP, Miller ME. Cochlear nerve aplasia and hypoplasia: predictors of cochlear implant success. Otolaryngol Head Neck Surg. 2017; 157(3):392–400

[41] Young NM, Kim FM, Ryan ME, Tournis E, Yaras S. Pediatric cochlear implantation of children with eighth nerve deficiency. Int J Pediatr Otorhinolaryngol. 2012; 76(10):1442–1448

[42] Acker T, Mathur NN, Savy L, Graham JM. Is there a functioning vestibulocochlear nerve? Cochlear implantation in a child with symmetrical auditory findings but asymmetric imaging. Int J Pediatr Otorhinolaryngol. 2001; 57(2):171–176

[43] Ozdoğmuş O, Sezen O, Kubilay U, et al. Connections between the facial, vestibular and cochlear nerve bundles within the internal auditory canal. J Anat. 2004; 205(1):65–75

[44] Vos SB, Haakma W, Versnel H, et al. Diffusion tensor imaging of the auditory nerve in patients with long-term single-sided deafness. Hear Res. 2015; 323:1–8

[45] Colletti G, Mandalà M, Colletti L, Colletti V. Nervus intermedius guides auditory brainstem implant surgery in children with cochlear nerve deficiency. Otolaryngol Head Neck Surg. 2016; 154(2):335–342

[46] Huang BY, Roche JP, Buchman CA, Castillo M. Brain stem and inner ear abnormalities in children with auditory neuropathy spectrum disorder and cochlear nerve deficiency. AJNR Am J Neuroradiol. 2010; 31(10):1972–1979

[47] Joshi VM, Navlekar SK, Kishore GR, Reddy KJ, Kumar ECCT. CT and MR imaging of the inner ear and brain in children with congenital sensorineural hearing loss. Radiographics. 2012; 32(3):683–698

[48] Jallu AS, Jehangir M, Ul Hamid W, Pampori RA. Imaging evaluation of pediatric sensorineural hearing loss in potential candidates for cochlear implantation. Indian J Otolaryngol Head Neck Surg. 2015; 67(4):341–346

[49] Xu XQ, Wu FY, Hu H, Su GY, Shen J. Incidence of brain abnormalities detected on preoperative brain MR imaging and their effect on the outcome of cochlear implantation in children with sensorineural hearing loss. Int J Biomed Imaging. 2015; 2015:275786

[50] Hong P, Jurkowski ZC, Carvalho DS. Preoperative cerebral magnetic resonance imaging and white matter changes in pediatric cochlear implant recipients. Int J Pediatr Otorhinolaryngol. 2010; 74(6):658–660

[51] Semenza C, Cavinato M, Rigon J, Battel I, Meneghello F, Venneri A. Persistent cortical deafness: a voxel-based morphometry and tractography study. Neuropsychology. 2012; 26(6):675–683

[52] Huang L, Zheng W, Wu C, et al. Diffusion tensor imaging of the auditory neural pathway for clinical outcome of cochlear implantation in pediatric congenital sensorineural hearing loss patients. PLoS One. 2015; 10(10): e0140643

[53] Schick B, Brors D, Koch O, Schäfers M, Kahle G. Magnetic resonance imaging in patients with sudden hearing loss, tinnitus and vertigo. Otol Neurotol. 2001; 22(6):808–812

[54] Linskey ME, Lunsford LD, Flickinger JC. Neuroimaging of acoustic nerve sheath tumors after stereotaxic radiosurgery. AJNR Am J Neuroradiol. 1991; 12(6):1165–1175

[55] Oas JG, Baloh RW. Vertigo and the anterior inferior cerebellar artery syndrome. Neurology. 1992; 42(12):2274–2279

[56] Kurtcan S, Hatiboglu MA, Alkan A, et al. Evaluation of auditory pathways using DTI in patients treated with Gamma Knife radiosurgery for acoustic neuroma: apreliminary report. Clin Neuroradiol. 2018; 28(3):377–383

[57] KuchtaJ. Central Auditory Implants. Books on Demand; 2010

[58] Brackmann DE, Hitselberger WE, Nelson RA, et al. Auditory brainstem implant: I. Issues in surgical implantation. Otolaryngol Head Neck Surg. 1993; 108(6):624–633

[59] Puram SV, Lee DJ. Pediatric auditory brainstem implant surgery. Otolaryngol Clin North Am. 2015; 48(6):1117–1148

[60] Marsot-Dupuch K, Meyer B. Cochlear implant assessment: imaging issues. Eur J Radiol. 2001; 40(2):119–132

[61] Vargas WS, Heier LA, Rodriguez F, Bergner A, Yohay K. Incidental parenchymal magnetic resonance imaging findings in the brains of patients with neurofibromatosis type 2. Neuroimage Clin. 2014; 4:258–265

[62] Aziz KM, Yu AK, Chen D, Sekula RF Jr. Chapter 204 - Management of cranial nerve injuries A2.In: Quiñones-Hinojosa, Alfredo. Schmidek and Sweet: Operative Neurosurgical Techniques.6th ed. Philadelphia: W.B. Saunders; 2012:2329–2338

[63] Shannon RV, Fayad J, Moore J, et al. Auditory brainstem implant: II. Postsurgical issues and performance. Otolaryngol Head Neck Surg. 1993; 108(6): 634–642

[64] Colletti V, Shannon RV, Carner M, Veronese S, Colletti L. Complications in auditory brainstem implant surgery in adults and children. Otol Neurotol. 2010; 31(4):558–564

[65] Cerini R, Faccioli N, Barillari M, et al. Bionic ear imaging. Radiol Med (Torino). 2008; 113(2):265–277

[66] Connor SE. Contemporary imaging of auditory implants. Clin Radiol. 2018; 73 (1):19–34

[67] Lo WW, Tasaka A, Zink B, Harris O. A simple CT method for location of auditory brain stem implant electrodes. AJNR Am J Neuroradiol. 1995; 16(3): 599–601

[68] Azadarmaki R, Tubbs R, Chen DA, Shellock FG. MRI information for commonly used otologic implants: review and update. Otolaryngol Head Neck Surg. 2014; 150(4):512–519

[69] Heller JW, Brackmann DE, Tucci DL, Nyenhuis JA, Chou CK. Evaluation of MRI compatibility of the modified nucleus multichannel auditory brainstem and cochlear implants. Am J Otol. 1996; 17(5):724–729

[70] Todt I, Tittel A, Ernst A, Mittmann P, Mutze S. Pain free 3 T MRI scans in cochlear implantees. Otol Neurotol. 2017; 38(10):e401–e404

[71] Walton J, Donnelly NP, Tam YC, et al. MRI without magnet removal in neurofibromatosis type 2 patients with cochlear and auditory brainstem implants. Otol Neurotol. 2014; 35(5):821–825

[72] Shew M, Bertsch J, Camarata P, Staecker H. Magnetic resonance imaging in a neurofibromatosis type 2 patient with a novel MRI-compatible auditory brainstem mplant. J Neurol Surg Rep. 2017; 78(1):e12–e14

4 Clinical Indications for ABI: Patient Selection and Alternatives

Mia E. Miller and Eric P. Wilkinson

Abstract

Traditional indications for auditory brainstem implant (ABI) in patients with neurofibromatosis type 2 (NF2) have been broadened to include other applications of the device in patients without an adequate cochlear nerve (CN) for implantation. Studies of auditory perception in many non-NF2 patients demonstrate superior outcomes to average NF2 patient function. As further clinical studies are completed in the US, ABI may become standard treatment for patient groups with limited hearing rehabilitation options, with ABI approval for CN aplasia likely to be the most imminent expanded indication.

Keywords: auditory brainstem implant, neurofibromatosis type II, sensorineural hearing loss, acoustic neuroma, vestibular schwannoma

4.1 Introduction

The auditory brainstem implant (ABI) was developed for patients with neurofibromatosis type 2 (NF2) because removal of bilateral acoustic tumors results in loss of the auditory nerve.[1,2] Since its first use in an NF2 patient by House and Hitselberger in 1979, the indications for ABI have expanded to include other patient populations in which stimulation of the auditory nerve by cochlear implantation is not possible. Acquired indications include complete cochlear ossification and skull base trauma resulting in severed cochlear nerves. ABI has also been found to be useful in pediatric patients with cochlear anomalies in which cochlear implants (CIs) are not beneficial; ABI is also the *only* treatment that can offer some hearing benefit for patients with congenital cochlear nerve (CN) aplasia.[3]

ABIs are FDA approved only for NF2 patients older than 12 years; however, expanded indications in non-NF2 patient groups, particularly in pediatric patients implanted before the age of 2, have demonstrated superior outcomes. Expanded ABI indications have been more widely implemented in Europe, and clinical trials are currently underway in the US for investigation of ABI use in patients with CN atresia.

Preservation of the CN during translabyrinthine and retrosigmoid resections of acoustic tumors has allowed for simultaneous CI in some cases; this is a viable alternative to ABI for NF2 patients, although CI function is variable and unpredictable, probably due to trauma to the CN from the tumor and from resection. Others have advocated early treatment of NF2 tumors with hearing preservation approaches when possible;[4] although maintaining auditory function after treatment is ideal, this alternative to ABI is not always achievable.

As groups in Europe, especially that of Vittorio Colletti in Verona, Italy, push the boundaries of traditional ABI indications with clinical studies demonstrating its efficacy in a variety of conditions, it becomes apparent that ABI is the gold standard for treatment of disorders in which the CN is absent or deficient.

Although still a very important tool in the management of patients with NF2, ABI may become a more accepted treatment for hearing rehabilitation when the cochlear nucleus is the most distal relay in the auditory pathway that is available to stimulate.

4.2 Clinical Indications

4.2.1 Regulatory Status of the Device

As previously mentioned, the first ABI was performed at the House Clinic in 1979. Subsequently, Cochlear Corporation helped design/manufacture the multichannel ABI in 1993. In March 2000, the Nucleus 24 ABI was submitted to the FDA, and the ENT Advisory Panel recommended Nucleus 24 ABI for use by individuals with NF2. The Nucleus ABI received approval for Premarket Approval Application (PMA) in October 2000 (PMA No. P000015). The Cochlear Nucleus Profile Auditory Brainstem Implant (ABI541) was granted PMA approval in 2016.

4.2.2 Current FDA Approval

In the original PMA, the ABI was approved for patients with NF2 who are at least 12 years old.[5] The FDA specified that implantation may occur during first-side or second-side tumor removal, or in patients with previously removed bilateral tumors. Patients must have appropriate expectations regarding the ABI and need to be motivated to participate in the rehabilitation process postoperatively. These same indications hold for the newer ABI541.

4.2.3 Current European CE Mark Approval

Although the MED-EL ABI device is not FDA approved, it is more widely used in Europe. In 2011, MED-EL introduced the Concerto ABI. ABI candidacy was originally approved in Europe for patients with NF2 who are at least 15 years old. MED-EL specifies that device implantation and tumor removal should take place in the same surgery.[6]

More recently, Ingeborg Hochmair, the CEO of MED-EL, informed us that CE mark approval has been obtained for ABI in children 12 months of age and older.

4.3 Patient Selection in Adults

4.3.1 Patient Selection in NF2

As discussed earlier, NF2 patients of 12 years or older must have realistic expectations and should be able to comply with auditory rehabilitation postoperatively in order to be selected for ABI. Although many patients are deaf at implantation or are undergoing surgical excision of a tumor in an only-hearing ear at the time of implantation, candidates may also be selected who have contralateral hearing but with reasonable expectation of hearing loss in the future. Although many patients do not use these "sleeper" ABIs for as long as they have useable hearing in the contralateral ear, sleeper ABI function has not been found to be significantly different from nonsleeper ABI function in NF2 patients.[7]

Patients implanted with ABI may undergo either a translabyrinthine or retrosigmoid approach for tumor resection and access to the lateral recess of the fourth ventricle and cochlear nucleus. Although the translabyrinthine approach has been traditionally used for ABI placement, proponents of the retrosigmoid approach cite possible advantages of decreased operative time and decreased risk of wound contamination with tympanomastoid flora.[8]

4.3.2 Patient Selection in Non-NF2 Indications for ABI

Although the most common indication for ABI today is still NF2, the ABI has more recently been used in other conditions in which either the cochlea or CN is not adequate for cochlear implantation. Colletti describes ABI use in 49 patients after trauma (with CN avulsion), with cochlear malformations, with auditory neuropathy, or with altered cochlear patency.[9] With the exception of patients with auditory neuropathy, these groups have superior ABI performance to NF2 patients with ABI (▸ Fig. 4.1 and ▸ Table 4.1)

Colletti et al explain that post-meningitic cochlear ossification results in poor CI outcomes,[10,11] with about half of the patients lacking open-set speech even with partial insertions or double-array electrodes. Neuronal degeneration associated with cochlear ossification may be the cause of this poor function. Cochlear ossification can also continue after implantation in these patients, resulting in declining CI function. These authors suggest that an ABI might provide better neural access to the auditory system in these cases.

Similarly, advanced otosclerosis may entail neoossification of the cochlea that poses similar challenges to cochlear implantation and may also result in facial nerve stimulation. Although most patients with otosclerosis do well with CI, those with advanced otosclerosis and poor CI function who require reimplantation have poor outcomes.[12,13] In those cases, ABI provided open-set speech in some patients.

Skull base trauma can result in labyrinthine fracture, inner ear concussion, perilymphatic fistula, and CN avulsion. Colletti points out that CN avulsion can result from acceleration/deceleration injuries and that the VIIIth nerve is particularly vulnerable due to its long central portion (8–10 mm).[14] Cochlear fracture or hemorrhage can also lead to ossification of the cochlear lumen that makes CI after hearing loss from trauma less effective than nontrauma CI.[15] Prior to implantation with ABI, trauma patients should have round window electrical stimulation that fails to elicit electric auditory brainstem responses (EABRs) and may also undergo a hearing aid trial.[16] Colleti et al proposed selection criteria for ABI after trauma (Box 4.1).

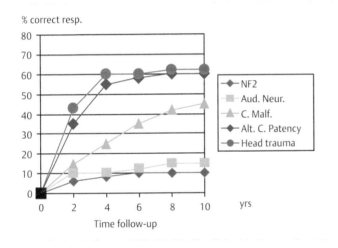

Fig. 4.1 Average performance (% correct on open-set speech over time [year]) for different non tumor (NT) (auditory neuropathy, altered cochlear patency, cochlear malformation, and head trauma) and neurofibromatosis type 2 (NF2) groups. (From Colletti V, Shannon RV, et al.[23])

Table 4.1 Results of open-set sentence recognition at the last follow-up (1–10 years) postoperatively in the different subgroups of NT adult patients

Cause	Number of subjects	Range (in %)	X	Md SD	T versus NT t test	Md SD
Head trauma	7	32–80	62	57	23.41	$p = 0.005$
Auditory neuropathy	4	12–18	15	16	2.52	$p = 0.07$
Cochlear malformations	6	37–61	44	61	11.2	$p = 0.006$
Altered cochlear patency	31	34–100	60	64	19.81	$p = 0.0048$

Abbreviations: Md, Median; NT, nontumor; T, Tumor; SD, standard deviation
Source: From Colletti V, Shannon RV, et al.[23]

Box 4.1 Selection criteria for ABI after skull base trauma (adapted from Colleti et al)[9]

- Evidence in CT scan and MRI of distortion of the cochlear anatomy due to fracture, ossification, or fibrosis of the cochleae;
- No response to round window stimulation with suspected CN avulsion;
- No severe residual neurological disorders, i.e., cerebral lesions with cognitive, behavioral, and communication deficits;
- Patient motivation.

4.4 Patient Selection in Children

4.4.1 Pediatric Patient Selection for NF2

ABI has been shown to be similarly effective in 12 to 18 years old teenagers as it is when used to rehabilitate hearing in adult patients with NF2.[16] In this group, family support, expectations, and motivation to participate in rehabilitation were important factors that separated users from non-users. In 2013, the FDA approved ABI use in clinical trials for children younger than 12 years old. Small pediatric studies have been done in the US and recent larger studies have been recently published on ABI in young pediatric patients.[17]

4.4.2 Cochlear Malformations

As suggested by Colletti et al,[9] ABI may also be useful in patients with cochlear malformations when CI does not provide them with good auditory function. It may be difficult or impossible to determine the location of the spiral ganglion in relation to the cochlear cavity at cochlear implantation in these patients, and anomalies of the facial nerve and increased risk of cerebrospinal fluid (CSF) leak with implantation pose specific surgical risks that may lead to failed CI. As long as cochlear implantation is feasible (e.g., not in Michel aplasia in which there is no cochlea to implant), we suggest

CI, and consider ABI in cochlear malformations only when CI is ineffective.

4.4.3 Cochlear Nerve Aplasia

Lack of auditory nerve is a clinical indication for ABI currently in clinical trials in the United States. CN aplasia is indicated by a narrow internal auditory canal on computed tomography (CT) and lack of CN on magnetic resonance imaging (MRI) (▶ Fig. 4.2). Preliminary results of a Phase I clinical trial indicate that four children who completed 1 year follow-up demonstrated speech detection thresholds of 30 to 35 dB and had pattern perception when presented with closed-set words.[18] Patients with CN aplasia have been implanted for some time in Europe. In 2008, Eisenberg et al reported on auditory testing at House Ear Institute of a 3-year-old patient implanted in Verona, Italy.[19] After 6 weeks of consistent stimulation, he had sound awareness and increased vocalization. Later testing showed him reaching closed-set speech at 6 months, and at 1 year he reached similar auditory function to CI patients implanted at a similar age.

In 2008, Colleti and Zoccante reported on 19 pediatric patients with CN aplasia implanted with ABI, 5 of whom had received a previous CI resulting in no auditory perception.[20] Although these authors did not separate CN aplasia patients

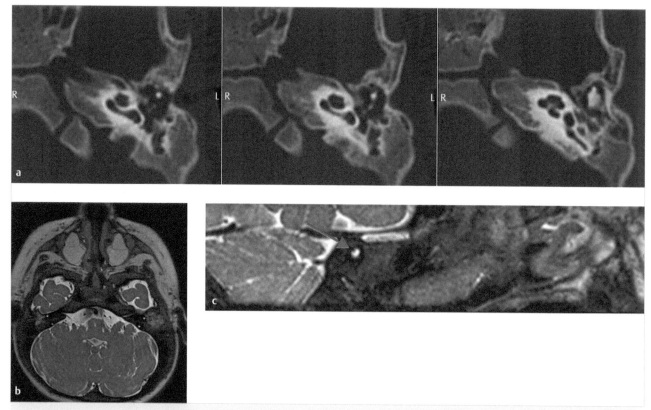

Fig. 4.2 **(a)** Computed tomography (CT) image of hypoplastic internal auditory canals (IAC), **(b)** Axial T2 MRI showing narrow IAC and **(c)** Sagittal T2 MRI showing only facial nerve in IAC (*arrow indicates facial nerve*).

Group 1: Well-Defined Congenital Indications
- Complete labyrinthine aplasia (Michel aplasia)
- Cochlear aplasia
- CN aplasia
- Cochlear aperture aplasia

Group 2: Possible Congenital Indications
- Hypoplastic cochleae with cochlear aperture hypoplasia.
- Common cavity and incomplete partition type I cases, if the CN is not present.
- Common cavity and incomplete partition type I cases, if the CN is present: even if the nerve is present, the distribution of the neural tissue in the abnormal cochlea is unpredictable, and ABI may be indicated in such cases if CI fails to elicit an auditory sensation.
- The presence of an unbranched cochleovestibular nerve (CVN) is a challenge in these cases. In this situation, it is not possible to determine the amount of cochlear fibers traveling in the nerve. If there is a doubt, a CI can be used in the first instance, and ABI can be reserved for the patients with an insufficient response.
- The hypoplastic CN presents a dilemma for the implant team.

A hypoplastic nerve is defined as less than 50% of the usual size of the CN or less than the diameter of the facial nerve. The radiology in these patients should be carefully reviewed with an experienced neuroradiologist. If a sufficient amount of neural tissue cannot be followed into the cochlear space, an ABI may be indicated.

from tumor patients, they did demonstrate that all pediatric patients receiving an ABI showed improved lipreading and environmental awareness of sound; they also demonstrated significant improvement in cognitive tests over those without ABI. Colletti, Wilkinson, and Colletti reported that 21 pediatric patients with failed CI and surgically confirmed absence of the CN who were reimplanted with ABI showed statistically significant improvement on auditory testing.[21]

In 2011, a consensus statement of several European ABI centers included congenital indications for ABI that are particularly relevant for this discussion.[22] In addition to CN aplasia, complete labyrinthine aplasia (Michel aplasia), cochlear aplasia, and cochlear aperture aplasia were included in well-defined congenital indications. It is clear in these diagnoses that a competent CN is not available for cochlear implantation. Both well-defined and possible congenital indications can be seen in Box 4.2. Review of these indications suggests that in cases where it is unclear if there is a competent CN, such as CN hypoplasia, CI can be attempted and improved responses to auditory stimuli have been achieved in some cases. In those where minimal progress is made, ABI can be performed secondarily.

Patients with CN aplasia should have a likelihood of a normal cochlear nucleus when being evaluated for ABI placement. This can be assumed from normal anatomy of the fourth ventricle and nearby brainstem on MRI. Similar to CI, ABI is likely to have better auditory outcomes and possibly result in speech understanding when patients are implanted at a younger age (i.e., before age of 2).[23]

Counseling of families with children with CN aplasia is particularly imperative and is also challenging. They need to understand that CI cannot function without the presence of a CN. At the same time, the level of function after ABI for these patients is variable and the families need to have realistic expectations about postoperative rehabilitation and function. Families should also understand that patients with developmental delays tend to perform more poorly on subjective measures of hearing performance, although they may enjoy their ABI and find it useful.[22]

4.4.4 ABI Programming in Pediatric Patients

Programming in pediatric patients is very difficult, as prelingual patients may not be able to help the programmer distinguish between auditory and non auditory sensations.[20] Moreover, a new auditory stimulus could be perceived as a negative one when heard by the patient for the first time and with later stimulation, the same electrode may produce only auditory stimuli. Programming generally begins 5 to 6 weeks after implantation, and after most-comfortable levels (MCL) are determined, successive electrodes from the center outwards are activated.[24] Children may show cessation of activity, cry, look at the mother, or hold the implant side in response to auditory stimuli. Electrodes that result in negative side effects (such as coughing related to vagal nerve stimulation) are turned off.

4.4.5 Barriers to Adoption of Expanded ABI Indications

The hesitancy of widespread adoption of ABI for non-NF2 indications is likely multifactorial. First, the great majority of experience with ABI is in the NF2 population, in which inconsistent hearing rehabilitation is achieved, probably due to trauma to the CN. Non-NF2 indications for ABI show significantly improved ABI function on average (▸ Fig. 4.1 and ▸ Table 4.1), but this improvement in function has not been widely established. Furthermore, in NF2 cases, a craniotomy is already indicated for tumor removal, and FDA guidelines indicate that ABI should be done at the time of the first- or second-side tumor removal. It does make sense to approach ABI with caution in patient groups who would not otherwise require a craniotomy. However, supporters of ABI for non-NF2 indications highlight that posterior fossa surgery is routinely used for vestibular neurectomy or other cranial nerve decompressions with minimal complications.[3] They also suggest that the retrosigmoid approach

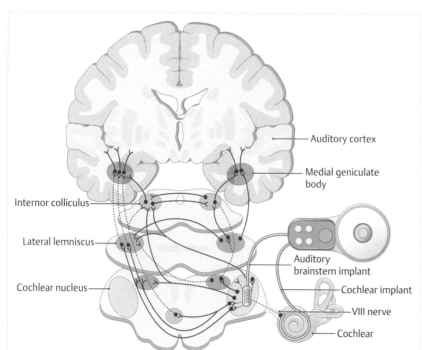

Fig. 4.3 Auditory pathways: relative positions of auditory brainstem implant and cochlear implant.

Labels in figure: Auditory cortex; Medial geniculate body; Internor colliculus; Lateral lemniscus; Cochlear nucleus; Auditory brainstem implant; Cochlear implant; VIII nerve; Cochlear

may be preferred in these patients because it is nondestructive, shorter in duration, and avoids entry into the mastoid air cells, minimizing risks of contamination and allowing for a watertight dural closure.

4.5 Alternatives to ABI

4.5.1 Hearing Preservation

Historically, a diagnosis of NF2 usually led to profound bilateral deafness. Contrast-enhanced MRI and genetic testing have led to earlier diagnosis in some cases, and treatment with hearing-preservation microsurgical approaches (middle fossa and retrosigmoid) has allowed some NF2 patients to maintain usable (Class A and Class B) hearing. In 2007, Slattery et al found that in middle fossa tumor removal of 35 children with NF2 (average age of 12.6 years old, average tumor size of 1.1 cm), more than half maintained hearing ≤ 70 dB pure tone average (PTA) and 47.7% maintained Class A hearing.[4] Interestingly, hearing preservation, if present, was nearly complete, as a great majority of the patients had Class A or D hearing postoperatively.

4.5.2 Cochlear Implantation

Surgical resection of acoustic tumors with preservation of the CN in NF2 patients has allowed cochlear implantation in some patients. In 2006, Lustig et al implanted seven patients who experienced some auditory perception, but only two out of seven had open-set speech.[25] The poorer performance of CI in NF2 has been found by others as well. The Sanna group demonstrated that of 15 patients with CI after vestibular schwannoma (VS) removal through an extended translabyrinthine approach (with intact CN), patients with NF2 (8/15) had 50% open-set discrimination, while patients with sporadic VS (7/15) had 71%

open-set discrimination, although this difference was not statistically significant.[26]

In general, CI performance after VS excision does not reach the level of standard CI users and depends on the integrity of the CN, which could be compromised by tumor growth, surgical trauma, or radiation. Controversy surrounds the lack of reliable intraoperative monitoring to determine whether the CN would be suitable to conduct electrical stimuli. ▶ Fig. 4.3 demonstrates the relative positions of ABI and CI in the auditory pathway in relation to the acoustic tumor.

Additionally, CI has also been reported in NF2 patients treated with stereotactic radiosurgery, with variable results.[27] CI has also been used to rehabilitate hearing in NF2 patients in the presence of a stable tumor, sometimes in conjunction with bevacizumab.[28]

References

[1] Edgerton BJ, House WF, Hitselberger W. Hearing by cochlear nucleus stimulation in humans. Ann Otol Rhinol Laryngol Suppl. 1982; 91(2 Pt 3):117–124

[2] Eisenberg LS, Maltan AA, Portillo F, Mobley JP, House WF. Electrical stimulation of the auditory brain stem structure in deafened adults. J Rehabil Res Dev. 1987; 24(3):9–22

[3] Colletti V, Carner M, Miorelli V, Guida M, Colletti L, Fiorino F. Auditory brainstem implant (ABI): new frontiers in adults and children. Otolaryngol Head Neck Surg. 2005; 133(1):126–138

[4] Slattery WH, III, Fisher LM, Hitselberger W, Friedman RA, Brackmann DE. Hearing preservation surgery for neurofibromatosis type 2-related vestibular schwannoma in pediatric patients. J Neurosurg. 2007; 106(4) Suppl: 255–260

[5] https://www.accessdata.fda.gov/scripts/cdrh/cfdocs/cfpma/pma.cfm?id=P000015

[6] http://www.medel.com/maestro-components-abi/

[7] Ramsden RT, Freeman SR, Lloyd SK, et al. Manchester Neurofibromatosis Type 2 Service. Auditory brainstem implantation in neurofibromatosis type 2: experience from the Manchester programme. Otol Neurotol. 2016; 37(9): 1267–1274

[8] Puram SV, Herrmann B, Barker FG, II, Lee DJ. Retrosigmoid craniotomy for auditory brainstem implantation in adult patients with neurofibromatosis type 2. J Neurol Surg B Skull Base. 2015; 76(6):440–450

[9] Colletti V, Shannon R, Carner M, Veronese S, Colletti L. Outcomes in non tumor adults fitted with the auditory brainstem implant: 10 years' experience. Otol Neurotol. 2009; 30(5):614–618

[10] Thomas J, Cheshire IM. Evaluation of cochlear implantation in postmeningitic adults. J Laryngol Otol Suppl. 1999; 24:27–33

[11] Rauch SD, Herrmann BS, Davis LA, Nadol JB, Jr. Nucleus 22 cochlear implantation results in postmeningitic deafness. Laryngoscope. 1997; 107(12 Pt 1): 1606–1609

[12] Ramsden R, Rotteveel L, Proops D, Saeed S, van Olphen A, Mylanus E. Cochlear implantation in otosclerotic deafness. Adv Otorhinolaryngol. 2007; 65: 328–334

[13] Rotteveel LJ, Proops DW, Ramsden RT, Saeed SR, van Olphen AF, Mylanus EA. Cochlear implantation in 53 patients with otosclerosis: demographics, computed tomographic scanning, surgery, and complications. Otol Neurotol. 2004; 25(6):943–952

[14] Colletti V, Carner M, Miorelli V, Colletti L, Guida M, Fiorino F. Auditory brainstem implant in posttraumatic cochlear nerve avulsion. Audiol Neurotol. 2004; 9(4):247–255

[15] Camilleri AE, Toner JG, Howarth KL, Hampton S, Ramsden RT. Cochlear implantation following temporal bone fracture. J Laryngol Otol. 1999; 113(5): 454–457

[16] Otto SR, Brackmann DE, Hitselberger W. Auditory brainstem implantation in 12- to 18-year-olds. Arch Otolaryngol Head Neck Surg. 2004; 130(5): 656–659

[17] Aslan F, Ozkan HB, Yücel E, Sennaroğlu G, Bilginer B, Sennaroğlu L. Effects of age at auditory brainstem implantation: impact on auditory perception, language development, speech intelligibility. Otol Neurotol. 2020; 41(1): 11–20

[18] Wilkinson EP, Eisenberg LS, Krieger MD, et al. Los Angeles Pediatric ABI Team. Initial results of a safety and feasibility study of auditory brainstem implantation in congenitally deaf children. Otol Neurotol. 2017; 38(2):212–220

[19] Eisenberg LS, Johnson KC, Martinez AS, et al. Comprehensive evaluation of a child with an auditory brainstem implant. Otol Neurotol. 2008; 29(2):251–257

[20] Colletti L, Zoccante L. Nonverbal cognitive abilities and auditory performance in children fitted with auditory brainstem implants: preliminary report. Laryngoscope. 2008; 118(8):1443–1448

[21] Colletti L, Wilkinson EP, Colletti V. Auditory brainstem implantation after unsuccessful cochlear implantation of children with clinical diagnosis of cochlear nerve deficiency. Ann Otol Rhinol Laryngol. 2013; 122(10):605–612

[22] Sennaroglu L, Colletti V, Manrique M, et al. Auditory brainstem implantation in children and non-neurofibromatosis type 2 patients: aconsensus statement. Otol Neurotol. 2011; 32(2):198–191

[23] Colletti V, Shannon RV, Carner M, et al. Progress in restoration of hearing with the auditory brainstem implant. In: Verhaagen J, et al. eds. Progress in Brain Research. Chapter 22. Vol. 175. Elsevier;2009

[24] Sennaroglu L, Sennaroglu G, Atay G. Auditory brainstem implantation in children. Curr Otorhinolaryngol Rep. 2013; 1:80–91

[25] Lustig LR, Yeagle J, Driscoll CL, Blevins N, Francis H, Niparko JK. Cochlear implantation in patients with neurofibromatosis type 2 and bilateral vestibular schwannoma. Otol Neurotol. 2006; 27(4):512–518

[26] Lassaletta L, Aristegui M, Medina M, et al. Ipsilateral cochlear implantation in patients with sporadic vestibular schwannoma in the only or best hearing ear and in patients with NF2. Eur Arch Otorhinolaryngol. 2016; 273(1):27–35

[27] Carlson ML, Breen JT, Driscoll CL, et al. Cochlear implantation in patients with neurofibromatosis type 2: variables affecting auditory performance. Otol Neurotol. 2012; 33(5):853–862

[28] Harris F, Tysome JR, Donnelly N, et al. Cochlear implants in the management of hearing loss in neurofibromatosis type 2. Cochlear Implants Int. 2017; 18 (3):171–179

5 Surgery for ABI: The Translabyrinthine Approach

Marc S. Schwartz, Eric P. Wilkinson, and Gregory P. Lekovic

Abstract

The translabyrinthine (TL) approach has been used since the 1960s to safely and reliably resect vestibular schwannomas (VS) and other tumors of the cerebellopontine angle (CPA). It provides direct access without the need for brain retraction. This is the initial approach utilized for auditory brainstem implant (ABI) surgery and remains the preferred approach in many centers, especially when ABI placement is done in conjunction with tumor resection. In this chapter, we describe the surgical principals and nuances of ABI via the TL approach.

Keywords: auditory brainstem implant, translabyrinthine, vestibular schwannoma, neurofibromatosis type 2

5.1 Introduction

The translabyrinthine (TL) approach was used for the placement of the first auditory brainstem implant (ABI) and it remains one of the main routes of surgical access to the cerebellopontine angle (CPA).[1,2,3,4] This approach traverses the mastoid and the inner ear, providing access to the internal auditory canal (IAC) and the adjacent intracranial area. Its advantages include complete bony resection before opening the dura and that cerebellar retraction is minimized. Fundamental principles of the TL approach include very direct access to the CPA and that resection of bone is preferable to manipulation of brain. The incision for the TL approach is made just behind the ear over the mastoid process, which lies just below the scalp.

The TL approach is ideal for the resection of many neurofibromatosis type 2 (NF2) related acoustic neuromas. Since portions of the inner ear are resected in the course of the procedure, the TL approach cannot be used if hearing preservation is a goal of surgery. Since by definition hearing preservation is not a goal of ABI surgery, this disadvantage is irrelevant in this particular setting.

Use of the TL approach requires understanding of the complex anatomy of the temporal bone, including the course of the facial nerve and the landmarks for the location of the IAC. As such, most centers utilize a team consisting of both a neurotologic surgeon and a neurological surgeon to carry out surgery via this approach. Typically, the bony approach is carried out by the neurotologic surgeon, and intradural tumor resection in the vicinity of the cerebellum and brainstem is carried out by the neurological surgeon.

Some surgeons prefer not to utilize the TL approach for vestibular schwannoma (VS) resection or other surgery of the CPA, such as ABI placement, preferring the retrosigmoid (RS) route. Disadvantages of the TL approach may include increased operative time, a relatively narrow corridor of access, and, arguably, a higher risk of cerebrospinal fluid (CSF) leak. With the TL route, the middle ear is widely opened and there is potentially a direct route for fluid to leak via the Eustachian tube and the nose. Typically, abdominal fat is harvested and used to obliterate the mastoid space, thus forming a barrier to leakage. With an experienced neurotologic surgeon, disadvantages may be minimized.

All operations carried out as part of the initial trials leading to approval of ABI use for patients with NF2 were carried out via the TL approach.[5] The TL remains the preferred approach for ABI placement in the setting of NF2 at many, if not most, large centers in the United States. In patients operated for ABI placement for deafness due to causes other than NF2-related tumors, the benefits of the TL approach may be less pronounced. Indeed, this approach may be contraindicated in nontumor patients who have maintained vestibular function despite deafness. The TL approach may also not be appropriate for young pediatric patients, who typically have small, undeveloped mastoids that do not provide sufficient operative exposure.

The TL approach allows for optimal placement of the ABI receiver immediately superior and posterior to the ear. The external ABI hardware thus sits in a natural position on the side of the head, anterior to and more optimal than the placement that can be achieved with the RS approach. The ABI electrode array is placed on the brainstem surface under direct, high power magnification using the operating microscope. The surgeon must have a detailed understanding of brainstem surface anatomy in order to identify the proper site of placement. Anatomic landmarks include the stump of the vestibulocochlear nerve, the glossopharyngeal nerve, and the choroid plexus from the fourth ventricle at the foramen of Luschka. It is also important to recognize that the anatomy of the brainstem can be very distorted by the CPA tumor resected prior to ABI placement.

The cochlear nucleus complex is found deep to the surface of the brain, along the superior-anterior wall of the lateral recess of the fourth ventricle, within the foramen of Luschka. The foramen of Luschka is one of the sites of egress of CSF from the ventricular system of the brain into the cisternal system on the outside of the brain. Under the operating microscope, the ependymal surface of the ventricular system has a distinct appearance, allowing it to be differentiated from the typical pial surface of the brain's exterior. The electrode array can be simply inserted into this "hole" with its active contacts placed in direct contact with the brain surface in the correct location.

Following insertion of ABI electrode array, it is held in place by packing the recess with Teflon (PTFE), muscle, fat, or other materials. Evoked auditory brainstem response (EABR) testing is then carried out to confirm correct placement. The wound can then be carefully closed after packing the operative cavity with abdominal fat harvested from the patient.

5.2 Anatomic Considerations

The major advantage of the translabyrinthine approach is that it provides direct access to the CPA and to the lateral side of the brainstem without the need for cerebellar retraction. This approach takes advantage of the sizable bony corridor, traversing the pyramidal shape of the temporal bone, including the mastoid sinus and the inner ear. Detailed anatomic understanding is a prerequisite for drilling through these structures. The time required and effort necessary to carefully dissect through the skull base may be seen as a disadvantage by many surgeons. The TL approach is, however, primarily carried out in the extradural space, with nearly all of the exposure done prior to opening the dura. As such, the risk of this approach is in many ways less than that of primarily intradural routes, such as the RS.

The limiting anatomic structures of the translabyrinthine route form a roughly triangular shape. These are the external auditory canal and mastoid portion of the facial nerve anteriorly, the dura of the temporal lobe superiorly, and the sigmoid sinus posteriorly and inferiorly. The sigmoid sinus should be understood as the critical structure influencing all approaches to the CPA. This is essentially a large vein running within the dura, and it carries much of the blood flow from the brain to the jugular vein and then on to the vena cava and heart. It is a bilateral structure with significant anatomic variability. Although usually even in size, it is not unusual for one to be much larger than the other. Small sigmoid sinuses can be sacrificed, but injury to an average-sized one can lead to significant postoperative problems. Injury of a large sinus will usually result in disaster. The TL approach is a presigmoid approach, that is, in front of the sinus, while the RS approach is obviously behind.

With the TL approach, temporal bone is drilled in order to directly expose the dura of the IAC and the adjacent CPA. The normal mastoid consists of a honeycomb of bone and air, allowing for identification of critical structures. Before itself being resected, the distinctly shaped hard bone of the labyrinth is the anatomic structure that acts as a landmark for identification of the other critical structures, most notably the facial nerve traversing the temporal bone on its course to its exit along the inferior skull and then the IAC itself (▶ Fig. 5.1).

As the final step of bony exposure, the facial nerve can be identified lateral to the tumor at Bill's bar, which is the landmark of its exit from the IAC to the labyrinthine portion of the temporal bone. After identification of the facial nerve, and after all drilling has been completed, the dura of the CPA can be opened directly adjacent to the tumor. The first critical intradural step is release of CSF. CSF release is critical to obtaining brain relaxation and to succeeding in the ongoing surgery. Release of fluid allows the brain to sag, which opens the cisternal spaces and creates enough room for tumor resection and ABI placement. As opposed to the RS approach, there is no need to retract cerebellum or to manipulate the brain to reach tumor or to release CSF.

After tumor resection is completed, hopefully with preservation of all neurologic and vascular structures other than the vestibulocochlear nerve, brainstem landmarks must be identified for ABI placement. The cochlear nucleus complex lies within the brainstem adjacent to the lateral recess of the fourth ventricle. This is inferior to the stump of the vestibulocochlear nerve, which enters the brainstem at the lowest part of the pons. The TL approach provides direct access to the CPA, with these structures near the inferior limit of the exposure. One disadvantage of the TL approach may be somewhat limited or awkward exposure of the site of ABI placement at the very inferior edge of exposure. The degree of difficulty is highly dependent upon individual anatomy. This may also be influenced 1either positively or negatively by distortion of the brainstem caused by large tumors, which is often the case with NF2.

The exact site of placement of the ABI electrode array is within the lateral recess of the fourth ventricle. Access to the lateral recess is via the foramen of Luschka. This is essentially a "hole" at the lateral aspect of the pontomedullary junction. The anterior border of the foramen is upper medulla at the level of the exiting glossopharyngeal nerve. The superior border of the foramen is formed by the pons, or, more properly, the middle cerebellar peduncle. The cerebellar hemisphere forms the foramen's posterior border. Inferiorly, the telachoroidea, formed by fusion of the surfaces of the brainstem and cerebellum, forms the final border. The enclosed nature of the placement site allows the array to be held in position by packing material such as Teflon felt behind it.

Closure of the TL surgical defect is concerned mostly with prevention of CSF leak. The approach involves opening of the middle ear space, and the middle ear is connected directly to the Eustachian tube. Thus, there is a natural route for fluid leakage into the nasal cavity. Abdominal fat is used to occlude the mastoid cavity. Even with fat packing, the risk of leakage is substantial. This is because intracranial CSF pressure is always elevated after craniotomy, and the ABI cable provides a natural conduit from intra- to extracranial, along which fluid is able to wick.

5.3 Preoperative Evaluation

In our practice, the TL approach for ABI placement is reserved for patients with NF2 undergoing resection of VS or other tumors or, rarely, in patients with NF2 having previously undergone tumor resection. We utilize the RS approach for non tumor patients, both adult and pediatric. Thus, preoperative evaluation of clinical factors is necessary in addition to anatomical ones.

Clinical considerations in these patients revolve primarily around NF2-associated tumors and their resulting intracranial sequelae. The most obvious consideration is that of bilateral VS. The ABI may be placed at the time of first or second-side tumor

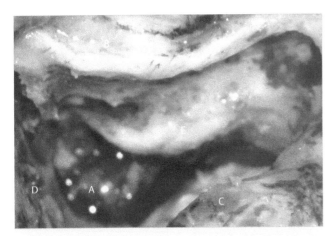

Fig. 5.1 Extradural translabyrinthine exposure, right side. Tumor is seen in the internal auditory canal (A). Frequently, there is a large amount of tumor in this region. The limits of the exposure are the posterior wall of the external canal (B), the sigmoid sinus (C), and the dura of the middle fossa (D). The descending segment of the facial nerve (E) also limits exposure anteriorly and inferiorly.

resection. Generally, the side of worse hearing is operated first, although occasionally the presence of a large and threatening tumor in the ear of better hearing makes this impossible. As TL resection is always hearing destructive and RS resection of a large, NF2-associated tumor provides little hope of this, the decision to operate on a patient's better-hearing ear is always difficult.

With the possible exception of giant tumors, data does not show that ABI performance is related to tumor size.[6,7] As such, surgeons should not be overly optimistic when facing small tumors. Giant tumors may be particularly problematic, as they are more difficult to remove from the brainstem atraumatically.

Tumor involving the facial nerve in its labyrinthine portion or at the geniculate should be noted, as this is proof of facial nerve tumor, which may complicate resection and postoperative recovery. Presence of collision tumors in the CPA should also be noted in order to plan accordingly. Furthermore, a large volume of contralateral CPA tumor can be expected to reduce the working space in the operative field as sagging of brain to the opposite side is prevented.

Study of the patient's temporal bone and skull base anatomy must also be undertaken. If not evident on thin-cut magnetic resonance imaging (MRI), temporal bone computed tomography (CT) may also be performed. Presence of a dominant sigmoid sinus raises both difficulty and risk of surgery. Contracted mastoid, high jugular bulb, and low tegmen should also be noted as these will impede visibility and increase the difficulty of both the approach and the subsequent intradural portion of the procedure. As many NF2 patients will have also undergone prior craniotomy, the effects of this on the proposed procedure should be considered.

Dysfunction of or risk to other cranial nerves is also possible with NF2 patients. Vocal cord function should be confirmed preoperatively via direct laryngoscopy even in the absence of clinical symptoms or obvious tumors on imaging. Failure to recognize pre-existing lower cranial nerve dysfunction, especially if it is on the contralateral side, may result in grave consequences for the patients' ability to protect their airway after surgery. Bilateral evaluation of trigeminal function as well as vision is also important. Patients without serviceable vision on the contralateral side are likely to suffer disproportionally in the event of facial and/or trigeminal dysfunction on the operative side.

Potential issues outside the CPA should also be considered. Hydrocephalus, venous sinus occlusion from tumors or prior surgery, or large supratentorial tumor burden may exacerbate postoperative CSF pressure elevation and may predispose toward CSF leak or other complication. If a ventriculoperitoneal shunt is to be performed, the side of placement should be considered carefully so as to interfere as little as possible with subsequent treatments. Adjustable shunt valves and ABI receivers cannot coexist on the same side.

Finally, preoperative spinal cord imaging is necessary in order to ensure that the cervical spinal cord especially is not at risk from operative positioning or other manipulation. Spinal cord or peripheral nerve dysfunction may interfere synergistically with vestibular dysfunction to impede mobilization during the postoperative period and thereafter.[8]

5.4 Operative Technique and Nuances

5.4.1 Anesthesia and Positioning

Standard endotracheal neuroanesthetic technique is used for craniotomy and ABI placement. While short-term chemical paralytics may be utilized for induction, these agents cannot be part of the ongoing anesthesia plan due to requirement for electromyographic (EMG) cranial nerve monitoring. All cases are carried out with Foley catheter, continuous arterial blood pressure monitoring via arterial line, and lower-extremity sequential compression devices.

Intraoperative monitoring includes that of the facial and glossopharyngeal nerves. EMG electrodes for the latter are placed in the soft palate.[9] While facial nerve monitoring can be dispensed within patients with pre-existing total facial nerve palsy, lower cranial nerve monitoring is always used. Additionally, the vagus nerve can be monitored using endotracheal tube electrodes, and the motor branch of the trigeminal nerve can be monitored as well. Cranial electroencephalogram (EEG) electrodes are placed for later EABR testing of ABI device response.

Spinal cord monitoring can also be utilized. We routinely use somatosensory evoked potential monitoring (SSEP) for cases of giant tumor or for previously treated tumors (either surgery or stereotactic radiation). If motor evoked potential spinal cord monitoring is used, it should be understood that further motor stimulation is absolutely contraindicated after the placement of the ABI electrode array on the brainstem. Additionally, it should be noted that use of monopolar cautery is also contraindicated after placement of the electrode array, or in the presence of a previously implanted contralateral ABI.[10]

The patient is positioned supine on the operating table with the head turned to the contralateral side. We do not use a cranial fixation device since the patient's head tends to fall naturally to the proper orientation on a flat operating table. The patient is, of course, properly padded and secured on the operating table, including the use of a soft gel pad behind the occiput. An area of abdomen is sterilely prepped and draped along with the operative site, which includes both the scalp and the external ear canal. We would recommend tilting the table far to each side before starting in order to ensure the patient is properly secured.

5.4.2 Approach and Tumor Resection

Details of the technique of TL resection of VS, including sporadic and NF2-related tumors, have previously been described.[11] It is beyond the scope of this chapter to reiterate all steps, considerations, and steps taken. Instead, we will focus on key issues particularly related to ABI placement.

A typical curved skin incision is made behind the ear, beginning at the mastoid tip, having an apex of about a fingerbreadth behind the ear, and ending superior to the ear. This anterior extension at the superior end is necessary to provide access to the mastoid. Care must be taken when planning the superior limb of the incision to avoid having the incision cross the eventual placement of the ABI receiver. This usually implies that the anterior limb cannot be made too far superiorly. If more superior

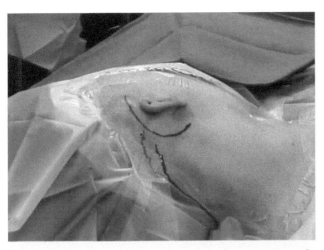

Fig. 5.2 Incision for translabyrinthine craniotomy for VS resection and placement of ABI. The superior limb cannot be so high so that incision overlies the ABI receiver. If necessary, the anterior end of the superior limb can be curved upward to provide better access to the site of the receiver.

exposure is required, the very end of the incision can be curved gently superiorly (▶ Fig. 5.2).

Little, if any, modification of bony exposure is needed for the extradural approach, with the understanding that complete bone drilling is necessary. Surgeons who might be tempted to provide less aggressive exposure, perhaps for a smaller tumor, should understand that extensive dural exposure is needed in order to access the region of the foramen of Luschka. The inferior trough of the IAC, especially, must be drilled well anterior to the level of the IAC itself. It is also necessary to completely decompress the inferior portion of the sigmoid sinus along its curved anterior course. Although we do not recommend depressing a high jugular bulb, it is critical to remove all bone from the dura posterior to such a bulb in order to fully expose the dura in this area. If this far inferior presigmoid dura is not widely exposed, the lateral recess cannot be accessed. As will be discussed below, it is also important to pack the Eustachian tube and middle ear early in this case. It is our practice to carry out these steps concurrent with the approach.

Tumor is resected in the typical fashion, with especial care taken along the brainstem and near the root entry zone of the vestibulocochlear nerve. Separation of tumor from the brainstem must be carried out as atraumatically as possible.[12] We avoid use of cautery and prefer to obtain hemostasis using thrombin-soaked gelfoam or other hemostatic materials. We also attempt to section the vestibulocochlear medially as early as possible so as to place cottonoids to further protect the brainstem surface.

If integrity of the facial nerve is not maintained, and if nerve repair is to be done, this should be completed prior to ABI placement. Also, it is our practice never to resect tumors of the lower cranial nerves in the course of surgery for VS. These tumors typically grow very slowly, and it is our experience that resection of these tumors inevitably leads to postoperative difficulties with swallowing or airway protection. This is true even for tumors seeming to be trivial to resect or for patients having pre-existing ipsilateral vocal cord paralysis.

The TL approach may be modified to a transotic (TO) or transcochlear (TC) approach in which a blind sac closure of the external auditory canal is performed along with additional drilling of the labyrinth. Typically, in the TO approach the facial nerve is left as an intact fallopian bridge, while in the classic TC approach the greater superficial petrosal nerve (GSPN) is cut and the facial nerve is translocated posteriorly, allowing more direct exposure to the anterior petrous region. In very large or recurrent tumors, or in collision tumors involving meningiomas and schwannomas, these modifications may be very helpful. The reader is referred to skull base surgery textbooks for more in-depth discussion of these surgical modifications.

5.4.3 ABI Placement

Proper and uncomplicated placement of the ABI is facilitated by understanding the discrete steps and by following these in a rational order. The key is for the surgeon to be fully prepared prior to unpackaging of the device and again to be fully prepared for device insertion. If routine steps are neglected early, even easy maneuvers may be made much more complicated when they are attempted with the ABI in place. Of note, it is critical to have two ABI devices available (including back-up device). This should be confirmed prior to beginning the case and certainly at "time out."

It is our preference to be fully ready for subgaleal receiver placement before tumor resection or even dural opening is carried out. Implantation of the extracranial receiver is essentially analogous to the same steps in cochlear implantation. A pocket is created deep in the scalp, above the initial incision. Subperiosteal elevation of scalp is carried out on the side of the head superior and posterior to the ear. Depending upon the device used and surgeon's preference, a trough can be drilled in the outer table to allow for the receiver to fit in this space. A dummy sizer facilitates proper sizing since at this point the ABI device will not have been opened on the operative field. Alternately, pocket preparation and drilling can be carried out after tumor resection, but it is never done after the electrode array has been deployed on the brainstem.

Following tumor resection, but before the ABI is unpackaged, as much "housekeeping" as possible is carried out. Cottonoids and other materials are removed from the operative field, and hemostasis is compulsively obtained. The field is made as "clean" as possible at this point, because doing so later will be much more difficult. A principle of ABI placement from this point onward is minimization of clutter and overall simplification.

The next step is localization of the foramen of Luschka. Especially in the setting of larger tumors, the stump of the vestibulocochlear nerve may be difficult to appreciate. The best landmark is the glossopharyngeal nerve, which exits the brainstem along the anterior border of the foramen.[13] After the nerve is identified in the cisternal space, it is followed medially. Often, the course of the nerve is obscured by the flocculus, which must be sharply dissected away. New cotton strips may be utilized to safely carry out this dissection. (▶ Fig. 5.3)

Choroid plexus is an unreliable indicator of the foramen. Although it can sometimes be identified in the expected location, just in view at the lateral end of the fourth ventricle, we have also been misled by ectopic rests of plexus in the CPA,

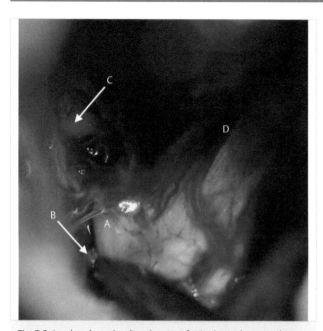

Fig. 5.3 Landmarks to localize the site of ABI electrode array placement, left side. The electrodes are placed along the surface of the lateral recess of the fourth ventricle (A). Choroid plexus (B) often can be identified in the fourth ventricle. This is located posterior to the glossopharyngeal nerve (C). In this case, a small tumor can be seen along the fibers of this nerve. The root entry zone of the facial nerve (D) is also labeled.

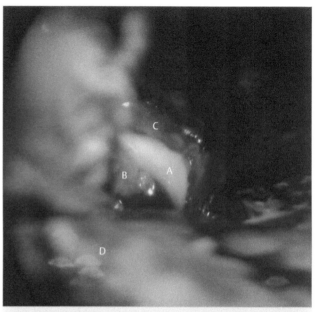

Fig. 5.4 Appearance of the lateral recess of the fourth ventricle, left side. The ependymal surface of the ventricle (A) is whiter and more reflective than the pial surface of the exterior of the brainstem. Choroid plexus (B) is seen in the recess and can obstruct it. Often, a vein lies across the brainstem surface as well (C). The sigmoid sinus (D) must often be compressed in order to obtain adequate access to the recess.

seemingly without any relation to the ventricular system. Especially in cases of very large tumors, the surface of brainstem at this area may be very distorted, without any obvious "hole" in the expected location posterior to the root entry zone of the glossopharyngeal nerve. In these cases, this area may display several suspect indentations. In these cases, it may be useful to ask the anesthesiologist to perform Valsalva on the patient. Escaping CSF indicates the foramen, which can be further explored. The identity of the lateral recess is confirmed by direct inspection. The ependymal surface of the insertion site has a distinct appearance which is easily recognized, at least after a surgeon's first successful case (▶ Fig. 5.4).

Once the lateral recess is identified, a micro cottonoid is used as a marker by placing it through the foramen. Use of cautery in this area should be avoided, and bleeding should be controlled by placement of hemostatic materials. Friable veins are typically found on the lip of the foramen. Arteries can nearly always be easily freed and repositioned atraumatically.

The ABI device is unpackaged only after identification of the proper brainstem insertion site. Also, at this time, all cottonoids are removed from the posterior fossa, with the exception of the single micro cottonoid marking the lateral recess. Decluttering, especially removing cottonoids with strings, is much more difficult after the ABI electrode array has been deployed. There is a strong tendency for strings and the ABI cable to become entwined, risking inadvertent explantation if left for later on.

Handling of the ABI differs between manufacturers. The receiver of the MED-EL device, which is MRI conditionally compatible at 1.5 Tesla, can be placed in its subgaleal pocket prior to insertion of the electrode array.[14] The magnet must be removed from the Cochlear device in order to make it MRI compatible, and for NF2 patients, who are likely to require frequent scans, it is usually implanted without the magnet.[10] For intraoperative testing, however, it is necessary to leave the magnet in place in order to ensure proper electromagnetic coupling between the external testing device and the receiver. Therefore, the Cochlear device is left outside the scalp at this time. We place a hemostat on the drapes directly superficial to the location of the subgaleal pocket and we attach the receiver using the magnet. The cochlear ABI has a ground electrode which is inserted deep to the temporalis muscle directly anterior to the ear.

The next step is the actual insertion of the electrode array into the lateral recess. Both devices have Dacron mesh backing overlying the array, and the surgeon may find it useful to carefully cut away excess material in order to facilitate proper placement. In the case of the cochlear ABI, we typically cut off the two small "wings" at the heel of the array.

Following such preparation, the array is lowered into the posterior fossa and then, under high-power magnification, gently placed into the lateral recess after first removing the micro cottonoid marking the site. The surgeon will note significant torque forces created by the cable, which interfere with easy placement. Fighting this torque is one of the main challenges facing the surgeon. The active surface of the array is ideally placed along the anterosuperior surface of recess, directly overlying the cochlear nucleus complex (▶ Fig. 5.5). The proper depth is such that the lateral most electrodes are in contact with the brainstem at the most superficial contact point possible.

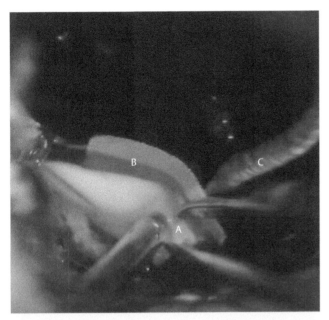

Fig. 5.5 Placement of the ABI electrode array in the lateral recess, left side. The array can be seen with electrodes contacting the anterosuperior surface of the lateral recess (A). Because this recess was widened, one Dacron wing (B) was left in place to help secure the array. The cable (C) often causes torque, which can make planned placement more difficult.

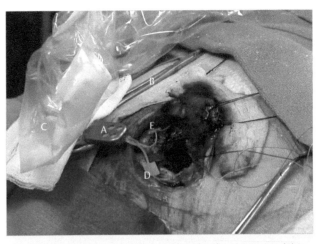

Fig. 5.6 EABR testing of the device, right side. The ABI receiver (A) is held by its magnet onto a hemostat (B) which has been attached to the surgical drapes. The testing device (C) is also coupled to the device by the magnet. A surgical sponge is placed between the receiver and testing device to mimic the thickness of the scalp. Also labeled are the device cable (D) and the ground electrode (E).

The surgeon must recognize tumor-related distortion of the brainstem, and must modify placement accordingly. This distortion can be translational, rotational, or both.

The following step is to secure the array in proper position. We utilize teased cardiac Teflon pledget material. Neurosurgeons will recognize this as the same material used for microvascular decompression.[15] Alternately, fat, muscle, or other materials can be used as well. Since the recess is cylindrical in configuration, the array can be packed securely against the brainstem surface. Direct approximation, without interposed material, is critical.

At this point, EABR testing of the device is carried out (▶ Fig. 5.6). The surgeon is provided feedback about areas of the array with better, worse, or absent responses. The positioning of the array can then be improved, either by "rotating" the array along the curved surface from superior to anterior or by increasing or decreasing its depth. It is usually necessary to remove packing before adjustments can be made. It must be noted that, at least with the Cochlear device, the array is larger than the target nuclei. As such, in most cases at least one corner of the array does not evoke good responses. Since each repositioning carries some risk as well as the potential for microinjury to the brainstem, this is definitely a situation of "perfect being the enemy of good."

With the Cochlear device, the receiver must still be placed into its subgaleal pocket. Prior to this, its magnet is replaced with a nonmagnetic disc. This is not a trivial step, especially since it is also critical not to dislodge the electrode array. After placement, the MED-EL ABI requires removal of a tab on the receiver. This converts the device from bipolar to monopolar stimulation mode.[14]

5.4.4 Closure

Closure proceeds in the usual fashion. It is anatomically not possible to obtain watertight dural closure with the TL approach, and presence of the ABI cable traversing the level of the dura increases the risk of both CSF leak and pseudomeningocele formation. If feasible, one or two 4–0 Nurolon sutures can be used to tack the presigmoid dura together, but this must be done with extreme care in order not to avulse the cable and array.

Abdominal fat is then used to pack the mastoid cavity, ensuring that fat surrounds the cable, which should not come in contact with the drilled surface of the temporal bone. As fat packing continues, the cable should also be allowed to lie in a position that avoids altering the angle of the cable at the interface with the brainstem. If a cranioplasty is carried out, this should also be done while avoiding damage to the receiver or to either the active or the ground cable. Scalp closure should be performed in layers with a similar degree of care.

5.5 Results

Most of the risk of TL ABI implantation in the setting of NF2 is attributable to tumor resection. In their description of the early use of ABIs implanted via the TL approach in 61 patients, Otto et al described CSF leaks in 3 patients (4.9%) and meningitis in 1 patient (1.6%).[7] In this series, no other complications were reported. Six patients did not obtain any useful stimulation (9.8%); in no case was any attempt made to reposition an array.

There are several other series of TL ABI placement in NF2 patients. Kanowitz et al reported the New York University experience in 2004.[16] In their 18 patients, there was a 5.5% risk each (1 patient) of CSF leak, superficial wound infection, and seroma formation requiring aspiration and pressure dressing. In addition, one patient (5.5%) did not obtain auditory stimulation. In 2012, Sanna and his colleagues reported their experience in

25 cases. While there were no CSF leaks in this series, one (4%) patient developed a collection requiring aspiration and another (4%) required explantation of the device due to wound infection. Four patients (16%) failed to receive auditory stimulation.

More recently, Ramsden et al detailed the TL ABI experience of the Manchester program.[17] Their surgical results are also similar, including a CSF leak rate of 6% and meningitis rate of 2% in their series of 50 ABI insertions. They also report a 14% risk of lower cranial nerve dysfunction, with a majority of these patients requiring temporary nasogastric tube feeding and one requiring temporary tracheostomy. One patient also required temporary tube feeding and tracheostomy after reoperation for attempted repositioning of the electrode array. This series also notes failure to obtain auditory stimulation in 9.8% of cases (4/41 activations).

Despite the many advances in surgical and other intraoperative technique, we have been unable to document significant improvements in auditory ABI results since the initial series. Our unpublished results have, however, shown improvements in both the achievement of auditory stimulation, with nonstimulation rates < 5%, and average number of useable electrodes. In addition, in the first author's personal series of 80 patients, there have been only 4 CSF leaks and no infections or meningitis.

References

[1] Ben Ammar M, Piccirillo E, Topsakal V, Taibah A, Sanna M. Surgical results and technical refinements in translabyrinthine excision of vestibular schwannomas: the Gruppo Otologico experience. Neurosurgery. 2012; 70(6): 1481–1491, discussion 1491

[2] Brackmann DE, Hitselberger WE, Nelson RA, et al. Auditory brainstem implant: I. Issues in surgical implantation. Otolaryngol Head Neck Surg. 1993; 108(6):624–633

[3] House WF, Hitselberger WE. Twenty-year report of the first auditory brain stem nucleus implant. Ann Otol Rhinol Laryngol. 2001; 110(2):103–104

[4] Schwartz MS, Kari E, Strickland BM, et al. Evaluation of the increased use of partial resection of large vestibular schwanommas: facial nerve outcomes and recurrence/regrowth rates. Otol Neurotol. 2013; 34(8):1456–1464

[5] US Food and Drug Administration. 2000. Nucleus 24 Auditory Brainstem Implant System. PMA #P000015. Docket number 00M-1659

[6] Matthies C, Brill S, Varallyay C, et al. Auditory brainstem implants in neurofibromatosis Type 2: is open speech perception feasible? J Neurosurg. 2014; 120(2):546–558

[7] Otto SR, Brackmann DE, Hitselberger WE, Shannon RV, Kuchta J. Multichannel auditory brainstem implant: update on performance in 61 patients. J Neurosurg. 2002; 96(6):1063–1071

[8] Schniepp R, Schlick C, Schenkel F, et al. Clinical and neurophysiological risk factors for falls in patients with bilateral vestibulopathy. J Neurol. 2017; 264 (2):277–283

[9] Singh R, Husain AM. Neurophysiologic intraoperative monitoring of the glossopharyngeal and vagus nerves. J Clin Neurophysiol. 2011; 28(6):582–586

[10] Schwartz MS, Otto SR, Shannon RV, Hitselberger WE, Brackmann DE. Auditory brainstem implants. Neurotherapeutics. 2008; 5(1):128–136

[11] Slattery WH III. The translabyrinthine approach. In Friedman RA, Slattery WH III, Brackmann DS, Fayad JN, Schwartz MS, eds. Lateral Skull Base Surgery: The House Clinic Atlas. New York: Thieme; 2012

[12] Behr R, Colletti V, Matthies C, et al. New outcomes with auditory brainstem implants in NF2 patients. Otol Neurotol. 2014; 35(10):1844–1851

[13] Rosahl SK, Rosahl S. No easy target: anatomic constraints of electrodes interfacing the human cochlear nucleus. Neurosurgery. 2013; 72(1) Suppl Operative:58–64, discussion 65

[14] Jackson KB, Mark G, Helms J, Mueller J, Behr R. An auditory brainstem implant system. Am J Audiol. 2002; 11(2):128–133

[15] Ammar A, Lagenaur C, Jannetta P. Neural tissue compatibility of Teflon as an implant material for microvascular decompression. Neurosurg Rev. 1990; 13 (4):299–303

[16] Kanowitz SJ, Shapiro WH, Golfinos JG, Cohen NL, Roland JT, Jr. Auditory brainstem implantation in patients with neurofibromatosis type 2. Laryngoscope. 2004; 114(12):2135–2146

[17] Odat HA, Piccirillo E, Sequino G, Taibah A, Sanna M. Management strategy of vestibular schwannoma in neurofibromatosis type 2. Otol Neurotol. 2011; 32(7):1163–1170

[18] Ramsden RT, Freeman SR, Lloyd SK, et al. Manchester Neurofibromatosis Type 2 Service. Auditory brainstem implantation in neurofibromatosis type 2: experience from the Manchester Programme. Otol Neurotol. 2016; 37(9): 1267–1274

6 The Retrosigmoid Approach in Auditory Brainstem Implantation

Robert Behr

Abstract

The retrosigmoid (RS) approach is the paradigmatic approach to the cerebellopontine angle for not only vestibular schwannomas but also a wide range of pathological processes. Indeed, it would be considered the standard and most common neurosurgical approach to this region. As shown more recently, auditory brainstem implants (ABIs) can be placed safely and effectively in adults via the RS approach with excellent results both for patients with neurofibromatosis type 2 (NF2) undergoing tumor resection at the same setting and for patients without tumors. For pediatric patients, the RS approach is the standard approach for ABI placement in all cases. The technique of ABI placement via the RS approach is discussed in this chapter, including use of the semi-sitting position (SSP) in select cases.

Keywords: auditory brainstem implant, retrosigmoid, semi-sitting position, vestibular schwannoma, neurofibromatosis type 2

6.1 Historical Remarks

The retrosigmoid approach was one of the earliest approaches in acoustic neuroma surgery. The earliest description of a vestibular schwannoma was probably given by Sandifort in 1777 (▶ Fig. 6.1).

It is widely known that Bell gave the first clinical description in 1830. However, the first comprehensive description of clinical symptoms and pathology was given by Jean Cruveilhier in 1835.[2]

The first successful surgical resection was accomplished by Sir Charles Balance in London in 1894.[3] He performed a two-step surgery and used the unilateral suboccipital approach and an osteoclastic trepanation. Also, Fedor Krause from Berlin propagated the unilateral suboccipital approach for these lesions as early as 1904.[4]

In the early 20th century, Cushing entered the field and performed a bilateral suboccipital approach for decompression and debulking of the tumor, which reduced the mortality and morbidity significantly.[5] Dandy, his pupil, went a step further and removed his first acoustic neuroma completely in 1917. He described his technique in 1925 using a unilateral suboccipital approach, debulking of the tumor, and painstaking resection of the capsule.[6]

Of course, also other approaches were used. Panse, for example, proposed the translabyrinthine access in 1904.[7] This technique was later modified and improved by House and his group.[8] He and Kurze and Rand also introduced the operative microscope in the acoustic neurinoma surgery in the mid-1960s.[9]

6.2 The Invention and Evolution of the ABI

It is very interesting and remarkable that only a bit more of a decade after the introduction of the operative microscope in vestibular schwannoma surgery, the first auditory brainstem implant (ABI) was successfully placed by House and Hitselberger in 1979.[10,11]

However, there wasn't much interest in ABI surgery at that time and therefore it took another decade until the interest rose again. This was mainly due to the technological development of the cochlear implant (CI) systems. At the beginning of the 1990s several CI providers (Cochlear, MED-EL, Advanced Bionics) produced ABIs and the first clinical experiences with multichannel ABI systems were obtained.[12,13,14]

6.3 Surgical Approaches to the Foramen of Luschka

From that time on, there was always a discussion about the most appropriate approach and positioning of the patient.

In the pediatric patient population, there is in principle no discussion about the access to the foramen of Luschka, the implantation site. The retrosigmoid approach and the lying position are the gold standard. In adults however, especially in NF2 patients, in principle two different approaches are possible. Next to the retrosigmoid, the translabyrinthine approach is widely used in acoustic neurinoma removal and ABI implantation. Contrary to the translabyrinthine approach, the retrosigmoid approach can be used in lying and in semi-sitting position (SSP), which has some advantages. In addition, the retrosigmoid approach in ssp seems to facilitate tumor resection, preservation of anatomical structures, and is related to improved hearing results with ABI.[15] Another option to reach the cochlear nucleus is the midline approach and subtonsillar dissection, which can also be used for bilateral implantation.[16]

6.4 Surgical Procedure for Retrosigmoid Approach

6.4.1 Positioning of the Patient

In the lying position (▶ Fig. 6.2), the patient is placed on the contralateral side to the tumor and the head is turned opposite to the tumor side and inclinated. It is fixed with a pin head holder like Mayfield clamp. The patient must be fixed and secured on the table since during operation the table should be turned deliberately around its length axis to gain a direct access to the cerebellopontine angle (CPA).

On the contrary, in the ssp the patient's head is turned to the tumor side (▶ Fig. 6.3) and inclinated. In both cases the large cervical veins should not be compressed.

In the ssp, either a precordial doppler device or a transesophageal ultrasound probe should be applied for detection of air embolism. In addition, an end-tidal CO_2 measurement is necessary.

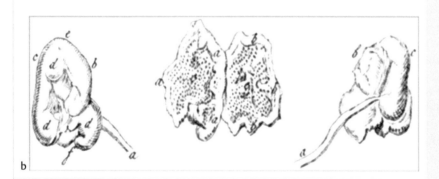

Fig. 6.1 (a, b) The first anatomic description of a vestibular schwannoma was made by Eduard Sandifort, of Leiden University, in 1777.[1]

It is advisable to check with magnetic resonance imaging (MRI) before the operation if there are additional schwannomas at the large peripheral nerves, for example, brachial plexus and lumbosacral plexus, large brachial nerves, and sciatic nerve, to prevent damage to these vulnerable structures by positioning. For example, a large tumor of the proximal sciatic nerve is dangerous in terms of compression lesion during ssp. It is also advisable to measure the somatosensory evoked potentials (SSEP) and motor evoked potentials (MEP) just before positioning of the patient and to repeat these examinations after positioning. Especially in NF2 patients, who may have tumors at cervical spine or have had operations and adhesions there, rotation and inclination of the head may cause

impairment of blood circulation or direct compression of the spinal cord. This can be detected before skin incision by the abovementioned monitoring procedures.

6.4.2 Skin Incision and Trepanation

We usually prefer a question mark-like skin incision to create a double layer flap for the housing of the implant (▶ Fig. 6.2 and ▶ Fig. 6.4). The base of the flap is always anterior to preserve a good blood supply from the temporal skin vessels. The occipital artery is always in danger of being sacrificed during the suboccipital and retrosigmoid dissection. So on the left side the incision is like a question mark, and on the right side, it is like a reversed question mark.

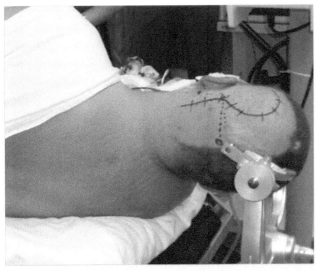

Fig. 6.2 Lying position, tumor left sided, head rotated to contralateral side. Question mark-like incision.

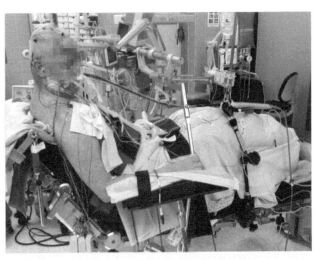

Fig. 6.3 Semi-sitting position (SSP). Head is turned to the tumor side.

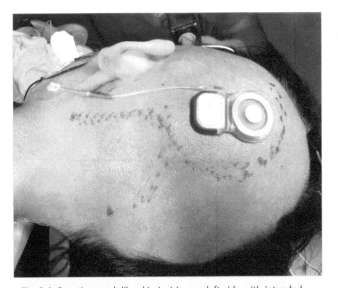

Fig. 6.4 Question mark-like skin incision on left side with intended placement of the implant.

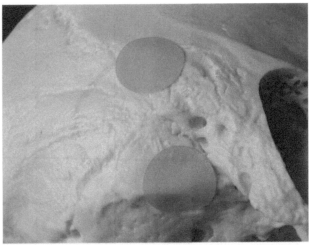

Fig. 6.5 Schematic placement of burr holes at asterion (above) and at the base of the posterior fossa. Blue line indicates the margin of bone flap.

After dissection of the skin flap which is gently retracted, a periosteal flap is created with its base opposite to the skin flap base. By these means a double-layered covering of the implant housing is possible.

Thereafter, the muscle layers over the posterior fossa are divided, for example, with monopolar cautery, and the periosteum is strapped medially and laterally to expose the bone. One landmark is the retromastoid incisure and the other the asterion. This is the area where three bony sutures join: the lambda suture, the occipitomastoid suture, and the parieto-mastoid suture. Once these landmarks are identified, a burrhole is placed just below the asterion and a second behind the mastoid incisure as much low to the base of the posterior fossa as you can get (▶ Fig. 6.5). An optional third burr hole may be placed more medially and perpendicular to a connecting line between the first two burrholes, forming a triangle. After dissecting the dura off the bone, it is cut out using a high-speed saw. The last cut should be the most lateral one, close to the expected location of the sigmoid sinus. In case the sinus is injured it can be accessed very quickly if there are no bone cuts left. In some cases, the trepanation must be enlarged osteoclastically to the base of the posterior fossa; no bony rim should be left in order to come as close as possible to the sigmoid sinus. Cranially, the junction between the transverse and sigmoid sinus should be visible; then you know that the trepanation is close to the tentorium (▶ Fig. 6.6). The bony rims of the trepanation should be thoroughly inspected if mastoid cells are opened. They have to be closed properly, mostly using bone wax or muscle with fibrin glue. Before opening the dura, the bony bed for the implant housing should be drilled. The main reason is that no

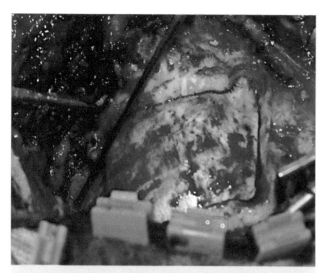

Fig. 6.6 Exposed dura in supine position. The blue structure on the right side of the trepanation is the transverse sinus. The pointer depicts the base of the posterior fossa.

bone dust should enter the intradural space. Therefore, a template is available for this purpose. The bed should be centered below the skin flap and above the transverse sinus. In adults it should be drilled deep enough to ensure a secure fixation with nonresorbable sutures. These can be inserted through a bony canal drilled with a small, 1 mm, diamond drill at the rims of the bony bed, or they can be fixed with micro titanium plates which are normally used for bone flap fixation. Especially in children who have thin bone, this is a good alternative.

As a second option for implantation of the housing, a subperiosteal, subcutaneous pocket, can be created and the device housing is slipped into this pocket without a fixation by a suture. Some colleagues drill a small well into the bone just to fit in a little bit of the electronic part of the housing, which is in general below the transmitter coil and the magnet. This method does not need a skin flap to cover the housing. Some implants are available with small pins which enhances the fixation by inserting into the bone. By this method the size of the wound and operating time are reduced. However, a disadvantage is that in case of a subcutaneous cerebrospinal fluid (CSF) leak, which is not seldom in children because they are not as compliant as adults, the housing starts floating in its pocket which may affect the lead by tension and torsion and cause dysfunction of the implant. Therefore, a secure fixation should be achieved.

6.4.3 Dura Opening and Tumor Approach

After cleaning the operative field by water irrigation, the dura can be opened. It is advised to palpate the tension of the dura beforehand and if it is quite strong, talk to the anesthetist to take some measures to lower intracranial pressure (ICP) and elevate the head of the patient by moving the table. Especially in the lying position and in children, the tension can be very strong which will cause herniation of the cerebellum during

dural opening. It is recommended to open the dura by only 1 cm at the base of the trepanation and fix the dura with a suture to the muscles or to the bone. This will keep the opening patent during suction of CSF. Under the use of the microscope for better illumination a small spatula is inserted and the cerebellar hemisphere is gently retracted. Once the arachnoid membrane is reached in the depth, mostly behind the lower cranial nerves, it is opened either by suction or with a pair of microscissors. Immediately after the opening of the arachnoid and draining of CSF, the cerebellum will relax and start pulsations. Now the dura can easily be opened in a semicircular fashion, with its two ends at the inferior sigmoid sinus and the junction of the transverse and sigmoid sinuses. The base of the dura flap is lateral, along the sigmoid sinus. The dura is fixed under gentle retraction and tension with two microsutures to the muscles. It should be protected with a sponge and kept wet throughout the whole procedure. The wound which is outside the center of interest should also be covered with wet patties as usual. With the use of a self-holding retractor device, the cerebellum is gently mobilized laterally. After draining enough CSF, this is normally possible without pressure, especially in the ssp. Now the arachnoid membranes can be dissected and the tumor visualized and resected step by step. Typically, this is done under monitoring of the facial and auditory nerves, if they are still functioning. The main steps are tumor debulking and then dissection of the tumor borders off the cranial nerves and the brainstem. This is facilitated in ssp since there is less need for suction of blood, irrigation fluid, and CSF, which are flowing out of the wound due to gravity. The tumor borders can be grabbed with a forceps, mobilized a little laterally, and with the second hand and a dissector the arachnoid membrane can be stripped over the tumor keeping the correct dissection plane. With this technique, the tumor can be resected in piecemeal with utmost protection of the neural and vascular structures. After completion of tumor resection outside the internal auditory canal (IAC), its medial bony wall is drilled and the tumor inside the IAC is removed. In our institution this part of the surgery is done by the ENT colleagues.[18]

In some situations, it may be necessary to open the IAC earlier, mainly if it is very difficult to localize the facial and/or auditory nerve, for example, in recurrences, after previous operation or radiation. Once visualized in the IAC, it may be easier to dissect the nerves also, medially to the IAC.

After drilling the IAC and tumor removal, it is highly important to inspect the bony walls of the IAC for opened cells. An endoscope with 30 degrees optic to look into the IAC is helpful. Opened cells have to be occluded properly to prevent transmastoid CSF leak.

When tumor removal is finished it is recommended to perform a bilateral jugular vein compression, especially in ssp, to identify small bleeding veins. In case of a dry field, the ABI implantation can be initiated, which however is not the topic of this chapter.

6.4.4 Closure after Tumor Resection and ABI Implantation

Once the tumor is removed and the ABI is placed and fixed properly, a last inspection should be done to identify minor bleedings. The dura is closed with either single or running sutures using a thin thread, for example, 5.0 Vicryl[R] or Prolene[R].

The dura penetrating ABI lead should be sutured tightly and covered either with muscle pieces and fibrin glue or TachoSil[R]. To prevent CSF leak, an additional sealing of the dura can be administered using, for example, Durasil[R].

The bone flap should be reinserted with titanium screws or similar devices. This is very helpful in cases of later revision. If there is no bone flap, the muscles will create massive adhesions with the dura and the lead of the ABI and a dissection will be much more difficult. With a reinserted bone flap, the dura can be re-exposed much easily with a better protection of the ABI lead. The soft tissues are closed in layers as usual. A drainage is not recommended because of CSF leak induction.

In adults use of compression bandage is not necessary. A sterile draping is sufficient. In children however, a soft compression bandage for 5 to 7 days is useful, since they are not as compliant and often increase ICP by crying and restlessness.

6.4.5 Postoperative Care

After the operation the patient is admitted to the intensive care unit (ICU) for at least one night. The head and chest are elevated by 30 degrees to reduce ICP and the medication consists of dexamethasone 4 to 8 mg three times a day and antibiotics for 3 to 5 days.

We regularly take a postoperative computed tomography (CT) scan at day 1 after the operation for early detection of postoperative complications or minor abnormalities which may become complications, for example, small hematomas, subdural air intrapment, intramastoid fluid accumulation etc. The positioning of the ABI electrode carrier is important, especially as a reference for later CT scans in case of a suspected migration.

If the patient is stable, he/she is admitted to the intermediate care unit for 1 to 3 days and later on to the normal ward. The stiches are taken out at day 10.

The first fitting of the ABI is normally performed 6 weeks after the implantation. For further details, see references of the manufacturer.

6.5 Discussion

The retrosigmoid approach is being used in acoustic neuroma surgery since the beginning of the 20th century.[3,4,5,6] In former times, suboccipital and retrosigmoid approaches were not always strictly distinguished, and some surgeons used even a bilateral approach in respect of decompression of the posterior fossa. In those times and even later, the dura was not sutured to create some space for the swelling of cerebellum.[17] The CSF tightness was achieved by the accurate suture of the muscle layers. With the proposal of the translabyrinthine approach by Panse in 1904,[7] a new possibility to remove vestibular schwannomas was presented. Since that time there have been long-lasting discussions on which approach is the best and what are the pros and cons.[18] In a retrospective review based on a database analysis of 5,064 patients from 35 studies, Ansari and coworkers[19] found no significant differences in incidence of residual tumor, mortality, tumor recurrence, major complications, and dysfunction of cranial nerves other than cranial

nerves VII and VIII. However, they found that the retrosigmoid approach was superior to other approaches in terms of facial nerve preservation in most important tumor sizes of 1.5 to more than 3 cm extracanalicular diameter. As to hearing, the middle fossa approach was better than the retrosigmoid in tumors smaller than 1.5 cm. Other tumor sizes showed no differences. However, hearing preservation is often not considered in ABI surgery. The retrosigmoid approach has a higher risk for CSF leak and headache. The latter, however, can be successfully prevented by reinserting the bone flap as a barrier against scarring of muscle and dura.[20] Since most of the ABI candidates have larger tumors and are already deaf or nearly deaf, the preservation of the VIIIth nerve is rarely a surgical goal. Only in very small tumors with residual functional hearing or if a CI implantation is planned, a middle fossa approach with the aim to preserve the auditory nerve may be considered. Especially on the left side, this approach is however associated with a higher risk of psychological dysfunctions.[21]

In the author's personal experience, another important advantage of the retrosigmoid approach is that it is much faster than the translabyrinthine approach. In an experienced hand, it can be accomplished from skin to dura in 30 minutes. This is an important issue because tumor removal and ABI implantation will also take a certain amount of time.

Also, Colletti and his group stated in an earlier paper[22] that the retrosigmoid approach is useful in NF2 and non-NF2 cases for tumor removal and ABI implantation. Especially if there is a chance for hearing preservation, this approach is recommended. In 2015, even the group at the Massachusetts Eye and Ear Infirmary/Harvard University supported the retrosigmoid approach as a safe and effective way to approach the foramen of Luschka for ABI insertion.[23]

In the pediatric patient group, the discussion about the approach is less diverse. Those surgeons and surgical teams who have a large experience in pediatric ABI recommend the retrosigmoid approach. It offers an excellent visualization of the operative field of interest, the foramen of Luschka and the surrounding nerves and vessels. After sufficient CSF drainage, the cerebellum is relaxed and needs almost no retraction. The spatula is needed, if at all, just to keep the lateral recess open for implantation. The trepanation is very fast and saves surgical time, and time of anesthesia is important especially in children. The reported complication rates attributed to the approach are very low and are mostly related to CSF extrusion. This issue, however, is related to the painstaking suture of the dura and entry of the lead through the dura. They can be augmented by using special dura sealants. Reimplantation of the bone flap is also a means to reduce some minor postoperative complaints.[24,25,26,27,28,29,30]

References

[1] Sandifort, E. Observationes Anatomico-Pathologicae vol. I. Leiden: Apud Eyk P. V. d., Vygh, D. University of Leiden. 1777.

[2] Cruveilhier, J. Anatomie pathologique du corps humain, ou Descriptions, avec figures lithographiées et coloriées, des diverses altérations morbides dont le corps humain est susceptible. Paris, Baillière, vol. 2, 1829–1842.

[3] Nehls DG, Spetzler RF, Shetter AG, Sonntag VK. Application of new technology in the treatment of cerebellopontine angle tumors. Clin Neurosurg. 1985; 32: 223–241

[4] Koos WT, Perneczky A. Suboccipital approach to acoustic neurinomas with emphasis of preservation of facial nerve and cochlear nerve function. In:

Rand RW, ed. Microneurosurgery. 3rd ed. St. Louis: Mosby CV Co.; 1985:335–365

[5] Cushing H. Tumors of the Nervus Acusticus and the Syndrome of the Cerebellopontine Angle. Philadelphia, W.B.: Saunders Co.;1917

[6] Dandy WE. An operation for total removal of cerebellopontine (acoustic) tumors. Surg Gynecol Obstet. 1925; 41:139–148

[7] Rand RW, Dirks DD, Morgan DE, Bentson JR. Acoustic neuromas. In: Youmans JR, ed. Neurological Surgery. 2nd ed. Philadelphia: Saunders WB Co.; 1982:2967–3003

[8] House WF. Transtemporal bone microsurgical removal of acoustic neuromas. Monograph I.. Arch Otolaryngol. 1964; 80:597–756

[9] Rand RW, Kurze TL. Facial nerve preservation by posterior fossa transmeatal microdissection in total removal of acoustic tumours. J Neurol Neurosurg Psychiatry. 1965; 28:311–316

[10] Edgerton BJ, House WF, Hitselberger W. Hearing by cochlear nucleus stimulation in humans. Ann Otol Rhinol Laryngol Suppl. 1982; 91(2 Pt 3) Suppl. 91: 117–124

[11] McElveen JT, Jr, Hitselberger WE, House WF, Mobley JP, Terr LI. Electrical stimulation of cochlear nucleus in man. Am J Otol. 1985 Suppl:88–91

[12] Behr R, Müller J, Shehata-Dieler W, et al. The high rate CIS auditory brainstem implant for restoration of hearing in NF-2 patients. Skull Base. 2007; 17(2): 91–107

[13] Mueller J, Behr R, Knaus C, Milewski C, Schoen F, Helms J. Electrical stimulation of the auditory pathway in deaf patients following acoustic neurinoma surgery and initial results with a new auditory brainstem implant system. Adv Otorhinolaryngol. 2000; 57:229–235

[14] Nevison B, Laszig R, Sollmann WP, et al. Results from a European clinical investigation of the Nucleus multichannel auditory brainstem implant. Ear Hear. 2002; 23(3):170–183

[15] Behr R, Colletti V, Matthies C, et al. New outcomes with auditory brainstem implants in NF2 patients. Otol Neurotol. 2014; 35(10):1844–1851

[16] Behr R. Bilateral auditory brain stem implantation with single implant. J Neurol Surg B Skull Base. 2015; S1(76):S113

[17] Irsigler FJ. Allgemeine Operationslehre. In: Olivecrona H, Tönnis W, Hrsg. Handbuch der Neurochirurgie. Band 4 1. Teil P 90.Springer Verlag; 1960

[18] Schwager K. [Acoustic neuroma (vestibular schwannoma) therapy from an oto-rhino-laryngological perspective]. HNO. 2011; 59(1):22–, 24–30

[19] Ansari SF, Terry C, Cohen-Gadol AA. Surgery for vestibular schwannomas: a systematic review of complications by approach. Neurosurg Focus. 2012; 33 (3):E14

[20] Harner SG, Beatty CW, Ebersold MJ. Impact of cranioplasty on headache after acoustic neuroma removal. Neurosurgery. 1995; 36(6):1097–1099, discussion 1099–1100

[21] Minovi A, Mangold R, Kollert M, Hofmann E, Draf W, Bockmühl U. [Functional results, cognitive and effective quality of life disturbances after trans-temporal resection of acoustic neuroma]. Laryngorhinootologie. 2005; 84(12):915–920

[22] Colletti V, Sacchetto L, Giarbini N, Fiorino F, Carner M. Retrosigmoid approach for auditory brainstem implant. J Laryngol Otol Suppl. 2000(27): 37–40

[23] Puram SV, Herrmann B, Barker FG, II, Lee DJ. Retrosigmoid craniotomy for auditory brainstem implantation in adult patients with neurofibromatosis type 2. J Neurol Surg B Skull Base. 2015; 76(6):440–450

[24] Jung NY, Kim M, Chang WS, Jung HH, Choi JY, Chang JW. Favorable long-term functional outcomes and safety of auditory brainstem implants in nontumor patients. Oper Neurosurg (Hagerstown). 2017; 13(6):653–660

[25] Sennaroğlu L, Sennaroğlu G, Yücel E, et al. Long-term results of ABI in children with severe inner ear malformations. Otol Neurotol. 2016; 37(7): 865–872

[26] Bayazit YA, Abaday A, Dogulu F, Göksu N. Complications of pediatric auditory brain stem implantation via retrosigmoid approach. ORL J Otorhinolaryngol Relat Spec. 2011; 73(2):72–75

[27] Colletti V, Shannon RV, Carner M, Veronese S, Colletti L. Complications in auditory brainstem implant surgery in adults and children. Otol Neurotol. 2010; 31(4):558–564

[28] Colletti V, Shannon R, Carner M, Veronese S, Colletti L. Outcomes in nontumor adults fitted with the auditory brainstem implant: 10 years' experience. Otol Neurotol. 2009; 30(5):614–618

[29] Colletti V, Fiorino FG, Carner M, Giarbini N, Sacchetto L, Cumer G. Advantages of the retrosigmoid approach in auditory brain stem implantation. Skull Base Surg. 2000; 10(4):165–170

[30] Noij KS, Kozin ED, Sethi R, et al. Systematic review of nontumor pediatric auditory brainstem implant outcomes. Otolaryngol Head Neck Surg. 2015; 153(5):739–750

7 Surgery for ABI: Retrolabyrinthine Approach

Ricardo F. Bento and Paula T. Lopes

Abstract

The retrolabyrinthine approach (RLA) to the cerebellopontine angle and posterior fossa is traditionally described to offer a quick and safe surgical access, as it reduces the operative distance and the need for cerebellar retraction with labyrinthine block preservation. However, its main landmarks may be well known to enable skilled neurotologists to gain access to lesions that are located in areas difficult to reach. In 2006, Bento et al were the first to describe the RLA to introduce an auditory brainstem implant (ABI) electrode in the foramen of Luschka. This chapter intends to present an overview, the surgical technique, complications, and our results.

Keywords: retrolabyrinthine, translabyrinthine, ear surgery, auditory brainstem implant

7.1 Introduction

In 1966 House described transtemporal surgical access to the cerebellopontine angle known as the translabyrinthine pathway, based on the removal of the entire labyrinthine block, providing a broad approach that allows identification of the facial nerve and less aggression to the brainstem, cerebellum, and vessels.[1]

However, this access approach sacrifices the patient's auditory and vestibular function.

In 1972, Hitselberger and Pulec proposed the retrolabyrinthine or infralabyrinthine approach, derived from the translabyrinthine approach, initially for the correction of functional problems of the trigeminal nerve and selective vestibular neurectomy and later used for decompression of vascular loops.[2]

The first auditory brainstem implant (ABI) surgery was performed in 1979 by Dr. William F. House and Dr. William Hitselberger at the Ear House Institute in Los Angeles, USA, in patients with type 2 neurofibromatosis whose tumor was removed and the electrode placed at the same surgical time.[3]

In 2001, Colletti et al used a classic retrosigmoid approach in two children with bilateral severe cochlear malformations and cochlear nerve aplasia for ABI.[4]

In September 2002, the retrosigmoid surgical approach was then extended by Bento et al for removal of acoustic small size schwannoma and also other tumors from the cerebellopontine angle in patients with hearing residual preservation.[5]

In 2012, Bento et al described the main landmarks of this route to place the brainstem implant. Since then, it has become a surgical practice.[6]

In 2013, the same group performed the first ABI in a child with bilateral cochlear nerve agenesis using this approach, and since then it has been the main approach chosen for this surgery to this time.[7]

In 2014, Bento et al also presented similar results as the ones obtained by translabyrinthine and retrosigmoid approaches for ABI surgery.[8]

The advantage of retrolabyrinthine technique is the preservation of the labyrinthine block in order to minimize the probable changes in balance in children. Currently, most surgeons are using the retrosigmoid approach in cases of auditory brainstem implantation, either for removal of the tumor (neurofibromatosis type 2) or in other indications such as cochlear nerve agenesis or trauma, ossified cochlea, and ear malformation.[9]

The presigmoid retrolabyrinthic approach presents as advantage the preservation of the labyrinthine, allowing the patient to maintain a normal vestibular function, and also providesadequate exposure of the bulbar nerves and foramen of Luschka. Other advantages of this route are the minimal retraction of the cerebellum, the small opening of the dura mater, less chance of liquoric fistula and bleeding because of vessel injury, shorter period of postoperative recovery in intensive care unit, and no necessity of drainage dispositive placement during this period.

The retrosigmoid approach offers some disadvantages such as the necessity for retraction of the cerebellum.

7.2 Retrolabyrinthine Surgical Technique

The patient is put under general anesthesia (without the use of muscle relaxing drug because of the monitoring of the cranial nerves VII, IX, X, and XI during the procedure).

The patient lies in supine position, with the head turned so that the involved ear side is up. Subcutaneous infiltration of lidocaine 2% associated with adrenaline in the concentration of 1:100,000 is performed, and an incision is made in the postauricular skin from above the helix of the ear to a point approximately 3 cm above the auricle, starting from the tangent plane to the posterior wall of the external auditory canal and about 5 cm from the postauricular groove to the tip of the mastoid. After postauricular incision, soft tissue is maintained above the periosteal and osteoperiosteal flap pedicle is created using the cortical bone close to the mastoid at the end of surgery[10] (▶ Fig. 7.1).

A C-shaped skin incision begins slightly superior to the pinna, extends posteriorly from the root of the zygoma to the inion, and ends 1 cm below and slightly anterior to the mastoid tip. The attachments of the sternocleidomastoid and splenius capitus muscles to the mastoid tip is exposed and maintained in position. During mastoidectomy, the groove of the digastric muscle is also exposed as one important anatomical landmark, close proximity to the stylomastoid foramen, from where the vertical segment of facial nerve emerge through.

Using an operating microscope and drill, a canal wall-up mastoidectomy is performed and the posterior bone external auditory canal is thinned but preserved. The incus, and lateral and posterior semicircular canals are identified along with the sigmoid sinus and facial nerve. The descending and mastoid segment of the facial nerve and the three semicircular canals are delineated. The bone is widely removed from the sigmoid venous sinus from the sinodural angle to the jugular bulb. If necessary, an island of bone is retained on the central portion of the sinus to facilitate a retractor placement (▶ Fig. 7.2). The dura of the posterior fossa is exposed and incised between the posterior canal, sigmoid sinus, and jugular bulb inferiorly, and is incised just anterior to the

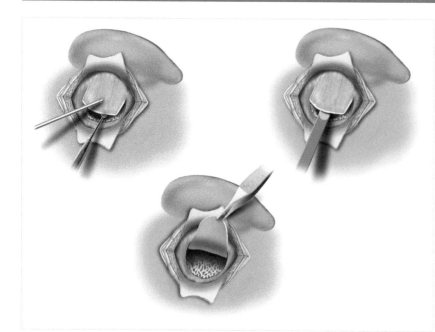

Fig. 7.1 After postauricular incision, soft tissue is maintained above the periosteal, and osteoperiosteal flap pedicle is created using the cortical bone close to the mastoid at the end of surgery.

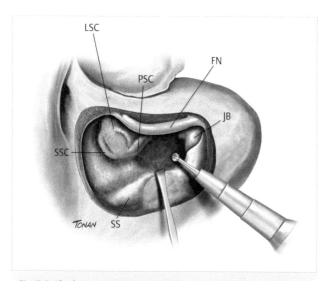

Fig. 7.2 The bone is widely removed from the sigmoid venous sinus from the sinodural angle to the jugular bulb. An island of bone is retained on the central portion of the sinus. FN, facial nerve; JB, jugular bulb; LSC, lateral semicircular canal; PSC, posterior semicircular canal; SS, sigmoid sinus; SSC; semicircular superior canal.

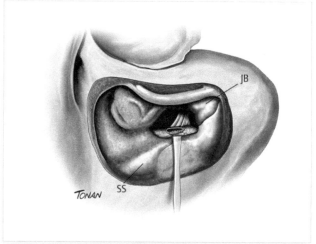

Fig. 7.3 Identification of posterior canal, sigmoid sinus, and jugular bulb as the main landmarks to expose the operative field. The dura of the posterior fossa is exposed between the posterior canal and the sigmoid sinus and is incised. Cerebellum is exposed and retracted and choroid plexus is visualized in front of foramen of Luschka. JB, jugular bulb; SS, sigmoid sinus.

sigmoid sinus. The main goal to achieve the visualization of the lower cranial nerves (IX, X and XI) is by drilling the jugular bulb inferiorly in order to obtain an adequate space between the posterior semicircular canal and the jugular bulb.

In very few cases (less than 10%) when you don't have a good exposure of the cranial nerves, the surgeon can drill the posterior semicircular canal posterior semicircular canal (PSC) and obliterate the cruras.

After the incision of the dura of the posterior fossa, the subarachnoid space is then opened to release spinal fluid in the cisterna. A small part of the cerebellum is exposed by

minimal retraction to show the exiting nerve roots in the cerebellopontine angle (▶ Fig. 7.3).

The cochlear nucleus complex, composed of the ventral and dorsal, is the site for the placement of the electrode. The ventral cochlear nucleus is the main neural impulse transmission nucleus of the VIII pair and its axons the main ascending pathway of the cochlear nerve. Both the ventral and dorsal are not visible during surgery and their location depends on the identification of adjacent anatomical structures. The dorsal nucleus is located superiorly to the lateral recess of the fourth ventricle, while the ventral nucleus is covered by the cerebellar peduncle.

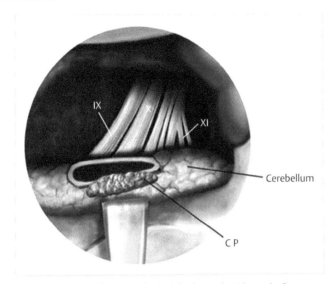

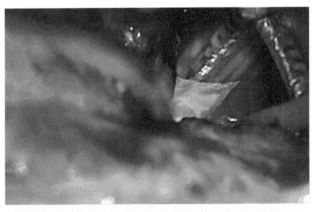

Fig. 7.5 Intraoperative image of the insertion of auditory brainstem implant (ABI) electrode into the foramen of Luschka.

Fig. 7.4 To approach the fourth ventricle, the arachnoid over the foramen is displaced, the flocculus and the choroid plexus retracted and the cranial nerves (IX, X, and XI) are identified. The electrode array is then inserted on fourth ventricle. CP, choroid plexus; Cerebellum, IX, X and XI cranial nerves.

Between the emergence of the facial (VII) and glossopharyngeal (IX) nerves lies the lateral recess or foramen of Luschka, just medially to the IX nerve emergence in the brainstem. The preferred location for placement of the electrode of ABI is the foramen of Luschka, where the ventral cochlear nucleus and lower part of the dorsal nucleus are located, as this region is less susceptible to nonauditory stimuli, such as facial and glossopharyngeal.

The most important landmarks used to identify the cochlear nucleus area is the IX nerve. The cochlear nucleus complex may be prominent as the VIII nerve approaches in direction of the IX nerve. The entry into the fourth ventricle through the Luschka foramen may be identified by the choroid plexus which covers the cerebellar flocculus, the most protruded structure visible from the foramen of Luschka. To approach the fourth ventricle, the arachnoid over the foramen is displaced and cut, the venous and arterial net are also detached and elevated and finally, the flocculus and the choroid plexus retracted. To this end, rostromedial retraction of the cerebellum is necessary. The choroid plexus projecting from the lateral recess (foramen of Luschka) and overlying the cochlear nucleus complex is followed and the entrance to the lateral recess is then found (▶ Fig. 7.4).

The opening of the lateral recess is confirmed by the outflow of cerebrospinal fluid. The cochlear nucleus complex is identified since it bulged in the floor of the lateral recess.

The electrode array is then inserted into the lateral recess with the aid of a small forceps.

The correct position of the electrode is estimated with the aid of the intraoperative electrically evoked auditory brainstem response and neural response telemetry.

The importance of the right positioning of the electrode is to avoid side effects of nonauditory neural stimulation. Electrodes placed in the foramen of Luschka have been shown to be effective in auditory stimulation with minimal side effects, besides being stable because of the limited space to place it (▶ Fig. 7.5).

Intraoperative electromyography and evocate potential are used to lead the surgeon during the electrode positioning

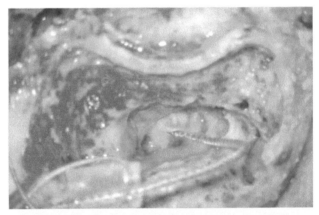

Fig. 7.6 Intraoperative image of the electrode of brainstem implant placed between the temporalis facia and the brainstem where the ventral cochlear nucleus and lower part of the dorsal nucleus are located.

procedure by receiving auditory responses at the time of placing it.

At the end, after the placement of the electrode, the dural defect is repaired using a graft of temporalis fascia and fibrin glue. The mastoid cavity is obliterated with a free fat graft taken from the anterior abdominal wall, from the left iliac fossa (▶ Fig. 7.6 and ▶ Fig. 7.7).

The osteoperiosteal flap is closed; first the periosteum, followed by the muscular suture with an absorbable surgical thread 3.0 wire, and the skin plane using nonabsorbable 4.0 wire. A compressive dressing is applied over the ear and maintained for 3 days.

7.3 Postoperative Concerns

The most apparent complications we try to avoid are the cerebrospinal fluid fistula, postoperative bleeding, meningitis, cerebellar syndrome, and intracranial hypertension. Concerned about the main complications reported, the first day postoperative may be at the intensive care unit.

To avoid the cerebrospinal fluid fistula, the closure needs fascia of the temporal bone glued with free fat. Also the newest osteoperiosteal graft is developed to decrease the risk. Some postoperative care is added, such as maintenance of total rest

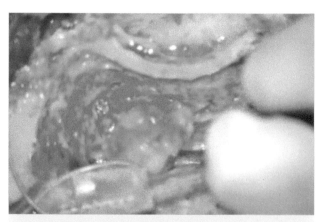

Fig. 7.7 Intraoperative image of the mastoid cavity obliterated with a free fat graft taken from the anterior abdominal wall, from the left iliac fossa.

for 72 hours, compressive dressing, laxative diet, and progression to relative rest for two more days, which allow the patient to evacuate, and continue rest on bed during this period.

Intravenous third-generation cefalosporin antibiotics is used 2.0 g every 12 hours during the hospital stay as postsurgical infection prophylaxis. Also, corticosteroids are used to reduce the inflammatory response to trauma caused by the surgery and antivertigo drugs are taken during the first days to reduce the symptoms of denseness caused because of the vestibular nerve manipulation.

7.4 Discussion

Our experiences about the surgical results show that synaptic input from the ABI electrode array placed along the surface of the cochlear nucleus through the retrolabyrinthine route had similar auditory responses to acoustic stimuli than compared to translabyrintine and retrosigmoid approaches.

Concerning mortality, the results obtained were satisfactory, with less morbidity and risk of death due to injury of blood vessel or cerebellum compression.[11]

Special topics may be considered before planning a surgery: A high jugular bulb can limit the space between the sigmoid sinus and the posterior semicircular channel is the most common reason and can be predicted with a high-resolution CT scan.

The opening of the posterior dura fossa should be broad, from the base of the jugular bulb to the internal auditory canal, extending posteriorly to the limit of the sigmoid sinus. This allows an adequate view by the lateral recess to the foramen of Luschka to insert the electrode array.

Minimum cerebellar retraction may be necessary and a delicate dissection of choroid plexus and arachnoid surrounding the bulbar cranial nerves should be done.

Landmarks for the correct localization of the foramen of Luschka are adjacently placed and are mainly the IX cranial nerve, the cerebellar flocculus, and choroid plexus. For this reason, there is no need for removal of the lateral and superior semicircular canals and to open the vestibule, and a small approach can be done even in small children.

One important advantage of this technique is that it can be easily changed to a translabyrinthine approach when a larger exposure is needed.

We also described this surgical approach by drilling the posterior canal which facilitates the procedure for surgical approach to the pontocerebellar angle, which can be used in addition for surgeries to remove big size tumors located there, which provide us with lower morbidity.

This surgical technique has been increasingly practiced as a surgical access route for patients who need surgeries at the cerebellopontine angle and who have some auditory residue to be preserved, with satisfactory results of auditory preservation and successful postoperative recovery.

Concerning morbidity and mortality, the results obtained were satisfactory, with no case of any neurological sequel in our series.

7.5 Conclusion

Considering ABI surgeries, this approach presented as a safe and reliable surgical technique in which there is no need to remove any semicircular canal or the vestibule. It has an extensive enough surgical field to allow for correct identification of the anatomic landmarks used as reference for the correct placement of the electrodes. So, a minimal approach can be taken. The drawback is that it cannot be used in cases with a large jugular bulb. The choice of the side to be operated on should take into consideration how large the jugular bulb is, by analyzing CT and MRI before planning the surgery. This facilitates the surgical procedure and a positive point is that this approach can be enlarged to a translabyrinthine one when necessary.

References

[1] Hitselberger WE, House WF. A combined approach to the cerebellopontine angle:a suboccipital-petrosal approach. Arch Otolaryngol. 1966; 84(3):267–285

[2] Hitselberger WE, Pulec JL. Trigeminal nerve (posterior root) retrolabyrinthine selective section:operative procedure for intractable pain. Arch Otolaryngol. 1972; 96(5):412–415

[3] Hitselberger WE, House WF, Edgerton BJ, Whitaker S. Cochlear nucleus implants. Otolaryngol Head Neck Surg. 1984; 92(1):52–54

[4] Colletti V, Carner M, Fiorino F, et al. Hearing restoration with auditory brainstem implant in three children with cochlear nerve aplasia. Otol Neurotol. 2002; 23(5):682–693

[5] Bento RF, De Brito RV, Sanchez TG, Miniti A. The transmastoidretrolabyrinthine approach in vestibular schwannoma surgery. Otolaryngol Head Neck Surg. 2002; 127(5):437–441

[6] Bento RF, Monteiro TA, Tsuji RK, et al. Retrolabyrinthine approach for surgical placement of auditory brainstem implants in children. Acta Otolaryngol. 2012; 132(5):462–466

[7] Bento RF, Monteiro TA, Bittencourt AG, Goffi-Gomez MV, de Brito R. Retrolabyrinthine approach for cochlear nerve preservation in neurofibromatosis type 2 and simultaneous cochlear implantation. Int Arch Otorhinolaryngol. 2013; 17(3):351–355

[8] BentoRF, LimaLRPJr, TsujiRK, et al. Tratado de ImplanteCoclear e Próteses Auditivas Implantáveis. Parte 6. Capítulo 58: Implante Auditivo de Tronco Encefálico: Bento RF, Santos AF, Goffi-Gomez MV. Editora Thieme Publicações Ltda. Rio de Janeiro, RJ, Brasil.; 2014:Págs. 37482

[9] Colletti V, Shannon RV, Carner M, Veronese S, Colletti L. Complications in auditory brainstem implant surgery in adults and children. Otol Neurotol. 2010; 31(4):558–564

[10] Bento RF, Tsuji RK, Fonseca ACO, Alves RD. Use of an osteoplastic flap for the prevention of mastoidectomy retroauricular defects. Int Arch Otorhinolaryngol. 2017; 21(2):151–155

[11] Goffi-Gomez MVS, Magalhães AT, Brito Neto R, Tsuji RK, Gomes MdeQ, Bento RF. Auditory brainstem implant outcomes and MAP parameters: report of experiences in adults and children. Int J Pediatr Otorhinolaryngol. 2012; 76(2):257–264

8 Auditory Brainstem Implantation in Children: Evaluation and Surgery

Levent Sennaroğlu and Burçak Bilginer

Abstract

Inner ear malformations frequently necessitate cochlear or auditory brainstem implantation (ABI) for hearing habilitation in children. ABI is indicated in certain severe inner ear malformations (IEM). In this chapter definite and probable ABI indications are explained in detail. In children with hypoplastic cochlear nerve there is still a debate on choosing the best method of rehabilitation. A review of literature is provided for this topic. Age limit in pediatric ABI has decreased considerably and this is also highlighted. Pediatric ABI necessitates a very good collaboration between otolaryngology, neurosurgery and audiology. Importance of the team work is explained. Main surgical approach is retrosigmoid approach. This is described in detail. Translabyrinthine and retrolabyrinthine approaches are also discussed and compared. Intraoperative monitoring is very important to determine the position of ABI electrode to provide maximum benefit. Finally, complications related to this approach are provided.

Keywords: auditory brainstem implantation, inner ear malformations, surgery, complete labyrinthine aplasia, cochlear aplasia, cochlear nerve aplasia, cochlear aperture aplasia, indications, cochlear nerve hypoplasia

8.1 Introduction

The first auditory brainstem implantation was performed in 1979 at House Ear Institute (HEI) in Los Angeles, by Drs. William House and William Hitselberger after removal of an acoustic neuroma.[1] In 2001, Colletti et al[2] reported their auditory brainstem implant (ABI) experience in two children with severe inner ear malformations and no apparent cochlear nerve (CN), for the first time in literature. Until that time, no appropriate habilitation was possible as cochlear implant (CI) surgery was contraindicated in these patients. Use of ABI for children opened a new era in the habilitation of patients, in whom CI surgery was contraindicated due to cochlear, labyrinthine, or CN aplasia. In their initial paper, they reported that both patients had achieved good environmental sound awareness and some speech detection. After a period of time, other centers also started to use ABI for rehabilitation of these children.

As Hacettepe team we started ABI surgery in children in 2006. Until now, we have performed 128 pediatric ABI surgeries. Hacettepe implant team organized the first consensus meeting in 2009 where indications were discussed and determined for pediatric ABI.[3] In 2013, long-term results of ABI in children were discussed in the second consensus meeting.[4]

8.2 Indications

ABI can be used in children with severe malformations and complete ossification of cochlea after meningitis. Inner ear malformations constitute the main group. ABI is not required in all cochleovestibular malformations. Patients with incomplete partition types II and III, and enlarged vestibular aqueduct almost always have cochlear and CN development to a certain extent and therefore, they can be (re)habilitated with CI. In a consensus paper, Sennaroglu et al divided the indications into two groups: definite and probable indications. Recently rudimentary otocyst was defined and added to definite indications.[3,5]

8.2.1 Definite Indications

- Complete labyrinthine aplasia (Michel aplasia): In this anomaly cochlea, vestibule, vestibular aqueduct, and cochlear aqueduct are absent.
- Rudimentary otocyst: Incomplete millimetric representation of otic capsule without an internal auditory canal.
- Cochlear aplasia: Cochlea is absent. The accompanying vestibular system may be normal or there may be an enlarged vestibule.
- CN aplasia: This is the absence of the CN.
- Cochlear aperture aplasia: This is the absence of the bony channel transmitting the CN from the internal auditory canal (IAC) to the cochlea.

8.2.2 Probable Indications

- Hypoplastic cochlea with hypoplastic cochlear aperture: Hypoplastic cochlea may have different audiological presentation. Some patients may be aided with hearing aids and they may have excellent speech and language development. If they are accompanied by hypoplastic cochlear aperture and narrow IAC on high-resolution computed tomography (HRCT), usually CN is hypoplastic or absent and they commonly have severe to profound hearing loss. In the latter group, the CN entering the cochlea may be hypoplastic and ABI may be indicated according to audiological findings.
- Common cavity and incomplete partition type I cases where CN is apparently missing: The nerve entering the common cavity is common cochleovestibular nerve (CVN). As cochlea and vestibule are separate in IP-I, the nerve entering the cochlea in IP-I is CN. If CVN and CN are present, they are candidates for cochlear implantation. If these nerves are absent, they are candidates of ABI.
- Common cavity and incomplete partition type I cases if the CN is present: Even if CVN and CN are present, the distribution of the neural tissue in common cavity or IP-I cochlea is unpredictable, and ABI may be indicated in such cases if CI fails to elicit an auditory sensation.
- The presence of an unbranched cochleovestibular nerve (CVN) is a challenge in these cases. In this situation, it is not possible to determine the amount of cochlear fibers travelling

in the CVN. If there is a suspicion, a CI can be used in the first instance, and ABI can be reserved for the patients in whom there is insufficient progress with CI.

- The hypoplastic CN presents a dilemma for the implant team. A hypoplastic nerve is defined as less than 50% of the usual size of the CN or less than the diameter of the facial nerve. Radiology of these patients should be carefully reviewed with an experienced neuroradiologist. If sufficient amount of neural tissue cannot be followed into the cochlear space, an ABI may be indicated.

Children with hypoplastic CN or thin unbranched CVN constitute the most controversial group in decision-making between CI and ABI. It must be kept in mind that children with hypoplastic nerves usually do not reach levels of those with normal cochlea, in terms of hearing and language development. It is obvious that radiology may not predict the presence of the CN accurately in these above-mentioned challenging five groups of patients. In all these subjects, audiological findings, as well as radiological findings, should be taken into consideration in order to decide between CI and ABI. If an experienced pediatric audiologist detects a slight response with insert of ear phones on either side of these cases, this information is very valuable in the side selection of CI. In such cases, family should be carefully counseled about the possibility of ABI surgery in future, if insufficient progress with CI is encountered during postoperative follow-up.

Some cases of pneumococcal meningitis produce total cochlear ossification where a CI cannot be placed satisfactorily into the scala timpani. Different surgical techniques (such as drill-out cochleostomy) have been described and electrode options (double or split array implants) are provided for total ossification. These usually result in suboptimal results. ABI is another option for patients with total ossification because the electrode can be placed in a normal location. In partial ossification however, every effort should be made to place the CI electrode in the scala tympani or vestibuli. If the electrode is not satisfactorily placed into either scala tympani or scala vestibuli, ABI may be another option.

8.3 CI versus ABI in Children with Hypoplastic Cochlear Nerve

Management of patients with hypoplastic CN is still controversial. Although it may rarely be possible to obtain good hearing and language development in certain cases with hypoplastic CN, majority of the patients have insufficient hearing, and limited language development with CI. These patients become candidates for ABI. It is important to correctly diagnose this subset of children and proceed with ABI directly when required; however, for the present time, preoperative and intraoperative audiological tests are not precise enough to enable correct diagnosis.

Bradley et al[6] reported their long-term experience in six children with hypoplastic CN. Preoperatively, they observed clear response to sound with hearing aids. Although initially all children demonstrated auditory thresholds within normal range, after using CI for 2 to 6 years, they demonstrated unsatisfactory outcome: five were at Categories of Auditory Perception (CAP) level 2 and one was at level 4. They concluded that even if they obtained thresholds similar to other CI users, the benefit of CI in children with hypoplastic CN is very limited.

Warren et al[7] reported three cases with narrow IACs bearing two nerves, one of them facial nerve and the other entering vestibule. Two of the families reported responses to auditory stimuli with amplification over time. They all underwent cochlear implantation. Early results after CI (4, 5, and 9 months, respectively) showed responses to auditory stimuli. They tried to explain the mechanism of sound transmission by a very tiny cochlear branch which could not be visualized due to extremely narrow distal IAC. It may also be possible that the nerve enters the vestibule and then turns toward cochlea. Regarding similar cases, our group observed that progress with CI usually reaches a plateau, and language development usually does not reach the level of CI use in normal cochlea. In general, hearing levels after CI may not be usually sufficient for appropriate language development.

Valero et al[8] recorded abnormal electrically evoked responses in the majority of CI recipients with hypoplastic CN. The atypical amplitude and latencies of these responses suggested nonauditory generators and should not be misread as typical evoked auditory brainstem response (EABR) peaks. There was no relationship between auditory pathway size and evoked brainstem response to determine whether they will be good CI candidates with these structural defects, and the unpredictable evoked responses observed here would make it difficult to predict auditory outcomes. Although there was limited initial improvement in speech perception outcomes, children with stenotic IAC and hypoplastic CN did not achieve comparable behavioral results with their CIs compared with children with an uncompromised CN. This poor outcome persisted in the long-term follow-up. Their scores at 120th month were comparable to 24th month scores of children with normal anatomy. They concluded that along with abnormal electrophysiological findings, children with hypoplasia of the CN are not good candidates for cochlear implantation. If the decision is made to proceed with cochlear implantation, families should be counseled that expectations of auditory and spoken language development should be tempered.

Buchman et al[9] reported CI results in patients with labyrinthine anomalies. They concluded that the peripheral neural populations in patients with CN deficiency are insufficient for the development of synchronized auditory stimulation in most instances. They proposed initial use of CI before ABI in these situations. One of the important findings of this study was that intracochlear eight nerve compound action potential (ECAP) testing results were associated with the development of speech perception abilities.

Song et al[10] reported their results of intracochlear EABR versus extracochlear EABR in predicting long-term outcomes of patients with narrow IAC. They concluded that intracochlear EABR measured either intraoperatively or in the early postoperative period may play an important role in deciding whether to continue with auditory rehabilitation with a CI or to switch to an ABI so as not to miss the optimal timing for language development. They concluded that for those cases in which cochlear implantation has been performed initially, considering the limited prognostic value of preoperative extracochlear electrophysiologic testing or imaging, intracochlear EABR measured either intraoperatively or in the early postoperative period may provide valuable prognostic information to predict long-term outcomes.

Song et al[11] concluded that residual response on pure tone audiometry and behavioral response to environmental sounds appeared to be more accurate markers for predicting the presence or absence of the CVN compared to imaging or electrophysiologic testing because all three patients who showed a response to sound stimuli demonstrated thin CVNs during surgery. Our team also reached to a similar conclusion, that is, behavioral audiological tests seemed to be more important in decision-making between CI and ABI. However, in our series, patients with hypoplastic CN demonstrated certain progress initially with CI, but could not carry on when more sophisticated learning processes were required.

Recently, Birman et al[12] reported better outcomes of auditory performance with CI in patients with aplastic/hypoplastic CN. Pediatric CI surgery in CN aplasia/hypoplasia is associated with variable outcomes. Overall, approximately 75% of children were able to use some verbal language. After CI, nearly 50% of those with CN aplasia and 90% of those with CN hypoplasia gained some speech understanding (CAP score 5–7). Their findings may be useful for preoperative counseling regarding the likelihood of CI outcomes in CN aplasia/hypoplasia. However, a comment that mentions "50% of cases with CN aplasia obtains CAP scores between 5–7" must be taken very cautiously.

Kutz et al[13] also reported their results after CI in children with hypoplastic CN. Seven children underwent CI in an ear without any CN on magnetic resonance imaging (MRI). One child developed early closed-set speech recognition. The other six children developed only speech detection or pattern perception. Two children with hypoplastic nerve were also implanted. One developed consistent closed-set word recognition and the other developed early closed-set word recognition. They concluded that CN deficiency is a common cause for profound sensorineural hearing loss and children with a deficient but visible CN on MRI can expect to show some speech understanding after cochlear implantation. However, these children do not develop speech understanding to the level of implanted children with normal CNs. Children with an absent CN determined by MRI can be expected to have limited sound and speech awareness after CI surgery.

Promontory stimulation or stimulation via round window is difficult to provide in cases with severe inner ear malformations (IEM). In Hacettepe University, we tested an Intracochlear Test Electrode (ITE) to simulate a CI to make the intraoperative decision between CI and ABI.[14] ITE has three intracochlear contact points of 18 mm length and one extracochlear ground electrode. Intracochlear part is inserted into the cochlea up to the ring as needed. It was used in 11 subjects with various inner ear malformations. In cases with normal anatomy or IP-II, excellent wave morphology was obtained. If there were no EABR, decision for an ABI was made. There were two cases with conflicting results. One was an IP-I with definite CN on MRI. The test result was negative but CI surgery was done and CI provided very good language development on long-term follow-up. The second conflicting result was from a child with common cavity. He had benefit from CI but he developed facial stimulation which was present on all contacts. During revision procedure, ITE was used but there was no response during surgery. In this particular patient with common cavity who had good progress with a CI, ITE failed to produce EABR. As a result, it appears that, if there is a positive response, ITE is reliable. A negative response, however, has to be considered very carefully and radiology and preoperative audiological test methods should be used together to make the decision between CI and ABI.

As can be seen, majority of the literature report unsuccessful outcome with CI in CN hypoplasia. As a result, it is still a problematic issue to decide between CI and ABI in patients with narrow IAC and hypoplastic CN. Intracochlear EABR might be a better indicator compared to preoperative electrophysiological tests.

8.4 Members of ABI Team

ABI surgery is a technically demanding operation. The team has to be experienced regarding the surgery, audiological follow-up, and rehabilitation of CI patients. An experienced pediatric neurosurgeon is key to achieve success and also to avoid possible complications as much as possible. He or she is responsible for accurate identification of the exact location of the foramen of Luschka. We have encountered many situations where the foramen was not apparent and careful dissection was necessary to identify its location. This is one of the most important factors to obtain successful outcome by preventing malposition of the electrode which may lead to unsuccessful results. An experienced neurosurgeon is the key to avoid this complication.

If the surgery leads to cranial nerve damage and/or brainstem injury which brings forth neurological sequela in otherwise healthy children, this would be a catastrophe both for the family and the team. Besides, this might create negative impact on public opinion regarding ABI surgery. It is very important to avoid any possible complications in these children by working with an appropriate team. Placing the implant in the brainstem involves the close collaboration of an experienced pediatric neurosurgeon, otologist, and audiologist. The otologist must be experienced in implant surgery. Intraoperative EABR test measurements allow placement of the electrode into the most appropriate location. This is not like CI surgery where intracochlear placement is very straightforward. Final position of the electrode plate is determined by intraoperative EABR measurements; experienced audiologist is very important for this part of the surgery.

8.5 The Age Limit for ABI in Children

According to the consensus statement, age limit for ABI in children is similar to CI patients.[15] Better language outcome is expected when the children are operated between 1 and 2 years of age. ABI surgery is more challenging than CI surgery because, young children have less blood volume and cerebrospinal fluid (CSF) in the posterior fossa. From the neurosurgical point of view, in the consensus paper, optimum lower limit was determined as 18 months but, depending on the experience of the center, it was also suggested that it may be done as early as on 12 months old. Our team operated on 12 children of around the age one without any complications. It is without any doubt that early intervention will have better audiological outcome. Although it can be argued that surgical risks will be less when the child is operated later on in their life, the language outcome will not be satisfactory because of the brain plasticity. This will lead to the discredit of the surgery as it will be thought that this intervention will not produce good hearing and language outcome. Therefore, ideal age appears to be between 1 and 2 years of age. As these are prelingually deafened children, this procedure should not be offered to patients older than 5 years old.

8.6 Preoperative Evaluation

All members of the team should evaluate ABI candidates in detail.

Radiological workup involves temporal CT and MRI. Diagnosis and indication for ABI are straightforward with CT in cases such as Michel deformity, rudimentary otocyst, and cochlear aplasia, which are definite indications for ABI.[3] Children with cochlear hypoplasia, hypoplastic cochlear aperture, and narrow IAC need more careful audiological and radiological evaluation with MRI. MRI, on the other hand, demonstrates the neural structures in the IAC. Any vascular abnormality around the lateral recess can be seen on MRI. The side with more developed inner ear or the cochleovestibular nerve should be preferred. As stated in the preceding paragraphs, MRI has limitations in the diagnosis.

Side selection is very important in ABI surgery. The team should try to choose the side which provides more information on the cochlear nucleus, hence, the side with more developed neural structures (e.g., facial nerve presenting unilaterally, or more prominent CVN or vestibular nerve may imply better developed cochlear nucleus area). If equal under all conditions, more developed inner ear should be chosen (if there is a cochlear aplasia on one side and a hypoplastic cochlea on the other side, the latter can be preferred). In addition, the side where the entrance of the lateral recess is more favorable, and the lateral recess is more accessible (where cerebellar retraction will be less) can be chosen.

8.6.1 Audiological Assessment Procedure

For preoperative evaluation of ABI candidates, all audiological test batteries should be conducted. This test battery includes both subjective and objective tests. It is apparent that in patients with complete labyrinthine aplasia and cochlear aplasia no response is expected. But even in these patients sometimes with maximum audiometric limits some response is observed in low frequencies which is in accordance with tactile sensation.

In subjective tests, the candidate should be evaluated with insert phones and if not possible, free field evaluation should be done. According to the age of the child, behavioral observation audiometry (BOA), visual reinforced audiometry, or play audiometry can be used.

For objective evaluation, it is appropriate to start with tympanometry and acoustic reflex tests to show middle ear status for all age groups, especially for infants and children. These tests should be followed by otoacoustic emissions (OAE), and auditory brainstem response (ABR) measurements.

Subjective tests are very important even when no response is obtained by other tests, including the objective ones. In this situation, subjective tests are the only method which give information about hearing status of the patient. Some patients with hypoplastic CN demonstrate behavioral response with pure tone or speech stimulation. These patients are counseled that the ear with best response with insert phone will be selected for CI, and the patient will be followed up for 6 to 9 months with CI. At the end of this period an EABR is also done to see if there is any response with CI. If there is no development in speech perception and no response on EABR, ABI will be offered to the family. It is also very important to take into consideration the observation of the family. In this situation we choose the opposite ear for ABI, thereby providing bilateral amplification to these children. In cases where there is a definite indication on one side, and a probable indication on the contralateral side, CI and ABI can be done simultaneously. Our team has performed six simultaneous CI and ABI surgeries until now.

8.7 Surgery

ABI surgery can be performed through translabyrinthine, retrosigmoid, or retrolabyrinthine approach.[16] In children main approach for ABI has been retrosigmoid approach. Temporal bone is much smaller in a child of 1 to 2 years of age when compared to an adult. As a result, translabyrinthine approach will provide much limited surgical exposure than retrosigmoid approach in a child. In addition, drilling of the temporal bone takes more time to expose the brainstem in comparison to retrosigmoid approach. Therefore, for the placement of ABI in a child, retrosigmoid approach is more advantageous. In addition, retrosigmoid approach makes it possible to bypass the mastoid air cells so that intracranial contamination by the middle ear flora can be prevented. This is another advantage when frequent otitis media in children are taken into account. The landmarks, advantages, and disadvantages of different approaches have been discussed in detail previously in another paper regarding ABI surgery in children.[16]

8.7.1 Retrosigmoid Approach

There are two different positions used for this approach, lateral oblique and semi-sitting positions. In children with severe inner ear malformations, lateral oblique position is preferred. In this position the patient's neck is slightly flexed and the ipsilateral shoulder of the patient is taped down and forward. In adults, Behr et al[17] prefer semi-sitting position. According to their experience, this allows the surgeon to remove blood and CSF from the surgical field easily; this aids in fixation of the array by fibrin glue in almost dry surroundings.

In Hacettepe University, retrosigmoid approach has been used in pediatric ABI cases, while the patient is in lateral oblique position. A straight vertical skin incision, about 7 to 8 cm in length, is performed behind the ear. Incision extends from 1 cm above asterion to a point inferior and posterior to the mastoid tip. A retrosigmoid craniotomy is performed. Superior and anterior limits are transverse and sigmoid sinuses, respectively. Bone removal is enlarged inferiorly toward the jugular foramen to decrease cerebellar retraction. In order to avoid bone dust

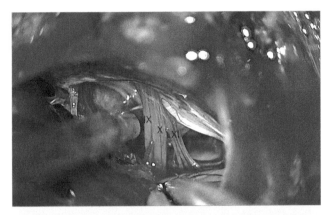

Fig. 8.1 Lower cranial nerves IX, X and XI.

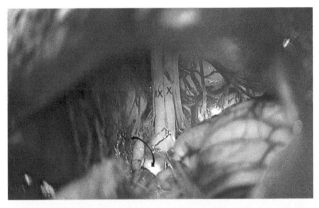

Fig. 8.2 Arrow pointing to the foramen of Luschka which is the open end of the lateral recess of the fourth ventricle.

from entering the intracranial space, implant bed is prepared before opening the dura. The implant bed is positioned vertically above the surgical field as far away from the incision as possible. One suture hole is drilled inferior to the implant bed to fix the device. Preparation of the implant bed is strongly advised by our team in all implant surgeries to lower the profile of the implant which decreases the likelihood of device failure in case of head trauma.[18] This is more important in pediatric ABI cases to avoid revision surgery which is more difficult in terms of removing the electrode from the brainstem when compared to standard CI surgery. If a Digisonic SP ABI is used, no implant bed is prepared but the implant is positioned away from the incision.

Then standard retrosigmoid approach is performed. Cerebellopontine cistern is opened to drain CSF. This will allow the surgeon to work easily without using any retractor. Anatomic structures in the cerebellopontine angle are identified. Lower cranial nerves are first exposed (▶ Fig. 8.1). In prelingually deafened children with malformations, vestibulocochlear nerve is usually hypoplastic or aplastic. Sometimes facial nerve is identified alone on the cranial part of the lower cranial nerves.

The next step is identification of the flocculus to reach the lateral recess. The choroid plexus protruding from the foramen of Luschka and the cochlear vein are landmarks for this step. The choroid plexus, which covers the foramen of Luschka, lies within a triangle formed by the VIIIth nerve, the IXth nerve, and the lip of the foramen of Luschka.[19] To approach the lateral recess, arachnoid over the foramen is cut, and the flocculus and choroid plexus are retracted either by suction or bipolar coagulator. The choroid plexus projecting from the lateral recess and overlying the cochlear nucleus complex is followed and the entrance to the lateral recess is found (▶ Fig. 8.2). The dorsal cochlear nucleus, which is the most accessible portion of the cochlear nucleus complex for electrical stimulation, is identified since it bulges in the floor of the lateral recess.[19]

In certain situations, lower cranial nerves cannot be identified. In three children operated in Hacettepe University, severe fibrosis made the identification of the nerves impossible. In order to avoid damage to the cranial nerves, individual nerves were not dissected. Instead, in these cases choroid plexus was identified close to the root entry zone of the IXth nerve and used as a landmark for the foramen of Luschka.

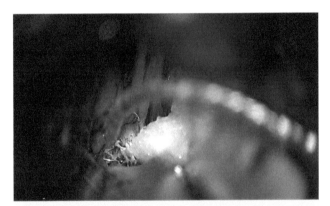

Fig. 8.3 Auditory brainstem implant electrode in place.

To determine the foramen of Luschka accurately, CSF pressure is raised by anesthesiologist to force CSF outflow from the lateral recess. The width of the recess is controlled with a blunt hook or dissector. Sometimes underlying veins and sometimes small arteries necessitate delicate dissection to open the entrance of the foramen of Luschka. In patients with a history of meningitis, fibrosis of the arachnoid which covers the entrance of the foramen of Luschka may complicate this part of the surgery. After opening and controlling of the recess, the receiver-stimulator is placed into the implant bed and fixed. The electrode is inserted gently into the recess (▶ Fig. 8.3). Care should be taken to avoid injury to numerous vessels around this area feeding the brainstem. If a small branch is bleeding it has to be controlled with Surgicel application or fine tipped bipolar cautery before undertaking insertion of the electrode paddle. It is very important to place the contact surfaces facing the cochlear nuclei. In our institution, the mesh around the electrode paddle is reduced in size as the recess is not as large as in adults. The final position of the electrode is verified with the help of EABR responses. According to test results, electrode paddle can be advanced vertically slightly in or out of the recess. It may also be moved slightly to the front and backwards. Usually, it is sufficient to see the outer rim of the electrode paddle. If we do not see the outer rim of the paddle it usually indicates too much insertion. To stabilize the electrode, two or three muscle tissues are placed into the recess behind the electrode pushing the electrode anteriorly to create better contact with the cochlear nuclei. Then the dura is closed tightly.

8.7.2 Translabyrinthine Approach

Translabyrinthine approach has been utilized for ABI in a child by Helge Rask Andersen and his team (not published, personal communication) and the electrode was successfully placed into the recess.

8.7.3 Retrolabyrinthine Approach

Bento et al[20] described the extended retrolabyrinthine approach (RLA) for ABI placement which was performed consecutively in three children without any further complications. They stressed the importance of radiological examination both in evaluation of the etiology and to choose the side to be operated on for RLA based on the size of the jugular bulb. They advised that the side with less prominent jugular bulb should be chosen. They stated that the approach is more familiar to the otologist. After a postauricular incision and mastoidectomy, they identified jugular bulb as the main landmark for access to the dura. It was exposed by removing bone from its entire circumference. Only the intracranial portions of the VIIth and VIIIth cranial nerves were exposed. Then cerebellar flocculus and lower cranial nerves were identified. After retracting the choroid plexus, they identified the foramen of Luschka and placed the ABI electrode. RLA was chosen due to their extensive experience in using this technique for vestibular schwannoma surgery in patients with useful hearing. RLA allowed direct visualization of the foramen of Luschka through a limited approach. There was no requirement for cerebellar retraction or even for opening the internal auditory meatus and semicircular canals. The disadvantage of this approach in children is that it cannot be used in a very young child with an extremely large jugular bulb. We used this approach in two cases with vascular anomalies which were preventing the retrosigmoid approach.

Although, all three approaches can be used in ABI surgery of children, retrosigmoid approach is still the most widely used technique when compared to the other two methods. With any preferred method, it should be noted that distorted anatomy at the cerebellopontine angle, at the cranial nerve entry zones, and brainstem due to absence of the cochleovestibular nerve makes surgery more difficult in certain cases.[1]

8.8 Intraoperative Monitoring

After placement of the electrode, electrical ABR is utilized to identify the localization of the cochlear nucleus. Different electrodes and electrode groups are stimulated one by one to check the position of the ABI electrode in relation to the cochlear nucleus. This will help to position the electrode array to maximize auditory stimulation while nonauditory stimulation is minimized. In children, the recess is not very large; therefore, after placement, usually only slight lateral movements are possible. If the electrode is too deeply inserted, there will be response only on the lateral channels. This necessitates minimal pulling out of the electrode. Similarly, if the response can only be obtained from the channels localized at the tip of the plate

electrode, it should be inserted slightly deeper into the recess. In adults, we encountered a few cases where the width of the lateral recess was twice the size of electrode. In these cases, the electrical ABR is very useful in confirming placement of the array. Slight adjustments in the position of the array should be made according to electrical auditory responses. The surgeon and the audiologist should be familiar with the numbers of individual active channels on the electrode array. A diagram showing the channels for both left and right sides should be kept in the operating room to avoid confusion about electrode orientation. Position of an individual active channel of an already inserted electrode on the left side is completely opposite on the right side.

In patients undergoing ABI surgery, an intraoperative EABR demonstrating III. and V. waves is a valuable finding. This shows that the electrode is in the correct location. Sometimes there may be no response or myogenic activity. Myogenic activity shows a possible future side effect. In this situation the position of the electrode array is adjusted according to the findings.

8.9 Initial Stimulation and Follow-Up

The first programming of the ABI electrode is done 3 to 4 weeks after the surgery. For the first four patients, we waited for 3 months after the surgery. But now the device is stimulated 3 to 4 weeks after the surgery. General anesthesia is not required; monitoring the child is sufficient.

Most comfortable levels (MCLs) are found by increasing the current level step by step. During this time, behavioral responses and side effects are observed. After MCLs are determined, all MCLs are decreased by 5 or 10 current unit (CU), and speech processor is activated. This decrement is done because the integrated level of all channels can be annoyingly loud for the first stimulation.

Initially, the channels in the center of the electrode are activated. If there are no side effects, then it is possible to proceed to neighboring ones. Usually 6 to 7 channels are activated in the first visit. The rest of the channels are activated during the second visit, which occurs usually 1 month after initial programming. If there is a side effect, the current level is lowered until hearing sensation without any side effects is achieved. If this is not possible, the channel leading to the side effect is closed. A few months later, the channel(s) causing side effects are activated once again. It has been observed that on many occasions, the channels initially causing side effects start to produce only auditory stimulation without any adverse reaction. The ones prompting side effects can be kept closed permanently.

Fitting infants and young children is a complex work due to the fact that no adult-like clear responses can be obtained from them. But in most of the cases they perform some behaviors with sound stimulation. These may be cessation of activity, looking at the mother, holding, or showing the implant side or crying. These programming sessions must be done by experienced pediatric audiologists. Side effects must be observed and monitored particularly during the first stimulation. These can vary from single cough to stimulation of vagus nerve which organizes heartbeat. So it is essential to perform this section in the presence of a medical doctor in case of cardiac arrythmia.

The initial program gives very important information for follow-up. These are all noted for future programming.

In Hacettepe University, we have done EABR before initial stimulation for the first patients. It has been observed that this does not add more information than the intraoperative EABR measurements. Today EABR is not performed anymore. We use intraoperative findings for the first programming session.

8.10 Audiological Outcome

Please refer to Chapter 14 for long-term results of pediatric ABI from our group.

8.11 Surgical Complications

Colletti et al[21] reported the complications of ABI surgery in their series composed of adults and children. They had no mortality. One child had a slow recovery after surgery; a CT scan revealed an intracerebellar clot. Revision surgery was performed, and clot was evacuated. He had a full neurologic recovery. Another child developed meningitis. This resolved uneventfully with medical treatment. As a minor complication they observed temporary asymptomatic cerebellar edema in the postoperative CT scans in nine children. They were all treated successfully with steroids and diuretics. Four children developed postoperative wound seroma which was successfully treated with aspiration and pressure dressing. Apart from these, infection of the incision, temporary dysphonia, and balance disorders occurred in some patients but resolved after treatment. The authors concluded that the surgery has less complications when compared to ABI operation of NF2 patients, and overall complication rate of ABI is not much greater than that of CI and is comparable to neurovascular decompression.

Bayazit et al[22] reported two cases of postoperative CSF leakage following ABI surgery in five children. Attention was drawn to possible long-term complications such as device failure, infection, biofilm formation, or extrusion, about which knowledge is still limited.

In our series of children, one of the initial three patients had postoperative rhinorrhea. He was revised immediately and the defect in the mastoid was repaired. Four patients had transient facial nerve palsy. This is most probably due to cerebellar retraction. Three resolved completely within 2 weeks. One had House-Brackmann grade II recovery. In one patient, severe cerebellar edema occurred intraoperatively which impeded rest of the surgery. Therefore, operation was stopped and completed in the second session uneventfully 3 weeks later. Seroma occurred in five patients due to CSF leakage. In four patients, it was easily controlled in a few days, with lumbar drainage and serial pressure dressings. However, in one patient, CSF leak continued despite these measures and prolonged the hospitalization period markedly. None of our patients had to be revised due to seroma; above-mentioned conservative treatment was successful enough to manage this complication. In these patients, CSF leakage was thought to occur around the electrode lead from subarachnoid space to subcutaneous tissue. It is important to place pieces of soft tissue around the electrode at the level of dura in order to attain effective sealing, and lumbar drainage is used now routinely to avoid CSF leakage. Both of these measures were successful and this complication was not experienced in the rest of the group.

The most serious complication in our series is a case of CSF flow disorder. This produced intermittent confusion leading to coma. Eventually, a peritoneal shunt was placed to stabilize CSF pressure and this made her situation more stable.

Overall results showed that this procedure can be performed with minimum surgical risks in centers with experienced otology, neurosurgery, and anesthesia facilities.

8.12 Conclusion

ABI in children provides auditory sensation when properly placed into lateral recess. Side effects due to the stimulation of the neighboring cranial nerves are common which can be overcome by decreasing current level or closing the channel permanently. Every effort should be made to decrease the intracranial complications by working in collaboration with experienced otologist, pediatric neurosurgeon, and anesthesiologist. Intraoperative EABR done by an experienced audiologist is very important to find the best location to stimulate cochlear nuclei. Satisfactory audiological outcome with language development is possible but handicaps impede success of outcomes. Probable indications still continue to be a challenge for the implant team.

References

[1] Toh EH, Luxford WM. Cochlear and brainstem implantation. 2002. Neurosurg Clin N Am. 2008; 19(2):317–329, vii

[2] Colletti V, Fiorino F, Sacchetto L, Miorelli V, Carner M. Hearing habilitation with auditory brainstem implantation in two children with cochlear nerve aplasia. Int J Pediatr Otorhinolaryngol. 2001; 60(2):99–111

[3] Sennaroglu L, Colletti V, Manrique M, et al. Auditory brainstem implantation in children and non-neurofibromatosis type 2 patients: a consensus statement. Otol Neurotol. 2011; 32(2):187–191

[4] Sennaroğlu L, Colletti V, Lenarz T, et al. Consensus statement: long-term results of ABI in children with complex inner ear malformations and decision making between CI and ABI. Cochlear Implants Int. 2016; 17(4):163–171

[5] Sennaroğlu L, Bajin MD. Classification and current management of inner ear malformations. Balkan Med J. 2017; 34(5):397–411

[6] Bradley J, Beale T, Graham J, Bell M. Variable long-term outcomes from cochlear implantation in children with hypoplastic auditory nerves. Cochlear Implants Int. 2008; 9(1):34–60

[7] Warren FM, III, Wiggins RH, III, Pitt C, Harnsberger HR, Shelton C. Apparent cochlear nerve aplasia: to implant or not to implant? Otol Neurotol. 2010; 31 (7):1088–1094

[8] Valero J, Blaser S, Papsin BC, James AL, Gordon KA. Electrophysiologic and behavioral outcomes of cochlear implantation in children with auditory nerve hypoplasia. Ear Hear. 2012; 33(1):3–18

[9] Buchman CA, Teagle HF, Roush PA, et al. Cochlear implantation in children with labyrinthine anomalies and cochlear nerve deficiency: implications for auditory brainstem implantation. Laryngoscope. 2011; 121(9):1979–1988

[10] Song MH, Bae MR, Kim HN, Lee WS, Yang WS, Choi JY. Value of intracochlear electrically evoked auditory brainstem response after cochlear implantation in patients with narrow internal auditory canal. Laryngoscope. 2010; 120(8): 1625–1631

[11] Song MH, Kim SC, Kim J, Chang JW, Lee WS, Choi JY. The cochleovestibular nerve identified during auditory brainstem implantation in patients with narrow internal auditory canals: can preoperative evaluation predict cochleovestibular nerve deficiency? Laryngoscope. 2011; 121(8):1773–1779

[12] Birman CS, Powell HR, Gibson WP, Elliott EJ. Cochlear implant outcomes in cochlea nerve aplasia and hypoplasia. Otol Neurotol. 2016; 37(5):438–445

[13] Kutz JW, Jr, Lee KH, Isaacson B, Booth TN, Sweeney MH, Roland PS. Cochlear implantation in children with cochlear nerve absence or deficiency. Otol Neurotol. 2011; 32(6):956–961

[14] Cinar BC, Yarali M, Atay G, Bajin MD, Sennaroglu G, Sennaroglu L. The role of eABR with intracochlear test electrode in decision making between cochlear and brainstem implants: preliminary results. Eur Arch Otorhinolaryngol. 2017; 274(9):3315–3326

[15] Sennaroglu L, Colletti V, Manrique M, et al. Auditory brainstem implantation in children and non-neurofibromatosis type 2 patients: a consensus statement. Otol Neurotol. 2011; 32(2):187–191

[16] Sennaroglu L, Ziyal I. Auditory brainstem implantation. Auris Nasus Larynx. 2012; 39(5):439–450

[17] Behr R, Müller J, Shehata-Dieler W, et al. The high rate CIS auditory brainstem implant for restoration of hearing in NF-2 patients. Skull Base. 2007; 17(2): 91–107

[18] Pamuk AE, Pamuk G, Jafarov S, Bajin MD, Saraç S, Sennaroğlu L. The effect of cochlear implant bed preparation and fixation technique on the revision cochlear implantation rate. J Laryngol Otol. 2018; 132(6): 534–539

[19] Colletti V, Carner M, Miorelli V, Guida M, Colletti L, Fiorino F. Auditory brainstem implant (ABI): new frontiers in adults and children. Otolaryngol Head Neck Surg. 2005; 133(1):126–138

[20] Bento RF, Monteiro TA, Tsuji RK, et al. Retrolabyrinthine approach for surgical placement of auditory brainstem implants in children. Acta Otolaryngol. 2012; 132(5):462–466

[21] Colletti V, Shannon RV, Carner M, Veronese S, Colletti L. Complications in auditory brainstem implant surgery in adults and children. Otol Neurotol. 2010; 31(4):558–564

[22] Bayazit YA, Abaday A, Dogulu F, Göksu N. Complications of pediatric auditory brain stem implantation via retrosigmoid approach. ORL J Otorhinolaryngol Relat Spec. 2011; 73(2):72–75

9 Pediatric Auditory Brainstem Implantation: Colletti Team Experience and Special Considerations

Vittorio Colletti, Marco Mandalà, Giacomo Colletti, and Liliana Colletti

Abstract

This chapter reviews our center's experience with auditory brainstem implantation in children over a 14 year period. The performance in children as a function of age at implantation as well as years after implantation, with or without other disabilities, is reviewed. Surgical implantation and postoperative programming of this patient cohort has allowed for development of useful principles and techniques, such as near-field compound action potential recording, the identification of the nervus intermedius as a critical landmark for the Foramen of Luschka, and experience with bilateral and revision surgery.

Keywords: cochlear implant, pediatrics, cochlear nerve deficiency, syndromes, nervus intermedius, revision, bilateral, complications, cranioplasty

9.1 Introduction

The surgical rehabilitation options for children with prelingual deafness include both the cochlear implant (CI) and the auditory brainstem implant (ABI). Continued studies are needed to assess the long-term benefit in auditory perception for prelingually deaf children fitted with these devices.[1,2,3,4,5,6,7,8,9,10,11,12,13,14]

Indeed, the population of children with no functional auditory nerve and who are not candidates for CIs constitutes a challenge. Their central auditory cortices may have never received input from the auditory periphery, and the remaining peripheral auditory system may be insufficient to support sound input from a prosthesis. Studies have shown encouraging results from children receiving an ABI.[15,16,17,18,19] This chapter discusses the outcomes obtained in a 74-child study group followed up to 15 years following ABI insertion. Additionally, we discuss our experience with bilateral ABI implantation in children, as well as cranioplasty techniques with resorbable mesh that may reduce the risk of cerebrospinal fluid (CSF) leak. We have learned through detailed review of our surgical video library that the nervus intermedius provides an important landmark leading to the foramen of Luschka (FL) and may assist in ABI placement. The use of near-field potentials in addition to traditional far-field evoked potentials has given us additional insight into improved positioning of the electrode paddles, and we have also gained some experience with revision ABI surgery in the case of device failure.

9.2 Total Experience and Selected Patient Study Group

From 2000 to 2014, 103 children (14 children with prior hearing and 89 children with congenital deafness), ranging in age from 8 months to 16 years, were implanted with ABIs via retrosigmoid approach, either Cochlear or MED-EL, at our institution or at other centers following our personal protocol. A thorough medical evaluation was performed before the decision for implantation, and patients were evaluated with computed tomography (CT) scan and magnetic resonance imaging (MRI).[20] All parents were informed of the risks and potential benefits of the ABI and provided informed consent as approved by the local hospital human subjects review board. Intraoperative and postoperative electrically evoked auditory brainstem responses (EABRs) were performed in all children.[21]

From the 103-patient surgical group, a 74-child study group implanted at our center for which full records were available included 57 cochlear nerve deficiency, 1 auditory neuropathy, 10 cochlear malformations, 3 bilateral cochlear post-meningitic ossification, and 2 neurofibromatosis type 2 and 1 bilateral cochlear fractures due to head injury. Among these children, 22 had been previously fitted elsewhere with CIs. The follow-up period ranged from 6 months to 15 years. Five children had less than 1 year of follow-up, 69 reached the 1-year postimplantation stage, 56 reached the 5-year follow-up stage, and 23 reached the 10-year follow-up mark, with 2 reaching 15 years of follow-up.

The assessment of auditory perception was performed in all children with the Categories of Auditory Perception (CAP) test,[22,23] an eight-point hierarchical scale of auditory performance.

9.3 Results

Seventy-four patients who underwent ABI at our institution were included in the study. The mean age was 3.8 ± 2.9 years. There were 40 males and 34 females. Clinical and demographical data of the study population are reported in ▶ Table 9.1. There were 38 patients with associated disabilities: 2 attention deficit hyperactivity disorders, 4 autistic spectrum disorders, 7 mild-moderate cognitive delays, 6 mild cognitive delays associated with motor deficits, 1 mild cognitive delay associated with visual impairment, 1 mild motor deficit, 2 oppositional defiant disorder, 2 specific language impairment, and 13 different syndromes (Crouzon, DiGeorge, Down, Goldenhar, Kabuki, lacrimo-auriculo-dento-digital [LADD], Moebius, Shprintzen, velocardiofacial). There were no intraoperative or perioperative permanent complications. One patient undergoing bilateral simultaneous ABI experienced pseudomeningocele formation, which was treated using revision surgery with fat grafting and resorbable cranioplasty plates, and is discussed later in this chapter.

The auditory performance is shown in ▶ Table 9.1, with CAP scores for the 74 children before implantation and at the last follow-up. All children showed improvement in auditory perception with implant experience. There was considerable variability in outcomes, and further analysis was undertaken to determine the causes. ABI outcome was analyzed as a function of the top score obtained, the age at implantation, the presence or absence of nonauditory disabilities, and etiology.

Table 9.1 Demographical and clinical data of 74 ABI children

		Statistical analysis (Mann Whitney test)
Number of subjects	74	/
Mean age at implantation (years)	3.81 ± 2.89	/
Sex (male/female)	40/34	/
Follow-up (years)	7.40 ± 3.90	/
Etiologies	• Cochlear nerve deficiency (57) • Auditory neuropathy (1) • Cochlear malformations (10) • Bilateral cochlear post- • meningitic ossification (3) • Neurofibromatosis type 2 (2) • Bilateral cochlear fractures (1)	/
Associated disabilities	38/74	/
CAP before implantation	0.15 ± 0.43 (median: 0)	p < 0.0001
CAP at last follow-up	3.64 ± 2.10 (median: 3)	

Abbreviations: ABI, auditory brainstem implant; CAP, Categories of Auditory Perception.

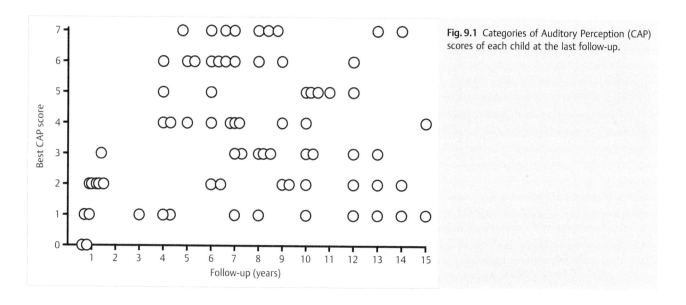

Fig. 9.1 Categories of Auditory Perception (CAP) scores of each child at the last follow-up.

▶ Fig. 9.1 shows the CAP scores of each child at the last follow-up. Among the nine children (12.1%) who ultimately were able to converse on the telephone (CAP level 7) the three postlingual children achieved this level by 3 years after ABI insertion, while the children with congenital deafness (CND without associated disabilities) achieved the same results later (at 6 years of follow-up). The 40% of the 10 children (13.5%) who achieved a CAP level of 6 achieved this level 3 years after ABI surgery. The 7 children (9.45%) who achieved the lowest open-set speech recognition CAP score of 5 took globally longer to achieve this level of performance—between 5 and 6 years. The 10 children (13.5%) who achieved closed-set discrimination of words (CAP level 4) took 4 to 6 years to achieve this score. A total of 26 children (35.1%) achieved some level of open-set speech recognition with the ABI (CAP levels 5, 6, and 7) and

almost half of the children (36/74 = 48.6%) achieved CAP scores of 4 or better.

Age at implantation is well known to be a critical factor in the success of CIs.[1,2,3,4,14]

▶ Fig. 9.2 shows the CAP score achieved as a function of the age at ABI surgery. Unsurprisingly, there is a trend for better performance in children implanted at a younger age (Kendall's $\tau = -0.23$, $p < 0.01$). This is particularly clear in children with no other disorders; many of these children implanted before 3 years of age were able to achieve a CAP score of 7 ($p = 0.0088$; ▶ Fig. 9.3).

Results in children with other congenital abnormalities ($n = 38$) and those without other complications ($n = 29$) were compared and the results are shown in ▶ Fig. 9.4. Children with no other disorders showed significantly higher CAP scores at the last

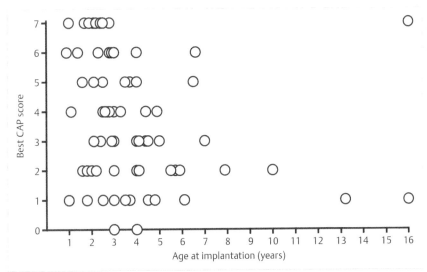

Fig. 9.2 Categories of Auditory Perception (CAP) score achieved as a function of the age at auditory brainstem implant (ABI) surgery.

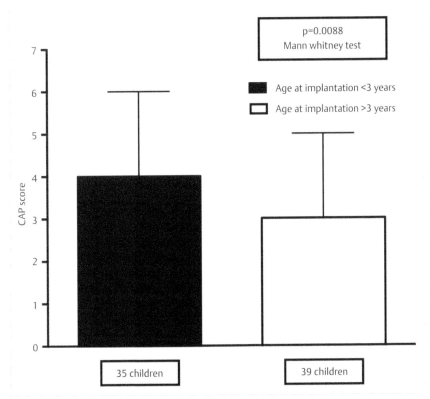

Fig. 9.3 Categories of Auditory Perception (CAP) scores (median and interquartile range) at the last follow-up for children implanted before or after 3 years.

follow-up ($p < 0.001$). Three years after ABI there was a three-category difference in the median CAP score between the two groups. The presence of additional disabilities was a significant predictor of the time to achieve CAP level 5 ($p < 0.0001$), regardless of whether the main deficit was of cochlear origin or nerve origin.

It is worth stressing that although children with other disabilities achieved low scores on the CAP, they still showed improved awareness of their environment and cognitive development.[7,8] In addition, while the median CAP score was only 2.5 for those children with additional disabilities, a few children in this category did obtain CAP scores of 4 or 5.

The effect of etiology of deafness was also reviewed. The 74 children were divided into five etiology groups: postlingual deafness due to trauma or severe ossification ($n = 4$), congenital deafness due to cochlear nerve aplasia ($n = 25$), cochlear malformations ($n = 10$), cochlear nerve aplasia with other nonauditory disabilities ($n = 32$), and NF2 and auditory neuropathy ($n = 3$). Children in the last category were considerably older at the time of ABI surgery (mean age 12.4 years) than children in other categories.

▶ Fig. 9.5 shows the CAP score for each etiology group as a function of years of ABI use. While there appear to be clear differences in the median CAP scores between etiology groups, the top and bottom curves have too few subjects to achieve statistical significance, and the middle three curves did not achieve significant differences due to the high variability in

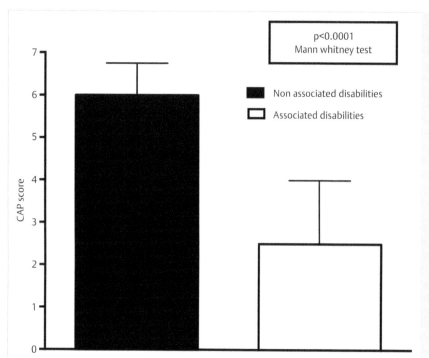

Fig. 9.4 Categories of Auditory Perception (CAP) score (median and interquartile range) of children with and without associated disabilities.

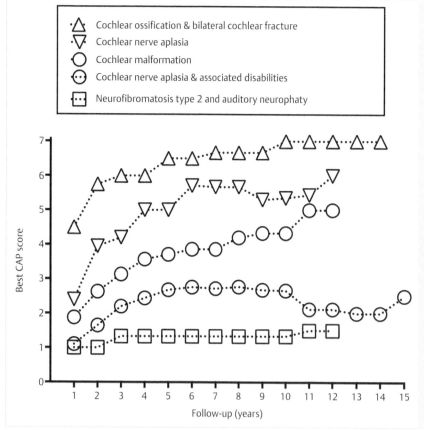

Fig. 9.5 Categories of Auditory Perception (CAP) score for each etiology group as a function of years of auditory brainstem implant (ABI) use.

performance within each etiology group. The four children who had prior hearing (three cochlear ossification, one trauma) clearly had the best outcomes, increasing in performance rapidly over the first 3 years and ultimately reaching the highest CAP level.

9.4 Discussion

In this study group, within 1 year of activation 83.8% of the children had obtained awareness of environmental sounds and 50% responded to speech sounds. Within 2 years of activation, 51.4%

of children were able to identify environmental sounds and discriminate speech sounds (CAP levels 3 and 4). Of the 64 children with 3-year follow-up data, 28.1% were able to understand common phrases without the aid of lipreading and 12.5% of the children could use the telephone with a known speaker.

This study confirms previous findings that the ABI is an appropriate device for auditory rehabilitation in children with cochlear and cochlear nerve malfunctions that cannot benefit from CIs. A comparison of the ABI outcomes obtained from this series of children versus a large group of children fitted with CIs clearly shows better performance outcomes obtained in a shorter time period in the CI group.[24] However, when CI results are compared with ABI children who have heard before, then performance is comparable and the developmental trajectory is comparable. In addition, when ABI performance is compared with congenitally deaf children who received a CI at the same age, then performance levels and trajectory over time are similar.[25] This group of ABI children had previous hearing but lost their auditory nerve from head trauma or severe ossification following meningitis. This result suggests that the ABI could be considered as salvage option for patients with progressive ossification.

Considering the cohort of children with cochlear nerve aplasia or hypoplasia who had a CI first, none showed satisfactory auditory development with a CI. In this cohort of children, the time spent trying out the CI was not only time (and expense) wasted, but also it may have prolonged the period of auditory deprivation. It is today well known that in the absence of auditory stimulation, neural structures show a failure to mature and can degenerate,[26,27] and, in addition, auditory cortical areas can be reallocated to other modalities.[28,29]

In light of this, when should a trial with a CI be skipped and move directly to an ABI? And second, under what conditions can one be confident that a CI will not provide useful hearing? Recent outcomes in children with CI have clear indicated etiologies where CI results can be poor.[6,12] In cases where no auditory nerve is visible on high-resolution MRI of the internal auditory meatus and when the EABR evoked by the CI is distorted or absent, auditory results were very poor. In such cases, an ABI may provide better performance than a CI. We recommend high-resolution CT imaging of the internal auditory meatus[20,30] and EABRs, stimulated either through an existing CI or from a wick electrode on the round window.

Today, there is compelling evidence that outcomes are better when CIs are provided as young as possible[1,2,3,4,14] and that it is of critical importance to have auditory input during the period of greatest neural plasticity in order to develop speech perception. Children who receive CIs below the age of 1 have clearly better and more rapid auditory development than children who receive CIs between 1 and 2 years of age.[31] If a CI is tried initially, clinicians must remain vigilant for the early signs of CI efficacy. If no progress is being made on simple auditory tasks, it may be necessary to move to an ABI as soon as possible to make the best use of that early neural plasticity. It is necessary to explant the CI, re-evaluate the child with neuroimaging studies and perform ABI surgery as soon as possible after the lack of progress with a CI has become evident. Children previously fitted with CIs and subsequently with ABIs may demonstrate a slower development of auditory perception, possibly because of the major difference in the neural pattern of activation from the two devices and possibly because the time window of plasticity has partially closed.

A topic of further concern is why some children fitted with the ABI can detect and discriminate environmental sounds but do not develop speech perception and language. Several of the following conditions may be responsible for the poor or low progression in speech perception abilities: incorrect positioning of the ABI array, incomplete development of the cochlear nuclei and auditory areas undetected by MRI, programming difficulties, or other negative psychological and cognitive factors. Most of the children with associated psychological and cognitive deficits could perceive the sounds and discriminate some speech patterns only a few months after ABI fitting. However, their overall auditory perceptual development has been very slow, and they continue to have trouble translating the electrical stimulation into speech and language development. Even if children are not able to achieve open-set speech recognition with the ABI, they may receive cognitive benefits. Access to auditory information from the ABI has been demonstrated[7,8] to influence the development of specific cognitive functions. Scores on two tests evaluating cognitive function (form completion and repeated patterns) increased significantly during the first 12 months of ABI use. These data demonstrated that the auditory stimulation of the ABI in preverbal children may facilitate the development of cognitive parameters related to selective visual-spatial attention and fluid (multisensory) reasoning.

The prevalence of surgical complications observed in the present group of 74 children fitted with ABI is comparable with what can be observed in children fitted with CI.[32] Clearly, the potential for complications is greater for an ABI than for a CI.

9.5 Special Situations

9.5.1 Nervus Intermedius as a Landmark

As a center implanting a high volume of children with ABI, we have accumulated an extensive experience with anatomic variations in the cerebellopontine angle (CPA). The identification of the FL can be challenging, due to absence of cranial nerves or even closure of the FL itself. Traditionally, the IXth cranial nerve and the choroid plexus have been used as guides to assist in the identification of the FL. However, after a thorough review of our surgical video documentation, we have completed a study with the nervus intermedius (NI) as a landmark that is interesting in itself due to its presence despite both periodic absence of cranial nerves VII and VIII (see ▶ Fig. 9.6).[33] In our surgical video database of 64 children, we found NI to be present in all subjects, even when cranial nerve VII took an aberrant course.

Indeed, the NI along with the lower cranial nerves appears to be one of the most consistent landmarks in the CPA, although it can have several bundles composing it.

9.5.2 Use of Near-field Compound Action Potentials

ABI electrode placement during surgery has traditionally been performed with far-field EABR measurements performed simultaneously with electromyography (EMG) measurements of the cranial nerve VII and the lower cranial nerves IX, X, and XI. This has been done in order to assess for the myogenic and other nonauditory side effects the ABI electrode may elicit. In our center, we

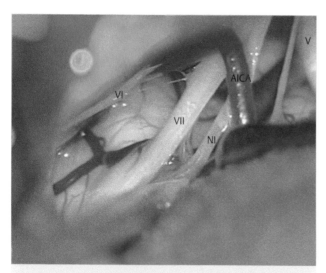

Fig. 9.6 Despite the absence of the VIII cranial nerve in the CPA in pediatric ABI surgery, the NI (nervus intermedius) is typically present and is often an additional landmark, along with the lower cranial nerves, to assist in the location of the Foramen of Luschka. V- Trigeminal nerve; VI- Abducens Nerve; VII- Facial nerve; NI- Nervus Intermedius; AICA- Anterior Inferior Cerebellar Artery.

have routinely performed near-field evoked compound nerve action potential (ECAP) measurements from the cochlear nucleus.[21]

ECAPs showed lower response thresholds and lower threshold of effects on adjacent cranial nerves. The ECAP electrical artifacts and saturation appeared similar to EABR responses, but ECAP provided a better signal-to-noise ratio.[21] ECAP serves as an additional tool in the precise placement of ABI electrodes.

9.5.3 Bilateral ABI

Among the 103 children implanted with ABIs by our team since 2000, 6 were bilateral: 4 were sequential and 2 were simultaneous. Our initial experience has been promising, and warrants further study. Bilateral simultaneous ABI surgery likely increases the risk of CSF leak in patients. Surgeons should be extremely cautious regarding recommending bilateral simultaneous ABI surgery and should consider sequential implantation (which has been well documented in the adult ABI population as well).[34]

9.5.4 Resorbable Mesh Cranioplasty and Fat Grafting

In patients undergoing bilateral simultaneous ABI, there is a danger of development of a subgaleal CSF collection (pseudomeningocele). Since the CSF pressure rises within the first 24 to 48 hours after CPA surgery and then declines, the first 24 to 48 hours after surgery is the critical time to prevent development of this fluid collection.[35] In one case of bilateral simultaneous ABI, a patient of ours experienced large pseudomeningoceles. In this patient, a lumbar drain was contraindicated due to Chiari malformation. Because of this, the patient required revision surgery with a technique that has become reliable for the treatment of recurrent CSF fistula after ABI surgery. The surgical sites were revised and the receiver-stimulators were placed back into the

proper position. New fat grafts were placed and resorbable cranioplasty plates of poly-L-D-lactic acid (PLDL) were placed over the fat grafts and flaps as well as the receiver-stimulators. This resulted in a resolution of the pseudomeningoceles, and it should be considered as a closure technique when the CSF pressure is suspected to be high or there is evidence of CSF leak.[34]

9.5.5 Revision ABI Surgery

In pediatric patients with ABI, malfunction of the receiver-stimulator or dislocation of the ABI array from the lateral recess occur rarely. We have treated a total of five children (three males, two females) implanted with the Cochlear ABI system via the retrosigmoid approach who underwent revision surgery with ABI explantation and simultaneous MED-EL device implantation. The length of use before revision surgery ranged from 5 to 12 years. Of the five children, one suffered from NF2 and tumor growth that required simultaneous tumor debulking, two had the electrode shifted from the lateral recess to the exit of the FL and two had device dysfunction. In all the children, intraoperative monitoring was performed and EABRs recorded.

All the patients showed fair to good restoration of hearing. The main issues seen at surgery were scarring making ABI paddle dissection difficult and new osteoneogenesis of the temporal bone encircling the cable, but no complications were experienced due to revision surgery. Despite its difficulty, it may be performed safely by experienced surgeons.

References

[1] Manrique M, Cervera-Paz FJ, Huarte A, Molina M. Advantages of cochlear implantation in prelingual deaf children before 2 years of age when compared with later implantation. Laryngoscope. 2004; 114(8):1462–1469
[2] Svirsky MA, Teoh S-W, Neuburger H. Development of language and speech perception in congenitally, profoundly deaf children as a function of age at cochlear implantation. Audiol Neurotol. 2004; 9(4):224–233
[3] Colletti L, Mandalà M, Zoccante L, Shannon RV, Colletti V. Infants versus older children fitted with cochlear implants: performance over 10 years. Int J Pediatr Otorhinolaryngol. 2011; 75(4):504–509
[4] Dettman SJ, Pinder D, Briggs RJS, Dowell RC, Leigh JR. Communication development in children who receive the cochlear implant younger than 12 months: risks versus benefits. Ear Hear. 2007; 28(2) Suppl:11S–18S
[5] Bayazit YA, Kosaner J, Cinar BC, et al. Methods and preliminary outcomes of pediatric auditory brainstem implantation. Ann Otol Rhinol Laryngol. 2014; 123(8):529–536
[6] Buchman CA, Teagle HFB, Roush PA, et al. Cochlear implantation in children with labyrinthine anomalies and cochlear nerve deficiency: implications for auditory brainstem implantation. Laryngoscope. 2011; 121(9):1979–1988
[7] Colletti L. Beneficial auditory and cognitive effects of auditory brainstem implantation in children. Acta Otolaryngol. 2007; 127(9):943–946
[8] Colletti L, Zoccante L. Nonverbal cognitive abilities and auditory performance in children fitted with auditory brainstem implants: preliminary report. Laryngoscope. 2008; 118(8):1443–1448
[9] Colletti L, Colletti G, Mandalà M, Colletti V. The therapeutic dilemma of cochlear nerve deficiency: cochlear or brainstem implantation? Otolaryngol Head Neck Surg. 2014; 151(2):308–314
[10] Colletti L, Wilkinson EP, Colletti V. Auditory brainstem implantation after unsuccessful cochlear implantation of children with clinical diagnosis of cochlear nerve deficiency. Ann Otol Rhinol Laryngol. 2013; 122(10):605–612
[11] Vincenti V, Ormitti F, Ventura E, Guida M, Piccinini A, Pasanisi E. Cochlear implantation in children with cochlear nerve deficiency. Int J Pediatr Otorhinolaryngol. 2014; 78(6):912–917
[12] Young NM, Kim FM, Ryan ME, Tournis E, Yaras S. Pediatric cochlear implantation of children with eighth nerve deficiency. Int J Pediatr Otorhinolaryngol. 2012; 76(10):1442–1448

[13] Couloigner V, Gratacap M, Ambert-Dahan E, et al. [A report of three cases and review of auditory brainstem implants in children]. Neurochirurgie. 2014; 60 (1–2):17–26

[14] McConkey Robbins A, Koch DB, Osberger MJ, Zimmerman-Phillips S, Kishon-Rabin L. Effect of age at cochlear implantation on auditory skill development in infants and toddlers. Arch Otolaryngol Head Neck Surg. 2004; 130(5):570–574

[15] Eisenberg LS, Johnson KC, Martinez AS, et al. Comprehensive evaluation of a child with an auditory brainstem implant. Otol Neurotol. 2008; 29(2):251–257

[16] Puram SV, Tward AD, Jung DH, et al. Auditory brainstem implantation in a 16-month-old boy with cochlear hypoplasia. Otol Neurotol. 2015; 36(4):618–624

[17] Sennaroglu L, Colletti V, Manrique M, et al. Auditory brainstem implantation in children and non-neurofibromatosis type 2 patients: a consensus statement. Otol Neurotol. 2011; 32(2):187–191

[18] Sennaroglu L, Ziyal I, Atas A, et al. Preliminary results of auditory brainstem implantation in prelingually deaf children with inner ear malformations including severe stenosis of the cochlear aperture and aplasia of the cochlear nerve. Otol Neurotol. 2009; 30(6):708–715

[19] Colletti L, Shannon RV, Colletti V. The development of auditory perception in children after auditory brainstem implantation. Audiol Neurotol. 2014; 19 (6):386–394

[20] Carner M, Colletti L, Shannon R, et al. Imaging in 28 children with cochlear nerve aplasia. Acta Otolaryngol. 2009; 129(4):458–461

[21] Mandalà M, Colletti L, Colletti G, Colletti V. Improved outcomes in auditory brainstem implantation with the use of near-field electrical compound action potentials. Otolaryngol Head Neck Surg. 2014; 151(6):1008–1013

[22] Archbold S, Lutman ME, Marshall DH. Categories of auditory performance. Ann Otol Rhinol Laryngol Suppl. 1995; 166:312–314

[23] Archbold S, Lutman ME, Nikolopoulos T. Categories of auditory performance: inter-user reliability. Br J Audiol. 1998; 32(1):7–12

[24] Niparko JK, Tobey EA, Thal DJ, et al. CDaCI Investigative Team. Spoken language development in children following cochlear implantation. JAMA. 2010; 303(15):1498–1506

[25] Eisenberg LS, Johnson KC, Martinez AS, Visser-Dumont L, Ganguly DH, Still JF. Studies in pediatric hearing loss at the House Research Institute. J Am Acad Audiol. 2012; 23(6):412–421

[26] Moore JK, Niparko JK, Miller MR, Linthicum FH. Effect of profound hearing loss on a central auditory nucleus. Am J Otol. 1994; 15(5):588–595

[27] Nadol JB, Jr, Young Y-S, Glynn RJ. Survival of spiral ganglion cells in profound sensorineural hearing loss: implications for cochlear implantation. Ann Otol Rhinol Laryngol. 1989; 98(6):411–416

[28] Lee DS, Lee JS, Oh SH, et al. Cross-modal plasticity and cochlear implants. Nature. 2001; 409(6817):149–150

[29] Giraud A-L, Lee H-J. Predicting cochlear implant outcome from brain organisation in the deaf. Restor Neurol Neurosci. 2007; 25(3–4):381–390

[30] Casselman J, Mermuys K, Delanote J, Ghekiere J, Coenegrachts K. MRI of the cranial nerves—more than meets the eye: technical considerations and advanced anatomy. Neuroimaging Clin N Am. 2008; 18(2): 197–231, x

[31] Mitchell RM, Christianson ER, Ramirez FM, et al. Auditory comprehension outcomes in children who receive a cochlear implant before 12 months of age. Laryngoscope. 2020; 130(3):776–781

[32] Colletti V, Shannon RV, Carner M, Veronese S, Colletti L. Complications in auditory brainstem implant surgery in adults and children. Otol Neurotol. 2010; 31(4):558–564

[33] Colletti G, Mandalà M, Colletti L, Colletti V. Nervus intermedius guides auditory brainstem implant surgery in children with cochlear nerve deficiency. Otolaryngol Head Neck Surg. 2016; 154(2):335–342

[34] Colletti G, Mandalà M, Colletti V, Deganello A, Allevi F, Colletti L. Resorbable mesh cranioplasty repair of bilateral cerebrospinal fluid leaks following pediatric simultaneous bilateral auditory brainstem implant surgery. Otol Neurotol. 2017; 38(4):606–609

[35] Laing RJ, Smielewski P, Czosnyka M, Quaranta N, Moffat DA. A study of perioperative lumbar cerebrospinal fluid pressure in patients undergoing acoustic neuroma surgery. Skull Base Surg. 2000; 10(4):179–185

10 ABI Engineering and Intraoperative Monitoring: Cochlear

Barry Nevison

Abstract

The auditory brainstem implant (ABI), while closely related in many ways to a cochlear implant (CI), is beset with its own unique technical, practical, and clinical challenges as it is implanted within the brainstem and involves stimulating a structure that can barely be seen during surgery. Through over 20 years of experience, the electrode array design and the surrounding surgical and clinical procedures have been tailored to meet the constraints imposed by the brainstem anatomy, implantability, electrical safety, long-term stability, and clinical effectiveness. This chapter details the ABI design along with its main technical features. It also addresses the way in which electrophysiology performed during device insertion, with careful selection and stimulation of discrete regions of the array, can be used to help ensure correct placement of the electrode over as much of the stimulable cochlear nucleus as possible. A procedure along with the key parameters for electrophysiological testing is described. With careful attention to the electrode placement, this helps to ensure each patient has the best chance of a positive clinical outcome, including useful auditory awareness and improved quality of life in patients without any other hope of hearing.

Keywords: brainstem implant, intraoperative monitoring, electrophysiology, EABR, cochlear nucleus, electrode array

10.1 Introduction

Ever since the first aspiration to achieve auditory awareness through electrical stimulation of the cochlear nucleus, both engineering design and anatomical understanding have grown hand in hand. The cochlear nucleus, our target for electrical stimulation, is hidden from view surgically and often pushed to one side or its recess compressed by a growing brainstem tumor making location and access sometimes quite difficult.[1] Despite this adversity, a brainstem implant can be inserted safely, fixed securely, and work reliably for the majority of recipients. All these factors come together to present quite a unique challenge surgically, mechanically, and practically. This chapter explores the unique ABI design focusing on the latest Nucleus ABI541 device that is commercially available. It also explains the electrophysiological testing that can be performed to try to work around the adversity of a hidden nucleus or strangely unfamiliar brainstem distorted by a large tumor. Placed optimally and operating effectively, the ABI can provide significant assistance to speech understanding.[2,3,4,5] Suboptimal placement or an electrode displaced by a moving brainstem can twist the outcome to nothing more than a range of unhelpful side effects. Clearly, this is a device with which experts in their respective fields need to work together.

10.2 ABI Design Engineering

The ABI takes its inspiration from the design principles of a cochlear implant (CI) yet comprises a quite different electrode array design due to its position within the lateral recess of the brainstem. Here it aims to stimulate the 2nd neuron of the auditory pathway at the exposed surface of the cochlear nucleus complex (CNC)—the point where the auditory nerve normally joins the brainstem. Remarkably the first reported use of an ABI was in 1978[6] when even CIs were in their infancy. Yet those early results proved not only that the cochlear nucleus was accessible surgically, but also that auditory sensations were indeed possible when modulated electrical current was applied.

Cochlear's involvement in the ABI development started in 1990. With a growing reputation for producing reliable CIs, Cochlear was approached by William Hitselberger and William House from the House Ear Institute in Los Angeles, California, to help create an implant based upon the commercial design of the Nucleus CI22 M CI that existed at that time. With the availability of many separate stimulation electrodes, this saw a design change from a three-electrode, single channel device to an eight-electrode, multichannel system comprising two staggered rows of four electrodes 1 mm in diameter mounted on a silicone elastomer carrier about 3 mm wide and 8 mm long. Almost simultaneously a slightly different design of ABI electrode was proposed by a team in Hannover, Germany lead by Roland Laszig.[7] The basic design mirrored developments at the House Ear Institute except that a 20-channel electrode array was proposed, necessitating much reduced electrode diameters to fit within the available paddle size. Two designs were accomplished, followed by two pilot studies and then two clinical trials between 1992 and 2000.[8,9]

This chapter will not dwell upon all the device iterations that occurred—especially with the early Hannover design. By 2000, a combined design of ABI electrode array was established and since then, the ABI electrode has remained largely unchanged. It is this design that over 1100 patients globally have received.

10.2.1 Physical Design

The Nucleus ABI541 is electronically identical to the CI500-series CI but physically there are two main differences pertaining to the electrode array and the electrode leadwire design (see ▶ Fig. 10.1). The electrode array, in particular, needs to be placed within the lateral recess of the fourth ventricle at a structure known as the cochlear nucleus. The exposed surface of the cochlear nucleus within the lateral recess measures, on average, 3 mm in width and 10 mm in length,[10] and this presents the "target area" for stimulation. To make use of as much of the exposed surface of the cochlear nucleus as possible, the ABI electrode array consists of a silicone electrode carrier, often referred to as the "paddle," 9.9 mm long by 3.5 mm wide and covered by a 7 × 3 staggered matrix of platinum electrode contacts measuring 0.7 mm in diameter. Each one of these contacts, which hopefully delivers some unique pitch sensation based upon the tonotopicity of the CNC, can be independently stimulated by a modulated electrical pulse train presented in a way so as to hopefully elicit an auditory sensation during the device "activation" or "switch-on"—a topic covered in Chapter 12.

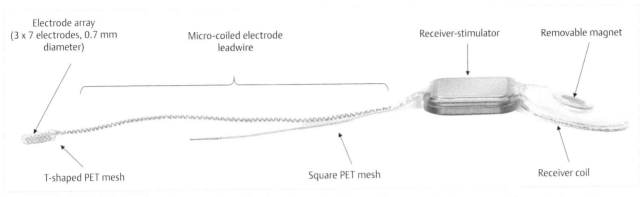

Fig. 10.1 Nucleus ABI541 auditory brainstem implant (ABI).

The electrode array is augmented by soft weave of polyethylene-terephtalat (PET) mesh on its rear surface, formed in the shape of a "T." This biocompatible material promotes adhesion of fibrous tissue. Since the lateral recess has no solid landmarks with which to safely stabilize the electrode once inserted, this fibrous tissue adherence acts as an important "glue" holding the device firmly in position, provided there is no movement of the electrode array within the first few days after surgery. The specific PET shape, that of a "T"-shaped wing, is designed so that as the electrode array is inserted, this wing can be looped back upon itself, not only providing a greater area for tissue growth, but also applying just a small amount of pressure to the lateral end of the electrode array within the entrance to the recess.

In the Nucleus ABI electrode array, the rear of the array also possesses a tiny positioning tube at its medial end. This tube allows the electrode array to be grasped by surgical instruments such as forceps or a claw, without damage, and then gently advanced into the opening of the recess.

The other notable difference of the ABI device compared to its CI cousin is the electrode leadwire which is both longer and more flexible. The increased length is simply to reach the target CNC in the brainstem, which is further away from the implant electronics package than the cochlea. The improved flexibility of the leadwire is achieved by using a smaller radius of wound wires within a narrower silicone leadwire. Not only does this promote improved handling, reducing the springiness of the electrode array, but it also minimizes fatigue stresses on the electrode wires themselves since this array will be sitting within a slightly moving brainstem for all of its working life.

Finally, a small revision was made to the implant design in around 2010 when a 10 mm square pad of PET mesh was attached to the leadwire more proximal to the electronics package. This mesh was added to address a few cases of cerebrospinal fluid (CSF) leakage occurring after surgery, the CSF wicking along the electrode leadwire. It was proposed by Derald Brackman from the House Ear Institute that adding a mesh pad where the electrode array comes through the dura would promote better fibrous tissue growth, form a better seal as well as improve options for stabilization of the array.

A final feature of the Nucleus ABI common to all generations of the product and not explicitly related to the electrode array is a removable magnet. This strong, rare-earth magnet, designed to hold the external sound processor's coil to the head during use, may pose an unwanted disturbance in the event

that subsequent magnetic resonance imaging (MRI) is required. While the ABI541 is approved for use in 1.5 Tesla MRI machines with a tight pressure dressing, imaging with any kind of magnet in situ becomes a problem due to the extensive artifact created. Removal of the magnet, either temporarily or permanently, can be undertaken as required. Once the magnet is removed, the ABI may also then be imaged at 3.0T if required.

10.2.2 Electrical Design and Safety

It has been detailed earlier that the electronic design of the ABI541 is identical to that of a CI, and indeed no specific changes were necessary due to the high degree of flexibility that the electronics provide. The electronic stimulator of the ABI is capable of delivering sequential biphasic current pulses where the pulse amplitude, the pulse width, the pulse rate, the active electrode, and the stimulation mode can all be set within wide parameters according to the needs of the individual patient.

Early patients receiving the ABI were stimulated using relatively modest stimulation rates of around 250 pulses per second (pps) in bipolar modes. It was quickly seen that while the electrode array might be in intimate contact with the neural substrate it was stimulating, electrical levels to reach audibility were quite large compared to a CI. These high stimulation levels necessitated careful assessment of the charge density around the electrode contacts. It was this consideration that lead to the current electrode diameters of 0.7 mm as this was the requirement to keep stimulation within the established safety margins as proved in experiments by McCreery et al[11] and summarized eloquently in a review paper by Shannon in 1992.[12] In fact the classic safety equation formula relating charge density (D) and charge (Q), namely $log\ D = k - log\ Q$, is now programmed into Cochlear's fitting software to ensure that if stimulation parameters do need to rise for some patients, at all times established safety levels are respected.

10.3 Electrophysiology to Support Optimal Intraoperative Electrode Placement

Insertion of an ABI electrode array into the lateral recess in such a way that it is optimally positioned over the exposed surface of the

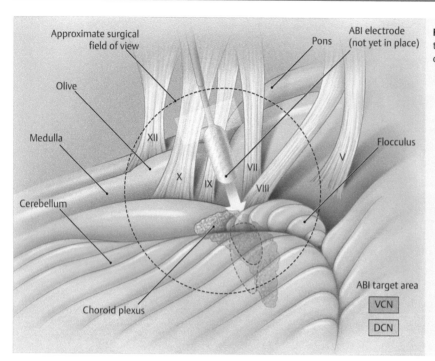

Fig. 10.2 Auditory brainstem implant (ABI) electrode array just prior to insertion with target cochlear nucleus hidden from view.

cochlear nucleus is hampered by the simple fact that in most cases the target area is just out of sight (▶ Fig. 10.2). While in some patients it may be possible to visualize the white bulge of the cochlear nucleus as it descends into the recess, in no case is it possible to assess its precise full size or indeed its exact orientation. This "half blind" approach can, however, potentially be aided by the use of electrophysiology,[13] which is now commonplace in ABI surgery.

The basic principle of the electrophysiological testing is quite simple. When the ABI electrode array has already been positioned in a location that looks anatomically correct with respect to the landmarks of the VIIth and IXth nerves, the choroid plexus, and any observed CSF flow from the lateral recess, the electrode array is stimulated while simultaneously recording the electrically evoked auditory brainstem response (EABR). In theory, if the electrode array is over the cochlear nucleus, then it should be possible to observe a number of small, positive, repeatable biological peaks on an evoked potential (EP) machine that characterize the firing of the cochlear nucleus and the ascending auditory pathway via the superior olive, lateral lemniscus, and inferior colliculus. Given that stimulation is occurring at the cochlear nucleus we might hope to record peaks corresponding to waves III, IV, and V from the classic five-peak ABR. Observation of these peaks, if in the right amplitude and latency, then acts as "proof positive" that the stimulated electrode, at least, is in close proximity to the cochlear nucleus. It logically follows that if a number of electrodes are stimulated across the array, then it should be possible to map-out the alignment of the array over the cochlear nucleus and then, if necessary, the device gently moved to optimize its location. ▶ Fig. 10.3 visualizes this alignment process.

10.3.1 Equipment Setup for EABR

In practice, measuring and interpreting the EABR reliably, and then giving appropriate direction to guide electrode placement

requires a number of technical and practical details to be taken into consideration. The equipment setup for EABR is shown in ▶ Fig. 10.4.

From an equipment perspective, it is necessary to use a commercial averager (aka "EP machine") to record the biological potentials from surface electrodes placed on the patient. It is also necessary to have an equipment capable of delivering a stimulus from the ABI device, which in the case of the Nucleus ABI consists simply of the standard programming hardware (a sound processor and coil which are placed over the implant during testing; plus a programming Pod interface) connected to a computer running Custom Sound EP software. Then, to ensure the EP machine records potentials linked with the stimulation, an all-important trigger cable connecting the stimulation and recording hardware is necessary to synchronize the two machines.

10.3.2 Recording Electrode Montage

The electrode montage frequently used for "traditional" EABR in a CI recipient would position the active recording electrode on the upper forehead, the indifferent electrode on the mastoid contralateral to the implant, and the ground electrode on the lower forehead. This montage has been adopted to minimize the amount of electrical stimulus artefact picked up by the EP machine—something that makes EABR considerably more challenging than an ABR. However, the above montage is based upon a CI electrode within the cochlea whereas we have an ABI electrode in the brainstem. This change of position and electrode array orientation have led to a more widely adopted montage using a true vertex positive electrode, a C7 negative electrode, and a ground at about the hairline, all on the midline.[14] This orientation not only helps to minimize electrical artifacts from the ABI during stimulation but is also sensitive to vertical electrical activity in the brainstem tracts that the

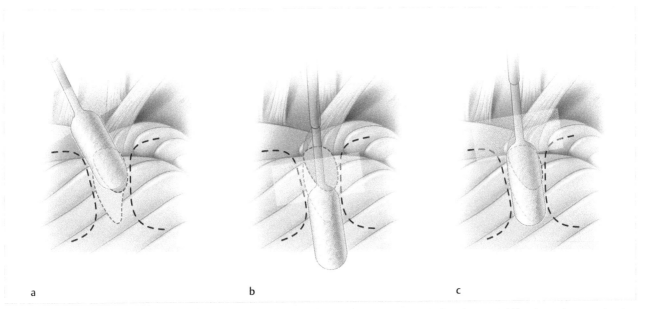

Fig. 10.3 Auditory brainstem implant (ABI) electrode positioning within the lateral recess (Note: cerebellum shown would be obstructing your view in practice). Example shows **(a)** too shallow, **(b)** too deep, and **(c)** optimal electrode positioning (NB: Electrode image shows contacts facing away from viewer; bold dotted line represents open portion of lateral recess).

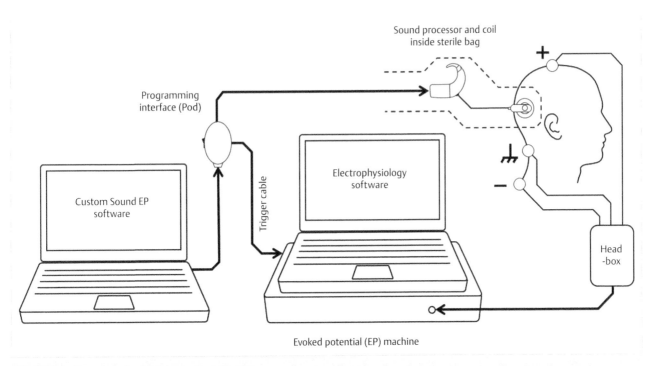

Fig. 10.4 Auditory evoked potential measurement setup.

biological potentials travel through as they ascend. In no way does this represent the only option for successful EABR. A montage that uses a high forehead positive, combined with an ipsilateral tragus negative and a low forehead ground, is increasingly being used. This has the slight advantage that its orientation is more favorable to the crossing depolarization of wave III of the EABR and, since it avoids the vertex, it lends itself

to the use of disposable rather than needle electrodes for the recording. Many electrophysiologists have quite firm views on electrode montage and electrode types, but in the author's experience, fresh disposable electrodes generally have lower noise and lower impedances than needles. This needs to be tempered against the need for electrode stability during a potentially long surgery. So in practice, if the surgery will be of long duration (e.g., over 5–6 hours) and the patient has a tumor to be removed, then needle electrodes are usually preferred. However, if the surgery might be shorter, disposable electrodes secured carefully with additional tape are adequate.

10.3.3 Configuring the EP Machine

The EP machine setup requires slight modification from those parameters used for recording an ABR. Listed in ▶ Table 10.1 is the author's preferred settings.

10.3.4 Configuring the Stimulation

This is an important factor in successful EABR because not only do the stimulation parameters significantly affect the success in terms of electrical artefact polluting the desired recordings, but also the methodology of which electrodes are stimulated completely dictates the guidance that can be used to reposition the electrode array.

One of the strengths of the Nucleus ABI stimulator electronics is that any combination of any electrode pair can be used for electrical stimulation. This is a huge advantage, because using electrode pairs that are only on the electrode array itself allows a very focused electrical field and only generates a relatively small electrical artifact when compared to monopolar (MP) modes. This is relevant from a practical perspective, because one of the key technical reasons why EABR can be unsuccessful is the way the EP machine's amplifiers (and filters) react to the huge electrical stimulus generated by the implant (potentially thousands of microvolts) while maintaining adequate sensitivity to then show the biological potentials of the EABR, which measure perhaps only 0.5 to 2 µV in amplitude. This issue can lead to a problem called "saturation" where little is visible in the recording except a slow decaying potential straddling the screen (or at least the first half of it). An effective way to minimize the electrical artifact is to stimulate in a narrow bipolar mode. While there are many combinations of electrodes that can be stimulated, the author prefers to use a longitudinal "skip one" mode (a kind of "BP + 1") which equates to what is labelled as BP + 5 in the test software due to the two-dimensional arrangement of electrodes. As it happens, all combinations of BP + 5 have the same orientation (as do BP + 2, BP + 8, etc.).

Apart from the stimulation mode, amplitudes of electrical current, which elicit a response from the cochlear nucleus, are

unusually high compared to a CI. This means that a typical starting stimulus for EABR may be 150 µs wide and 150 CLs/current levels (approximately 250 µA) in amplitude, when delivered at the low repetition rates that are typical of an EABR (e.g., 35 Hz). Current (mainly) and/or pulse width (less often) are then adjusted to find a level at which a biological response is seen from the cochlear nucleus, as evidenced by a "good-looking" EABR waveform. Note that typically we are not trying to find thresholds, but just evidence of a good, repeatable morphology from which optimal location can be inferred.

The author's preferred initial EABR stimulation parameters are listed in ▶ Table 10.2.

10.3.5 Obtaining and Interpreting a Response

The lateral recess is often narrow and opened only sufficiently to allow the electrode array to advance inside. So for many ABI surgeries the only direction in which the electrode array can really be moved is either more medially or more laterally ("in" or "out"). To facilitate this decision, three pairs of electrodes are tested, E4–E10, E10–E16, and E16–E22—right down the middle of the array. If, say, E16–E22 gave good recognizable EABRs while E4–E10 and E10–E16 did not (as per ▶ Fig. 10.3a), then this would suggest that a slightly deeper position might be more optimal. If no electrodes gave a good response then the side electrodes (e.g., E8–E14 and E9–E15) or the corners (E2–E8, E3–E9, E14–E20, and E15–E21) might also be tested.

When a large lateral recess is encountered, not only can depth be varied but so too can the angle or rotation of the array. Similar to above, it would be routine to not only test the three electrode combinations down the middle of the array but also, at least, the four corners.

When making the decision to move the electrode, especially if that involves superior or inferior movement or perhaps rotation, it is necessary to understand the physical arrangement of

Table 10.1 Evoked potential machine setup parameters for EABR

Parameter	Custom Sound EP Software Setting
Stimulation mode	BP + 5
Stimulation rate	35 Hz
Starting pulse width	150 µs
Starting current level	150 CL (intraop only)—never start at these levels if performing any postoperative assessment
RF free period	10 ms
Number of sweeps	1,500 (i.e., a few more than you plan to average)
Averaging type	Basic and reverse polarity (alternating only once recognizable waveform is observed)

Abbreviations: EABR, evoked auditory brainstem response; EP, evoked potential; RF, radio frequency.

Table 10.2 Electrical stimulation parameters for EABR

Parameter	EP Machine Setting (terminology may differ by machine)
Electrode montage	Cz positive, C7 negative, Hairline ground
Amplifier gain	×100,000
Amplifier filter settings	1 Hz (high pass filter) to 5 kHz (low pass filter) with notch filter deactivated
Recording window length	10 ms
Stimulus offset (delay)/pre-trigger	1 ms (this brings the stimulus artefact more onto the screen; in some EP machines this might need to be a negative number to achieve the desired effect)
Blanking	None
Triggering	External, 5V TTL, positive edge
Artefact rejection	Off (or armed only from 3 ms after the stimulus with a rejection level at 20–50 µV)
Screen display scale	0.2 µV per vertical division initially
Averages	1,000

Abbreviations: EABR, evoked auditory brainstem response; EP, evoked potential.

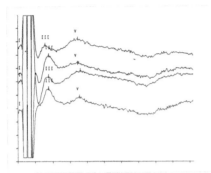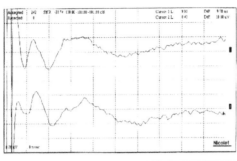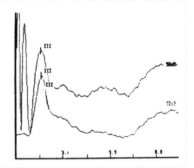

Fig. 10.5 Examples of confirmatory evoked auditory brainstem response (EABR) waveforms.

the electrode in relation to direction. A correctly inserted electrode array on the right side will have electrode row 3, 6, 9, 12, 15, 18, and 21 superiorly. Conversely a left-sided implant will have electrodes 2, 5, 8, 11, 14, 17, and 20 superiorly.

There is sometimes discussion about whether EABR is helpful in the operating room or indeed whether, in the end, it correlates in any way to the patient outcome. The best way of thinking about its value is probably like this:

If the surgery is taking place in a case where there is no distortion of the brainstem, and if all the necessary landmarks for correct identification of the CNC fall into place and especially if the root entry zone of the lateral recess comprising the initial bulge of the ventral cochlear nucleus is visible, then arguably the role of any electrophysiology performed is very much secondary to the clear anatomical landmarks; although obtaining a good EABR would nevertheless be reassuring.

If, on the other hand, the surgery occurs in a patient with a distorted brainstem due to a large tumor that has required removal, and if the location of the various landmarks for the lateral recess have been displaced and are difficult to recognize, then for sure the presence of an EABR is extremely reassuring. Indeed, in this scenario, the absence of an EABR should be considered a point to reflect carefully on the visible anatomy in case an alternative location can be found.

In principle, it is much more pleasing to have good EABRs across the majority of the electrode than to have just a few. As for the link between the number and quality of the EABRs and the subsequent performance, there seems to be some positive correlation.[15] The extent to which that correlation is not higher is likely due to the complexity of the CNC with its numerous neuron types as well as, possibly, the effect that surgery may have on the stimulability of those neurons—especially in cases of an excised tumor. For sure, absence of an EABR is not "game over" when other anatomical landmarks are clearly identified. Equally, good EABRs do not guarantee an auditory outcome since small electrode array movement or other degenerative effects might still occur post surgery.

10.3.6 Intraoperative Response Waveforms

Given that electrical stimulation of the CNC occurs at the 2nd neuron and having skipped the spiral ganglion and auditory nerve, the "perfect" EABR might be expected to comprise three peaks corresponding to waves III, IV, and V on the traditional five-peak ABR. In practice, however, there seems to be some variation from single to even quadruple peaks. A selection of typical EABRs is shown in ▶ Fig. 10.5. The variation is interesting but probably less important from an electrode placement perspective since there is rarely ever much difference in the waveforms that an individual cochlear nucleus generates. Driving this variation will be factors such as the anatomy of the dorsal and ventral cochlear nuclei with their innervation pathways to both ipsilateral and contralateral sides of the brainstem. So too will be the various nerve cell types with both excitory and inhibitory behavior. So too will be the quality of contact between the electrode and the cochlear nucleus which will affect how broad an electrical field is necessary to stimulate this body. And then overlaid on all of that will be the stimulability of the CNC due to the effects of an excised tumor which possibly has caused localized neuronal atrophy or even nerve death if local blood supplies have been compromised. In the author's experience, so long as there is evidence of at least two peaks (one generally less distinct) in the first 3.8 ms from the electrical stimulus, it is possible to be confident of auditory pathway activation. The most prominent peaks typically occur at around 1.5 to 1.9 ms and at 2.8 to 3.8 ms. But other peaks as early as 0.7 ms and somewhere in the gap between 1.9 and 2.8 ms are also occasionally observed.

Obtaining a "good-looking" EABR is reassuring, of course, but of equal importance is to not obtain anything that looks unlike an EABR. The entry zone of the lateral recess is within only a few millimeters to the facial nerve (VII) and the glossopharyngeal nerve (IX). Even the vagus nerve (X) is less than 1 cm away. Stimulation of the VIIth or IXth nerves typically generate large amplitude (many 10's of μV) biphasic waveforms becoming visible on any EP recording at 5 ms or later. Presence of these waveforms during an EABR test is certainly something to be explored and electrode position altered accordingly.

10.4 Discussion

The current design of the ABI is well suited for its position within the lateral recess delivering stimulation to the CNC. Furthermore, the use of electrical ABR is an effective method to gain confidence in the anatomy and positioning of the electrode array, and hopefully this leads to the best outcome with the fewest possible side effects to manage. But yet these are not all the issues that might concern us.

The design of the ABI electrode, with its PET mesh backing to promote fibrous tissue integration helping to provide stability within the brainstem, has both positive and negative consequences. Clearly, a stable electrode, and one that obtains that stability as soon as possible after surgery, is desirable. But yet, in the unlikely event that an implant should either fail technically or migrate, fibrosis around the device results in an electrode array that does not necessarily want to move. And now, a feature designed to help is a feature that rather hinders. The effort involved in freeing up the electrode array such that it can either be replaced or repositioned is not straightforward in some cases. This fact should not only inspire potential solutions for movable electrodes, but until that time arrives, one should, at a bare minimum, encourage careful counseling before a recipient chooses such a device. For the moment, the best protection against part of this issue (device failure) is to ensure that devices used for brainstem implantation really are the most reliable they can be.

This discussion about the interplay of stability, migration, and failure becomes all the more focused and relevant when younger patients without life-threatening indications are being considered, as some have been,[2,16,17,18,19] since here we would be implanting a generally healthy population with a device that would be expected to work reliably for a lifetime measured not in years but in decades.

10.5 Conclusions

The Nucleus ABI541 implant is the result of over 20 years of development and clinical experience-its properties, electrode contacts, PET mesh shape, and leadwire design tailored to the requirements imposed by brainstem anatomy, implantability, electrical safety, long-term stability, and clinical effectiveness. Broadly speaking, the ABI is a precise solution to a specific need in patients with a disconnection between their auditory periphery and the brainstem. And yet it remains frustratingly imperfect when viewed through the lens of clinical performance which, while undoubtedly beneficial for many and undoubtedly improving both communication and quality of life, still lags considerably behind what is expected and routinely achieved through a CI. So, despite the technology between CI and ABI being similar in many respects, the precise interaction between electrical stimulation and sound coding applied at the first auditory neuron is anything but straightforward when applied to the second auditory neuron. It reminds us that we still have more to learn and perfect. So development of the ABI has surely not reached its summit.

Aided by electrophysiology the electrode can certainly be implanted with some precision over the CNC insofar as it is our current goal. But issues of stability, optimal contact, re-implantability, and optimal sound coding remain on the tick-list for future developments, as too does the need for much greater understanding of the CNC itself from anatomical and physiological perspectives.

References

[1] Rosahl SK, Rosahl S. No easy target: anatomic constraints of electrodes interfacing the human cochlear nucleus. Neurosurgery. 2013; 72(1) Suppl Operative:58–64, discussion 65

[2] Siegbahn M, Lundin K, Olsson GB, et al. Auditory brainstem implants (ABIs)—20 years of clinical experience in Uppsala, Sweden. Acta Otolaryngol. 2014; 134(10):1052–1061

[3] Grayeli AB, Kalamarides M, Bouccara D, Ambert-Dahan E, Sterkers O. Auditory brainstem implant in neurofibromatosis type 2 and non-neurofibromatosis type 2 patients. Otol Neurotol. 2008; 29(8):1140–1146

[4] Schwartz MS, Otto SR, Shannon RV, Hitselberger WE, Brackmann DE. Auditory brainstem implants. Neurotherapeutics. 2008; 5(1):128–136

[5] Otto SR, Brackmann DE, Hitselberger WE, Shannon RV, Kuchta J. Multichannel auditory brainstem implant: update on performance in 61 patients. J Neurosurg. 2002; 96(6):1063–1071

[6] Hitselberger WE, House WF, Edgerton BJ, Whitaker S. Cochlear nucleus implants. Otolaryngol Head Neck Surg. 1984; 92(1):52–54

[7] Laszig R, Kuzma J, Seifert V, Lehnhardt E. The Hannover auditory brainstem implant: a multiple-electrode prosthesis. Eur Arch Otorhinolaryngol. 1991; 248(7):420–421

[8] Ebinger K, Otto S, Arcaroli J, Staller S, Arndt P. Multichannel auditory brainstem implant: US clinical trial results. J Laryngol Otol Suppl. 2000(27):50–53

[9] Nevison B, Laszig R, Sollmann WP, et al. Results from a European clinical investigation of the Nucleus multichannel auditory brainstem implant. Ear Hear. 2002; 23(3):170–183

[10] Klose AK, Sollmann WP. Anatomical variations of landmarks for implantation at the cochlear nucleus. J Laryngol Otol Suppl. 2000(27):8–10

[11] McCreery DB, Agnew WF, Yuen TG, Bullara L. Charge density and charge per phase as cofactors in neural injury induced by electrical stimulation. IEEE Trans Biomed Eng. 1990; 37(10):996–1001

[12] Shannon RV. A model of safe levels for electrical stimulation. IEEE Trans Biomed Eng. 1992; 39(4):424–426

[13] Nevison B. A guide to the positioning of brainstem implants using intraoperative electrical auditory brainstem responses. Adv Otorhinolaryngol. 2006; 64: 154–166

[14] Waring MD. Properties of auditory brainstem responses evoked by intraoperative electrical stimulation of the cochlear nucleus in human subjects. Electroencephalogr Clin Neurophysiol. 1996; 100(6):538–548

[15] Anwar A, Singleton A, Fang Y, et al. The value of intraoperative EABRs in auditory brainstem implantation. Int J Pediatr Otorhinolaryngol. 2017; 101:158–163

[16] Colletti V, Shannon R, Carner M, Veronese S, Colletti L. Outcomes in nontumor adults fitted with the auditory brainstem implant: 10 years' experience. Otol Neurotol. 2009; 30(5):614–618

[17] Colletti L, Shannon RV, Colletti V. The development of auditory perception in children after auditory brainstem implantation. Audiol Neurotol. 2014; 19 (6):386–394

[18] Sennaroğlu L, Sennaroğlu G, Yücel E, et al. Long-term results of ABI in children with severe inner ear malformations. Otol Neurotol. 2016; 37(7): 865–872

[19] Grayeli AB, Bouccara D, Kalamarides M, et al. Auditory brainstem implant in bilateral and completely ossified cochleae. Otol Neurotol. 2003; 24(1):79–82

11 ABI Engineering and Intraoperative Monitoring: MED-EL

Marek Polak

Abstract

Subjects with a nonfunctioning auditory nerve do not benefit from cochlear implantation. In such cases, if the subject is older than 12 months of age, an auditory brainstem implant (ABI) may be an option to treat the hearing impairment.

This chapter provides details of the state-of-the-art MED-EL ABI system, along with providing an overview of the tools developed to aid the surgeon in determining the functionality of the auditory nerve prior to implantation.

An ABI placing system based on electrophysiologic guidance was developed to determine the number of electrodes required to stimulate the auditory system and the optimum placement of the implanted electrode array.

This chapter also provides an overview of the use of intraoperative electrophysiology to aid electrode placement using both an ABI placing system and the ABI itself. This procedure involves recording electrically evoked auditory brainstem responses (eABR), which allows for the electrode array to be placed onto the cochlear nuclei (CN) by distinguishing between auditory and nonauditory responses.

Keywords: intraoperative monitoring, electrically evoked auditory brainstem response, eABR, evoked potentials, auditory brainstem implant, ABI, electrode array, HDCIS

11.1 Introduction

The auditory brainstem implant (ABI) was originally developed at the House Ear Institute in 1979 for NF2 patients who lost their VIII nerve function bilaterally after surgery to remove vestibular schwannomas (VS).[1,2,3,4] The first implantation of the MED-EL Combi 40 + ABI was performed in 1997 by Prof. Behr at the University of Wurzburg, Germany. In 2014, MED-EL introduced the fourth generation of ABI implant, the SYNCHRONY ABI system.

Technically, the ABI shares a common design concept with the cochlear implant (CI). As shown in ▶ Fig. 11.1, the ABI consists of three components: (1) audio processor, (2) receiver-stimulator, and (3) electrode array. An audio processor picks up sounds from the environment and digitizes them; a receiver-stimulator is placed under the skin and receives electrical signals along

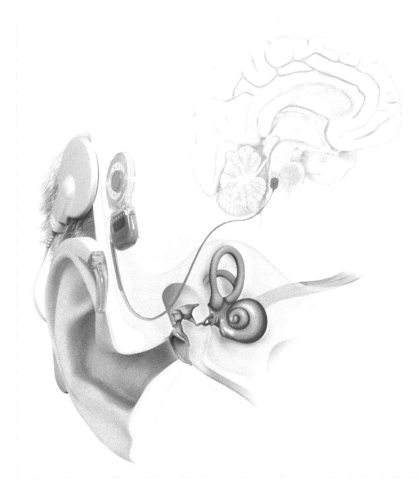

Fig. 11.1 An auditory brainstem implant (ABI) setup. Audio processor and transmitting coil, shown on the left, worn externally. The implant with the receiving coil is placed under the skin. The ABI electrode (right) goes through the dura and is placed on one of the cochlear nuclei (CN) of the brainstem.

with obtaining power from the audio processor via a transmitting coil. The signals are decoded and delivered in a controlled manner through a surface electrode array to the cochlear nuclei (CN) in the brainstem, thereby bypassing the nonfunctioning auditory nerve. Such stimulation produces responses that the brain can interpret as sounds.

11.2 State-of-the-Art MED-EL ABI System

As shown in ▶ Fig. 11.2, the MED-EL ABI array comprises 13 platinum disc electrode contacts (12 stimulation electrodes and 1 reference electrode), with a diameter of 0.6 mm each, which are embedded in a silicone carrier (5.5 × 3.0 × 0.6 mm). The overall size of the array allows the pad to fit within the lateral recess of the fourth ventricle and to adapt to the surface of the CN. On the opposite side of the silicone carrier, there is a polymer mesh backing which promotes fibrous ingrowth and secures the electrode in the desired location, thereby increasing stability of the electrode array on the surface of the CN. The electrode array is pre-shaped by cross-running platinum wires. This allows for an element of individual shaping so that it adapts to the contour of the CN.

Besides the implant, the system consists of an externally worn audio processor, with a coil that is held over the implant via magnetic attraction. Additionally, the implant system comprises Maestro fitting software with MAX interface box as well as various tools and accessories.

The Mi1200 SYNCHRONY (PIN) implant received the CE mark in June 2014. The SYNCHRONY (PIN) receiver-stimulator uses the i100 electronics with a reduced thickness of 4.5 mm for the stimulator. The HDCIS coding strategy (modified Continous interleaved Sampling coding strategy with the Hilbert Transform envelope extraction) with a maximum stimulating rate of 50,704 pps is used.[5] Monopolar stimulation is used postoperatively. The speech outcomes in ABI adult patients by use of this coding strategy are discussed in a report by Behr et al.[6]

The Mi1200 SYNCHRONY (PIN) consists of a hermetically sealed stimulator, a coil with a magnet at its center, a reference electrode, an electrically evoked action potential (EAP) reference electrode, and a variant of an active electrode. The stimulator consists of the implant circuitry and a microchip, encapsulated in hermetically sealed titanium housing, covered in silicone, with a reference electrode and an EAP electrode mounted on the housing. Two variants of the titanium housing exist:
- With a flat bottom—the Mi1200 SYNCHRONY,
- With two pins, protruding from the flat bottom, which are used to further ease the immobilization of the device— Mi1200 SYNCHRONY with suffix PIN. The two pins secure the implant against translational and rotational motion. These pins add 1.4 mm to the bottom of the device.

An important feature of the SYNCHRONY ABI is the possibility of receiving a magnetic resonance imaging (MRI) of up to 1.5 Tesla without having to remove the magnet. The magnet is diametrically magnetized and rotatable within its housing, and the whole magnet assembly is also removable (in this case, it is necessary to use a nonmagnetic spacer instead). The torque forces related to the performance of an MRI on the rotatable magnet are considered negligible. Therefore, the magnet does not become discharged and no magnetic discharge is possible during

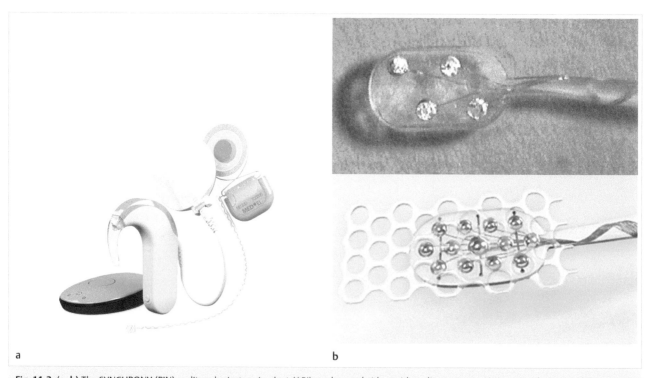

a   b

Fig. 11.2 (a, b) The SYNCHRONY (PIN) auditory brainstem implant (ABI) can be used either with audio processors Sonnet 2 or button audio processor Rondo 3. ABI electrode paddle and ABI placing electrode are highlighted.

an MRI treatment, which increases patients' comfort whenever an MRI is needed.

A typical MRI distortion of the SYNCHRONY ABI is approximately 3 cm around the implant case. Although the use of a nonmagnetic spacer instead of the magnet results in less MRI distortion, the option of keeping the magnet in place during an MRI is preferable. Importantly, this means that no additional surgery for magnet removal and placement is required, and with the use of an MRI and a high-resolution computed tomography (CT), it is often possible to obtain necessary information from the distorted area. Positioning the implant in a more horizontal and posterior way as well as a distance of at least 9 cm between the magnet and the external ear canal have shown to improve the visibility of the internal auditory canal.[7,8]

11.3 ABI Indication

The initial indication was etiology related. ABI candidates needed to be 15 years of age or older with NF2 and both cochlear nerves nonfunctional, or anticipated to be rendered nonfunctional by the presence or removal of a tumor. In 2017, the indication criteria were expanded to include candidates that are aged 12 months or older who would not benefit from a CI due to a nonfunctioning auditory nerve. The cause of nonfunctioning auditory nerves may be congenital due to auditory nerve aplasia or auditory nerve hypoplasia or accrued during the life span due to cochlear nerve disruption caused by head trauma, non-NF2 tumors, or severe cochlear ossification.

11.4 Tools in Questionable Candidacy for CI or ABI

The goal of the developed tools is to minimize the time of hearing deprivation in questionable candidates, who normally would not be implanted or implanted with uncertainty, and to help the implant team to decide which implant is the best choice for each candidate. Both of the tools discussed below and the evoked auditory brainstem responses (eABR) stimulation were developed for the Maestro MED-EL clinical system, version 9.0 and higher, and require only a dedicated evoked potential measuring system (i.e., no other equipment is needed).

In some instances candidates show no response or a questionable response to sound while diagnostic imaging tests suggest normal or abnormal anatomy. This may include individuals with a narrow internal auditory canal, or individuals with either malformed or patent cochlea. For this purpose, the preoperative promontory stimulation system was developed. The benefits of this test were shown in initial studies with a success rate of 80 to 90% in children implanted with a CI.[9,10] In our case, a transtympanic electrode is placed on the round window niche. Biphasic electrical pulses are delivered to the transtympanic electrodes. At the time of stimuli, the MAX interface triggers the evoked potential device and the eABR response is obtained from the surface electrodes. If the eABR shows a positive response, the implant team may decide to proceed with cochlear implantation. If no responses are obtained, the candidate may be considered for an ABI, or further tests may be required. The transtympanic electrode is avail-

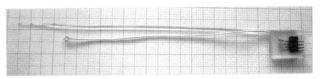

Fig. 11.3 Cochlear test electrode array. The electrode array is used for testing nerve functionality in subjects that are suitable for cochlear implant (CI) or auditory brainstem implant (ABI).

able in two different sizes in order to accommodate different middle ear space sizes.

In situations where an individual shows no response to the sound or the individual is expected to have no response to the sound, imaging tests show normal or abnormal anatomy, and the individual has already been selected for either a CI or an ABI, an intraoperative test of nerve functionality may be used. This test includes placement of the cochlear test electrode array into the scala tympani (▶ Fig. 11.3).

The cochlear test electrode consists of four electrode contacts. It is intended to be inserted into the cochlea during surgery. The length of the electrode is 18 mm, as indicated by the marker ring. Three of the electrode contacts are placed directly into the cochlea, with the fourth electrode contact placed under the temporalis muscle. Biphasic pulses can be applied using all electrode combinations. The biphasic pulses are generated using the MAX interface and delivered to the cochlea. At the time of stimuli, the MAX interface triggers the evoked potential device and eABR response is obtained from the surface electrodes.

This tool is suitable for individuals with questionable functionality of the auditory nerve, individuals with a narrow internal auditory canal and patent or malformed cochlea, in tumor patients to monitor nerve functionality during the tumor removal, or in situations where any other tests/methods failed to show CI candidacy including the use of eABR with the promontory stimulation system.[11,12,13]

To improve the reliability of the recordings from both of these tools, a new eABR artifact cancellation method was implemented.

11.5 Intraoperative eABR Protocol

Although the electrode array is designed to cover the complete area of the CN, the optimal electrode location can be difficult to ascertain due to anatomy distortion following VS removal or anatomy abnormalities that are typical in children with auditory nerve hypoplasia or nerve aplasia.

For the purpose of aiding electrode positioning during implantation, an ABI placing system and an intraoperative eABR protocol were developed. Waring[14] introduced the eABR as a tool to determine the optimal position of an ABI in the foramen of Luschka. Since then, eABRs have become a gold standard in selecting the optimal position for an ABI electrode array during surgery.

The electrode array and the lead of the ABI placing electrode (▶ Fig. 11.2) have the same dimensions as the ABI electrode array. The paddle has four electrode contacts and don't have any polyester mesh.

The eABR measurements are performed using the ABI placing system with the ABI placing electrode prior to device implantation. Anatomical landmarks need to be established prior to placement of the ABI placing electrode. The electrode paddle is inserted into the lateral recess, aimed at a position where both the ventral and the dorsal CN can be stimulated. By stimulating the brainstem with bipolar biphasic current pulses, the eABR potentials can be assessed.

The intraoperative eABR protocol starts with stimulation of contacts 1 and 4 at 100 current units (CU, 1 CU ≈ 1 μA). The pulse duration is set to 60 μs. The stimulating level is increased until response is recorded up to 500 CU. Once the eABR is obtained, the same stimulating level is applied for stimulation of contacts 2 and 3. If no response is obtained for contacts 1 and 4 at 500 CU, the stimulating level can be increased to 750 CU. The stimulation of contacts 2 and 3 is then performed. After the eABR is recorded, the outcomes are discussed with the surgeon who may decide to reposition the ABI electrode array. Contacts 1 and 4 and 2 and 3 are then stimulated at the same stimulating levels. This process is repeated until responses for both contact settings are obtained. The stimulating level may be increased by up to 1000 CU. ▶ Fig. 11.4 depicts the contact pairs selected in the protocol.

Once the eABR signals become identifiable, the ABI receiver-stimulator package is placed and fixed into a milled bone well in the temporo-occipital bone in the same way as a CI.

Thereafter, the placing electrode is exchanged with the ABI electrode array. And in a similar manner, we begin by recording the eABR. We start with the electrodes in the middle of the electrode array, 6, 5, and 9, and then we move to the most lateral electrode 1 and the most medial electrode 12 (▶ Fig. 11.4). Starting with electrode 6, we stimulate it with 100 CU. The stimulating level is increased until a response is recorded (up to 500 CU). Once the eABR is obtained, the same stimulating level is applied for stimulation of electrode 5. If no response is

obtained for electrode 6 at 500 CU, the stimulating level can be increased to 750 CU. The stimulation of the remaining electrodes is then performed. After the eABR is recorded, the outcomes are discussed with the surgeon who may decide to reposition the ABI electrode array. All electrodes are stimulated at the same stimulating levels. This process is repeated until responses for all electrodes, or at least all middle electrodes (electrodes 6, 5, and 9), are obtained. The stimulating level may be increased by up to 1000 CU.

The polymer mesh, which is embedded in the silicone of the ABI active electrode array, is cut to fit in the lateral recess, and the ABI active electrode array is placed into the estimated correct location, where the ABI placing electrode evoked eABR signals. Therefore, the insertion depth into the lateral recess is the same for both electrodes.

After completion of the final eABR check, the ABI active electrode is fixed on the brain's surface. The main fixation is achieved by gluing the electrode lead to the rostral surface of the cerebellum. Fixation of the electrode array should be performed with TachoSil in combination of fibrin glue. Thereafter, the wound is closed.

The placing electrode can be used first to find an approximate electrode position, that is, for mapping the area or to localize the best response. Another strategy may be to wait and open the implant after an eABR response is obtained; it is easier to manipulate than the ABI implant, and based on the placing electrode, you can decide how much mesh you need to cut. Furthermore, it is particularly useful in abnormal anatomies, where several landmarks can often be missing. Because of the fact that ABI candidates are mainly difficult cases, having two different measuring systems is particularly beneficial (i.e., use of placing electrode or ABI implant itself).

11.6 Benefits of Intraoperative eABR

In 17 young children implanted with ABIs, with a mean age of 2 years and 4 months (range: 8–64 months), eABR measurements were performed intraoperatively and at activation. All children implanted between 2012 and 2013 at the Policlinico Borgo Roma, Verona, Italy by Prof. Colletti were included in this study.[15]

Results from this study showed that an eABR could be obtained intraoperativeley from all of the children. Responses were recorded in 75 to 100% of all electrodes. It was possible to record eABR at initial stimulation in all of the children. The eABR was obtained in 79.7% of all electrodes (range: 25–100%) with a mean eABR threshold of 22.3 nanocoulombs; (range: 8.3–46.2%). eABR without any nonauditory stimulation was recorded across all electrodes in 11 children. Mixed eABR and nonauditory responses were recorded on 2 to 6 electrodes in six children. The nonauditory response was observed only on children and electrodes with mixed eABR and nonauditory responses.

11.7 eABR Morphology

Examples of eABR recordings can be seen in ▶ Fig. 11.5. For both intraopertative and postoperative eABR, eABR amplitudes

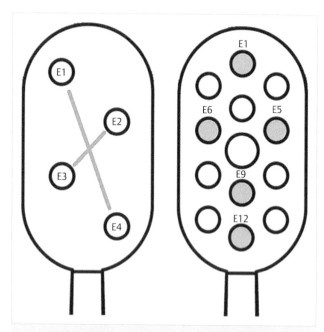

Fig. 11.4 Intraoperative protocol: Electrode stimulation options with the placing electrode and auditory brainstem implant (ABI) electrode array.

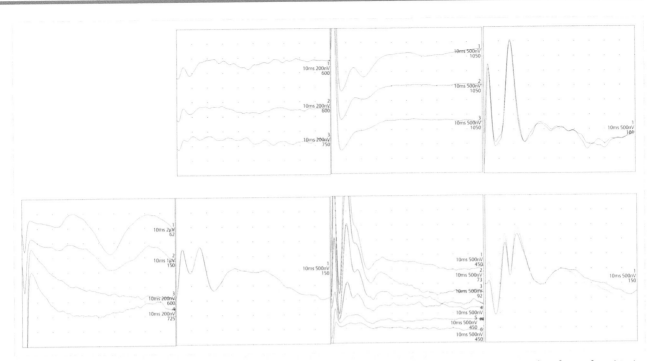

Fig. 11.5 Examples of intraoperative and postoperative evoked auditory brainstem responses (eABR) recordings varying in number of waves from 1 to 4. (From Polak M, Colletti L, et al.[15])

Table 11.1 Mean eABR latencies with an ABI. Recordings are performed from the contralateral mastoid (−), vertex (+), and lower forehead (ground).

	Range [ms]
Peak 1	0.4–0.9
Peak 2	1–2.5
Peak 3	1.7–4.5
Peak 4	3.5–5

Abbreviations: ABI, auditory brainstem implant; eABR, evoked auditory brainstem responses.

varied between 0.15 and 4.2 μV. Responses were recordable from 0.4 ms to approximately 5 ms. Wave P2 was most robust, appearing from 1 to 2.5 ms, and was present for all eABR recordings. Wave P1 occurred between 0.4 and 0.9 ms. Wave P3 occurred between 1.7 to 4.5 ms and wave P4 between 3.5 and 5 ms. The P3 and P4 waves were present only in the presence of P1 and P2. ▶ Table 11.1 depicts the mean eABR latencies. The shortest eABR was a 2 wave response occurring within 1 ms, while the longest eABR was a 4 wave response within 5 ms. The nonauditory responses, confirmed by the observation and/or subjective response, were recordable from 2.5 to 10 ms, typically after 4 ms.

The data confirm that intraoperative eABR is a reliable tool to judge ABI electrode placement. In addition to the correct electrode placement, further eABR based fitting techniques help children with ABI to achieve faster auditory perception and development (equivalent of 6 months old child's auditory developmental period).[15] Lastly, intraoperative eABR can be used to judge the development and the anatomy. This may be particularly interesting in children.

11.8 Conclusion

There are numerous factors affecting the outcomes of individuals implanted with an ABI.[6] It was shown that even adults with a tumor may achieve hearing abilities that are equal to that achieved using a CI.[6,16] The proper selection of candidates, early and safe implantation, choice of ABI implant system, correct electrode placement, and further ABI fitting techniques have a significant influence on hearing performance with an ABI.

The tools developed and discussed in this chapter may help aid the decision in selecting ABI candidates and allow for earlier implantation. Furthermore, intraoperative protocols and use of the placing electrode may improve the correct electrode placement. Intraoperative and postoperative eABR measurements or eABR based fitting may help to further improve the speech abilities and hearing performance of ABI implanted children and adults.

References

[1] Edgerton BJ, House WF, Hitselberger W. Hearing by cochlear nucleus stimulation in humans. Ann Otol Rhinol Laryngol Suppl. 1982; 91(2 Pt 3):117–124

[2] Hitselberger WE, House WF, Edgerton BJ, Whitaker S. Cochlear nucleus implants. Otolaryngol Head Neck Surg. 1984; 92(1):52–54

[3] Brackmann DE, Hitselberger WE, Nelson RA, et al. Auditory brainstem implant: I. Issues in surgical implantation. Otolaryngol Head Neck Surg. 1993; 108(6):624–633

[4] Shannon RV, Fayad J, Moore J, et al. Auditory brainstem implant: II. Postsurgical issues and performance. Otolaryngol Head Neck Surg. 1993; 108(6): 634–642

[5] Hochmair I, Hochmair E, Nopp P, Waller M, Jolly C. Deep electrode insertion and sound coding in cochlear implants. Hear Res. 2015; 322:14–23

[6] Behr R, Colletti V, Matthies C, et al. New outcomes with auditory brainstem implants in NF2 patients. Otol Neurotol. 2014; 35(10):1844–1851

[7] Todt I, Rademacher G, Mittmann P, Wagner J, Mutze S, Ernst A. MRI artifacts and cochlear implant positioning at 3 T in vivo. Otol Neurotol. 2015; 36:972–6

[8] Schroder D, Grupe G, Rademacher G, et al. Magnetic resonance imaging artifacts and cochlear implant positioning at 1.5 T in vivo. Biomed Res Int. 2018; 2018:9163285

[9] Kileny PR, Zwolan TA, Zimmerman-Phillips S, Telian SA. Electrically evoked auditory brain-stem response in pediatric patients with cochlear implants. Arch Otolaryngol Head Neck Surg. 1994; 120(10):1083–1090

[10] Aso S, Gibson WP. Surgical techniques for insertion of a multi-electrode implant into a postmeningitic ossified cochlea. Am J Otol. 1995; 16(2):231–234

[11] Lassaletta L, Polak M, Huesers J, et al. Usefulness of electrical auditory brainstem responses to assess the functionality of the cochlear nerve using an intracochlear test electrode. Otol Neurotol. 2017; 38(10):e413–e420

[12] Özbal Batuk M, Çınar BÇ, Özgen B, Sennaroğlu G, Sennaroğlu L. Audiological and radiological characteristics in incomplete partition malformations. J Int Adv Otol. 2017; 13(2):233–238

[13] Dahm V, Auinger AB, Arnoldner C et al. Simultaneous vestibular schwannoma resection and cochlear implantation using electrically evoked auditory brainstem response audiometry for decision-making. Otol Neurotol. 2020; 41

[14] Waring MD. Auditory brain-stem responses evoked by electrical stimulation of the cochlear nucleus in human subjects. Electroencephalogr Clin Neurophysiol. 1995; 96(4):338–347

[15] Polak M, Colletti L, Colletti V. Novel method of fitting of children with auditory brainstem implants. Eur Ann Otorhinolaryngol Head Neck Dis., 2018; 135(6):403–409

[16] Matthies C, Brill S, Kaga K, et al. Auditory brainstem implantation improves speech recognition in neurofibromatosis type II patients. ORL J Otorhinolaryngol Relat Spec. 2013; 75(5):282–295

12 Programming, Rehabilitation, and Outcome Assessment for Adults: I

Daniel S. Roberts, Lawrence Kashat, Jordan M. Rock, and Steven R. Otto

Abstract

Loss of integrity of the auditory nerve after surgical removal of vestibular schwannomas (VS) in neurofibromatosis type 2 (NF2) is a frequent occurrence. In cases where patients completely deafened either by the natural history of NF2 or by surgery, the auditory brainstem implant (ABI) may be used to bypass the auditory nerve and directly stimulate the cochlear nucleus complex. Patients have significantly benefited from ABI and useful auditory sensations have resulted in the majority of patients.[1,2] The multichannel version of the ABI (Nucleus®, Cochlear Corporation, Englewood, Colorado) successfully completed US Food and Drug Administration (FDA) clinical trials in July 2000 and received approval for commercial release. ABIs have also been produced by other implant manufacturers including MED-EL, which are not approved for use in the US. This chapter summarizes the performance of patients with NF2 implanted with an ABI and focuses on the programming and auditory rehabilitation.

Keywords: auditory brainstem implantation, ABI, neurofibromatosis type 2, NF2

12.1 Outcomes

Establishing reasonable expectations for patients is paramount from counseling perspective in auditory brainstem implant (ABI) recipients. It should be clearly defined that ABI provides most patients with some degree of environmental sound awareness and in conjunction with lipreading is typically is a beneficial rehabilitation strategy.[3,4,5,6] Notably, a minority of patients obtain open-set speech understanding.[3,7,8]

Over 350 patients with NF2 have been implanted with the multichannel ABI system at House Clinic between 1992 and the present (▶ Fig. 12.1) and approximately 1,300 patients have been implanted worldwide.[2] With few exceptions at our center, the performance of ABI does not typically reach the results of cochlear implantation. Approximately, 80% of our implant recipients are device users and higher percentage (92%) received auditory sensations. Most patients recognize environmental sounds and speech understanding is enhanced by an average of 35% when ABI sound is combined with lipreading. In our clinic, approximately 25% of ABI users have achieved open-set speech discrimination (at least 20% correct without lipreading cues on the City University of New York [CUNY] Sentence Test).[9,10]

Reports from some European centers suggest notably better audiometric outcomes compared to data from the United States. Among NF2 recipients, open-set speech perception was noted in 37 and 41% of patients within 2 years of activation.[8,11] These outcomes have significantly improved upon data from the United States and factors accounting for these improved outcomes are an area of active investigation. One interesting consideration is whether phonetic differences between languages play a role in open-set outcome results[7,12,13,14] (▶ Table 12.1).

A comprehensive analysis of the available literature suggests preponderance of patients' benefit from a rehabilitation standpoint. We performed a comprehensive analysis of all the world literature. Key words for our literature search included auditory

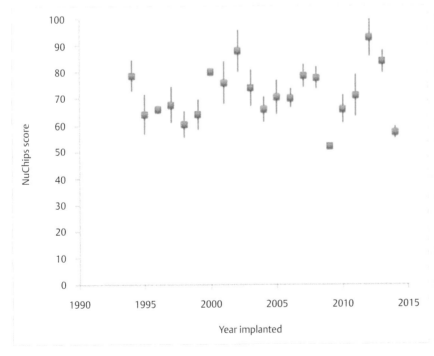

Fig. 12.1 Auditory brainstem implant (ABI) performance over a 20-year period (1994–2014) at the House Ear Institute for 130 adult NF2 patients with a minimum of 2-year follow-up. (Average +/– SEM) (unpublished data).

Table 12.1 Summary of prospective and retrospective original studies of adult ABI patients

First author	Number active electrodes mean (range)	Number of patients (N)	Daily user (%)	Patients with environ. sound awareness (%)	Open-set scores	Age at implant mean (range) (years)	Follow-up duration mean (range) (months)	Nation	Duration hearing loss mean (range) (months)	Tumor size mean (range) (mm)
Roberts, DS[15]	10.14 (0–18)	7	NR	NR	NR	32.5 (17–52)	6.6 (3–9)	USA	NR	NR
Nakatomi, H[3]	At activation: 9 (5–12) Most recent: 6.7 (1–12)	11	NR	100%	20%	46 (25–66)	NR	Japan	46.5 (0–204)	17.5 (0–35)
Thong, J[12]	14 (9–18)	8	38%	75%, 6 months 63%, 2 years	0% (65% at 1–2 years w/lipreading)	31.2 (22–54)	11 (4–18)	China	NR	30 (15–55)
Puram, SV[16]	12.5 (8–21)	5	NR	100%	NR	20–68	2.5	USA	NR	NR
Lundin, K[17]	NR	11	73%	Did not assess	Did not assess	NR	NR	Sweden	NR	NR
McKay, CM[18]	NR	5	NR	NR	NR	NR	NR	UK	NR	NR
McSorley, A[19]	NR	23	54%	NR	NR	NR	6 (1.5–15)	UK	NR	NR
Herrmann, BS[20]	9.5	4	75%	100%	NR	32 (16–48)	NR	USA	NR	NR
Behr, R[21]	Total electrodes = 8.4 (5–12) # Distinct pitch electrodes = 8.2 (5–11)	26	NR	All patients for study eligibility	Minimum 30% to be included in the study	>60% open-set= 36.3 (19–63) <60% open-set= 30.6 (21–68)	NR	Multi-nation	Statistically improved scores if < 1 year	NR
Mandalà, M[34]	17.2 (surgery+EABR/ECAP) vs. 13.1 (surgery+EABR/EMG alone)	9 exp. & 9 cont.	NR	NR	78.9% in surgery+EABR+ECAP 56.7% in surgery+EABR only	47.3–51.9 (mean)	>48 months	Italy	>10 years	NR
Siegbahn, M[7]	13.3 (at activation) →11.6 (most recent follow-up)	20	65%	9/20 patients	1/20 patients	5.5 (15–75)	0–16 years	Sweden	NR	NR
Matthies, C[8]	Positive correlation noted between # active electrodes and speech discrimination scores	18	NR	NR	24 months–12 of 16 patients (32.5% at 12 months, 41% at 24 months)	37.6 (19–66)	1–5 years	Germany	NR	Tumor volume did not correlate with speech scores
Matthies, C[11]	8.8 (5–12)	32	NR	NR	12 months–37%	38.4 (19–66)	1 year	Multi-nation	NR	NR

(continued)

Table 12.1 Summary of prospective and retrospective original studies of adult ABI patients. (continued)

First author	Number active electrodes mean (range)	Number of patients (N)	Daily user (%)	Patients with environ. sound awareness (%)	Open-set scores	Age at implant mean (range) (years)	Follow-up duration mean (range) (months)	Nation	Duration hearing loss mean (range) (months)	Tumor size mean (range) (mm)
Sanna, M[22]	12 → 13 (most recent follow-up)	24	79%	82%	8 of 23	35 (18–69)	2 years	Italy	NR	3 cm
Colletti, V[23]	NR	34 with VS (T) 48 nontumor (NT)	NR	NR	T: 16% (5–31%) NT: 53% (10–100%)	NR	Min 1 year	Italy	T: 5.1 (3.2–8.5) NT: 9.6 (1.2–19.8)	NR
Maini et al[24]	NR	10	70%	NR	~0% →8% (later follow-up)	31.5 (17–46)	5 years (1–12)	Australia	NR	NR
Bento, RF[25]	3 pts >12; 1 patient with only	4	NR	NR	NR	25–28	NR	Brazil	NR	Intrancranial – 3.5 cm
Otto, S[26]	Penetrating electrodes range: 0–7	10		NR	2.6%	36.9 (19–53)	NR	USA	NR	NR
Grayeli, AB[14]	NR	31 23 = NF2 8 = NT	NF2 = 70% NT = 75%	NR	NF2 = 8 pts > 50% NT = 5 pts > 50%	NF2 = 36 (17–59) NT = 52 (37–71)	NF2: 43 (12–120) Nontumor: 39 (6–100)	France	NR	NR
Colletti, V[27]	NF2: 5–21 Nontumor: 11–14	Total: 39 25 nontumor and 14 NF2	NR	NR	Nontumor: 59% Tumor: 11%	NR	1 year or greater	Italy	NR	4–52 mm
Colletti, V[13]	NR	20, 10 NF2, 10 NT	NR	NR	Nontumor: 65% Tumor: 10%	NR	NR	Italy	NR	NR
Kanowitz, SJ[28]	8 pts w/N22 – 4.3 3 pts w/N24 – 11.3	18	61%	NR	0%	33.5% → 45.33%	21 (2–78)	USA	NR	25 mm (9–50)
Lenarz, M[29]	NR	14	100	NR	NR	NR	NR	Germany	NR	NR
Nevison, B[5]	12.4 → 8.6	27	NR	NR	Improved w/ lip-reading & ABI	33.1 (13–58)	NR	Multi-nation	NR	2.71 cm
Otto, SR[6]	NR	61	NR	>50% for most patients	Rare	12–71	NR	USA	NR	NR
Vincent, C[30]	NR	14	NR	20–100%	5 of 9 patients (10–30%)	27 (14–56)	25	France, Italy	NR	NR
Lenarz, T[4]	NR	14	93	NR	Rare and late	40 (24–61)	19 (1–41)	Germany	30 (2–144)	NR

Abbreviations: ABI, auditory brainstem implant; EABR, evoked auditory brainstem response; ECAP, evoked compound nerve action potential; EMG, electromyography; NF2, neurofibromatosis type 2; VS; vestibular schwannomas.

brainstem implant, neuroprosthetic device, auditory neuropathy, deafness, deafness treatment, acoustic stimulation, auditory cortex, brain mapping, evoked potentials, recovery of function, psychoacoustics, and humans. Our search generated 117 articles of which 26 were included in our literature review (▶ Table 12.1). Articles were included in our analysis if they were original prospective or retrospective studies which included a primarily adult population. The majority of patients experienced some component of sound perception. Associated with lipreading, ABI is a beneficial strategy. A minority of patients achieved open-set speech recognition (▶ Table 12.1).

Factors leading to high performance of the ABI remain an area of active investigation and the specific factors that may lead to enhanced performance remain to be fully characterized.[31] Large case series are not available for analysis and multivariate analysis has not been performed to date. Several variables are suggested to be important factors for performance. These include the number of electrodes utilized during programming, tumor characteristics such as tumor size at the time of resection or prior history of radiation, the influence of time after implantation to maximal performance, differences in device design and processor function, and differences in surgical technique. It is also likely that some of the factors that are reported to be important for cochlear implantation performance, such as duration of deafness, are also important factors for ABI. Differences in patient selection may also be an important variable which may differ between implantation centers.

12.1.1 Electrode Number—Evolution of the ABI

William House and William Hitselberger developed the first ABI and implanted the first patient in 1979[1] with a modified cochlear implant fitted with two ball electrodes placed on the cochlear nucleus. The device used in the early 1990s included three platinum plates mounted on Akron mesh backing. Stimulation of electrodes produced auditory sensations in most patients, which were comparable to the results with the original ABI.[9] Over time, the device was modified to include eight electrodes

through a collaboration with Cochlear Corporation and the eight-electrode device was implanted between 1993 and 1999, leading to FDA approval in 2000.[2] Early in the experience with the eight electrode multichannel ABI, it was demonstrated that high performance with the ABI was possible. In a series of 20 patients, 3 patients achieved sound-only sentence recognition scores between 49 and 58% with the notable ability to speak on the telephone.[32] These results were further supported with long-term data, where the 8-electrode multichannel device proved capable of providing some patients with an ability to understand speech by using the sound from the ABI without the assistance of lipreading cues.[6]

The device that has been implanted at our center from 2000 to present includes 21-electrode contacts in the array. With this retrospective historical data, an important question is whether or not the increase in electrode contacts is important. Data from the House Ear Institute indicates that performance improved after 1999, when the number of electrodes was increased to 21 electrodes from 8 electrodes (NUCHIPS testing, and univariate analysis, unpublished data) (▶ Fig. 12.2). Clearly, other variables such as improvements in surgical techniques or other factors could also account for these findings.

Among high performers, analysis was performed with the goal of determining the number of active electrodes that are needed for open-set performance. In an analysis of 22 patients, all patients had seven or more active electrodes. The correlation of performance to a greater number of active electrodes was a weak correlation ($R^2 = 0.2554$) (▶ Fig. 12.3). Similarly, in a multicenter retrospective study of 26 patients who performed highly with 30% or better on correct identification of sentences testing, there was no correlation between performance and electrodes utilized.[21]

12.1.2 Tumor Characteristics—Size and History of Radiation

Tumor characteristics could also account for differences in outcomes. Specifically, tumor size where larger tumors equate to poor performance is hypothesized. A secondary consideration

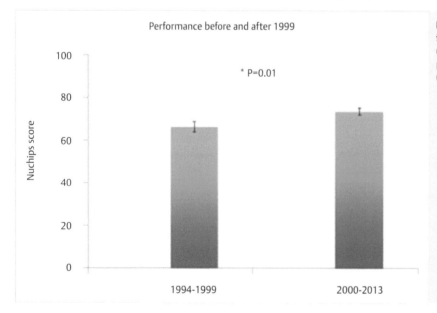

Performance before and after 1999

Fig. 12.2 Auditory brainstem implant (ABI) performance 1994–1999 ($n = 31$) and 2000–2013 ($n = 73$) at the House Ear Institute for adult NF2 patients with a minimum of 2-year follow-up. (Average +/− SEM) (unpublished data).

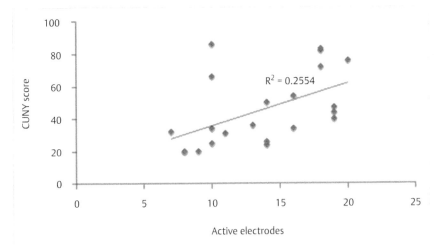

Fig. 12.3 Correlation between active electrodes and City University of New York (CUNY) scores among open-set performers ($N = 22$) (unpublished data).

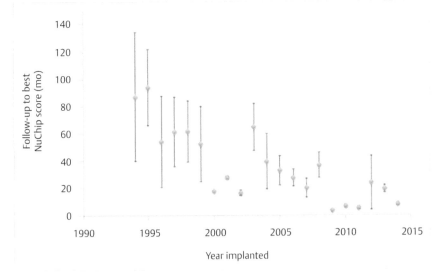

Fig. 12.4 Auditory brainstem implant (ABI) performance as a function of follow-up time and year of implantation over a 20-year period (1994–2014) for 130 adult NF2 patients with a minimum of 2-year follow-up. (Average $+/-$ SEM) (unpublished data).

would be a prior history of stereotactic radiosurgery prior to implantation. In an early study of outcomes at our institution of 17 ABI implants, tumor size was not correlated to patient outcomes.[33] A similar finding was also demonstrated among high-performing ABI recipients. Tumor size was also not correlated to audiometric performance.[21] We have analyzed patients who received stereotactic radiosurgery prior to tumor resection. Patients with a history of stereotactic radiosurgery had a higher incidence of failure to achieve auditory sensations from their ABIs (30%) than those who did not (8%). When active ABI users were compared to historical controls, there was no difference between audiometric outcomes (NUCHIPS testing). Patients who had previously received ipsilateral stereotactic radiosurgery ($N = 8$) achieved a NUCHIPS score of 80% $+/-6.9$ Standard Error of the Mean (SEM) versus 71% $+/-1.39$ ($N = 130$) for historical controls (unpublished data). Follow-up times between both groups were comparable (radiosurgery 38 months $+/-14.4$ SEM; historical controls 42 months $+/-3.7$ SEM). Based on these data, it is likely that previous ipsilateral stereotactic radiosurgery does not influence audiometric outcomes if auditory sensations may be initially achieved after implantation.

12.1.3 Time to Optimal Performance

While the majority of the improvements were seen during the first year, many patients continue to improve over a decade. In the recently unpublished analysis of the results at the House Ear Institute, the average duration of best performance using NUCHIPS testing was 36 months. ▶ Fig. 12.4 illustrates the overall trend of longer follow-up times to better ABI performance. While clearly this data is possibly skewed toward successful implant recipients who seek further programming modifications, the overall trend suggest that sustained utilization of the device leads to better outcomes. Similar improvements with sustained use have also been reported in other studies.[8,12,24]

12.1.4 Device Differences

Differences in implantable devices may account for possible differential outcomes. A majority of ABI procedures use either the Cochlear Corporation device or the MED-EL device. A principal difference in devices is the number of electrode channels. The Cochlear device utilizes 21 electrodes while the MED-EL device uses 12. The MED-EL device also differs from the Cochlear device in that the MED-EL device has enhanced cable flexibility and a smaller surface area profile of the electrode array (electrode array size is 8 × 3 mm for Cochlear vs. 5 × 3 mm for MED-EL). Stimulation strategy also differs between the two devices. The MED-EL device also contains a four-channel test electrode, which allows for the electrically evoked auditory brainstem response (EABR) testing to occur intraoperatively prior to the final placement of the electrode array. It is unclear whether these device differences may be correlated to performance; however, it should be noted that the highest number of high performers have occurred after implantation with the MED-EL device.[31]

Another consideration is use of EABR at the time of activation which may be performed for all devices. One retrospective study evaluated 202 patients with ABIs fitted with EABR during the implant fitting and compared outcomes with patients who also underwent electrical compound action potential recording (matched to a control group of 9 patients who only had the EABR recorded).[34] Of note, electrical compound action potential during ABI significantly improved the definition of the potential threshold, number of auditory and extra-auditory waves that were generated, and led to an improvement in open-set speech scores.

12.1.5 Surgical Procedure

Surgical approach is hypothesized to contribute to patient outcomes.[31] Suitable candidates are patients who are undergoing translabyrinthine or retrosigmoid VS. The retrosigmoid approach in the semi-sitting position with a MED-EL ABI device (not FDA approved in the United States) is primarily utilized by European centers while a translabyrinthine approach has been primarily used at the House Ear Institute.[16,35] The retrosigmoid approach is particularly useful in cases where the sigmoid sinus is located anteriorly. The retrosigmoid approach combined with the semi-sitting position is argued to be superior because the semi-sitting position may facilitate brain relaxation and bloodless dissection. The semi-sitting position is believed to reduce intraoperative bleeding by reduction of venous pressure. Positioning may subsequently improve hemostasis, reducing the requirement for electrocautery, and improving health of the neural tissue in the auditory brainstem nucleus. The semi-sitting position must be performed with the rare added risk of air embolism.[36] In a meeting of the ABI neurosurgeons in 2012, surgical factors were highlighted as a key component for differential outcomes. However, it is unclear what specific surgical difference could possibly account for these observations.[31]

12.1.6 Patient Selection

Originally, the ABI device was designed for patients with NF2. FDA criteria include bilateral VIIIth-nerve tumors, age 12 years or older, psychological suitability, willingness to comply with the follow-up protocol, and realistic expectations. At the House Clinic, implantation may occur at the time of first- or second-side acoustic neuroma removal or in patients whose tumors have previously been removed. Implantation during removal of the first tumor ("sleeper" implantation) allows patient to gain experience with the device and may enhance performance if the patient loses all hearing. Suitable candidates are patients undergoing translabyrinthine or retrosigmoid VS removal who have (1) non-serviceable hearing or an only-hearing ear with a symptomatic tumor or (2) serviceable hearing in the contralateral ear but a contralateral tumor of sufficient size to indicate that hearing will potentially be lost (a so-called "sleeper" ABI). Implantation on the first side gives the patient two chances at obtaining an optimally functioning system should the procedure in the first side is not successful which may occur in up to 8% of cases. With respect to speech perception performance in our first-side implantees, data from our center suggests that these patients improve by an average of 20% in their scores between the time when they were first implanted and the time when their second schwannoma was removed, even if they had considerable hearing remaining on their second tumor side. So, in effect, recipients are 20% further along in terms of performance if they become completely reliant on their ABI for hearing compared to recipients who waited until implantation at the time of a second VS resection.

From the outcomes standpoint, it is not fully known whether residual hearing at the time of implantation influences audiometric outcomes. Limited early experience with the ABI in 15 patients indicates that preoperative hearing level was not correlated to audiometric performance.[33] In a more recent analysis, speech recognition was correlated with duration of deafness. Patients who were deafened for less than 1 year had a greater likelihood of high performance compared to those who were deaf for greater than 1 year.[21] A central question is whether different ABI implantation centers differ in patient selection through any of these measures.

12.2 Programming and Rehabilitation

Over the course of 30 + years at House Ear Institute/House Clinic, we have been involved in the management of over 350 adult ABI recipients and conducted thousands of hours of sound processor programming. This has been primarily with the Nucleus ABI manufactured by Cochlear Corporation (Centennial, CO), the only device with FDA approval in the US. Much of the information that follows may also be applicable to ABI devices from other manufacturers.

Fundamental to a successful ABI program is the thorough and appropriate preparation of patients and their families. There is no substitute for realistic expectations and informed consent, especially in individuals who already may have other serious problems related to NF2.

Experience in programming CIs is a prerequisite to programming ABIs. Also, it is essential to take the manufacturer's Auditory Brainstem Programming Course and to follow the manufacturer's published guides. Initial programming sessions should be undertaken with the assistance of an experienced ABI audiologist, preferably a representative of the ABI manufacturer.

Electrical stimulation of the auditory brainstem can result in very different percepts than electrical stimulation of the cochlea, and these responses typically change over time. Therefore, programming ABIs is not the same as programming CIs. However, many of the techniques and procedures used with CIs can be effectively adapted to, and serve as a basis for, programming

ABIs. Programming ABIs requires additional steps, time, care, and flexibility to assess, interpret, and appropriately accommodate patient responses. This fact should be considered in all phases of ABI recipient management.

While ABI performance can be excellent, it generally doesn't start that way, or match typical CI performance. Considerable publicity exists about outstanding CI results, and ABI candidates should be clearly informed about this difference preoperatively. Reassurance that improvement requires time and experience but can continue for many years has been very encouraging to ABI recipients concerned about their progress. Giving up too soon means patients will miss out on the considerable benefits that accrue to more persistent ABI users.

It bears repeating that we are dealing with direct electrical stimulation of the brain. Although ABI stimulation has been demonstrated to be safe over the long term, manufacturers have specified additional measures to protect ABI recipients and clinicians, and those measures should be carefully followed.[37] In doing so, the ABI is still benefitting users almost 40 years after its initial use, and its indications have broadened to include infants without viable auditory nerves.

12.2.1 General Plan for Programming

Prior to initial testing, audiologists should carefully organize equipment and materials and ensure that emergency equipment/procedures/personnel are in place. Follow manufacturer's instructions implicitly. Printed patient instructions should be at hand, as well as a brief summary of possible outcomes and general goals and procedures of the test session. These should be reviewed immediately prior to initial testing. The outcomes should be the same as those discussed preoperatively. It should be stated to everyone present at the initial activation that the primary goal is to achieve a sound processor program that is comfortable for the patient to listen to, and that optimizing performance will continue over many follow-up visits.

With respect to scheduling, it has worked well to allow one and a half days over consecutive days for the initial activation of ABIs, including follow-up appointments with surgeons. Since ABI recipients typically have NF2, things may need to proceed more slowly than with CI recipients. Generally, it has worked well to try to achieve an initial complement of usable electrodes as soon as possible on the first morning so that recipients can try the sound processor over lunch on the first day. In the afternoon, any difficulties encountered over lunch can be addressed, and further testing can be done to expand the number of usable electrodes. Time also should be spent on a careful assessment of electrode-specific pitch percepts and this information employed in assigning electrodes appropriately to frequency analysis bandwidths. The patients can then be sent for an overnight trial of their equipment.

During a half day appointment on Day 2, any overnight difficulties can be addressed, threshold and comfortable loudness levels re-measured, and the patients prepped for taking their equipment home. Baseline speech perception testing may also be initiated. Although patients initially may feel they are guessing at responses, reassure them that the testing is to establish a performance baseline for documenting later improvements.

Traditionally, follow up every 3 months for the first year after device activation has worked well in order to accommodate changes in electrical hearing that are common with ABIs. After the first year, at least annual follow-up appointments work well. Patients should be reminded of the importance of these "tune-ups" to keep them hearing optimally. Follow-up visits typically are adapted to suit the needs of the returning patients. Some patients require more repetition of earlier testing, some do not. It is best to be conservative and do more testing rather than less to validate earlier results and make sure than any electrical hearing differences are accommodated appropriately.

12.2.2 Programming Session

The overriding aim of the ABI test session should be to focus on the patients and their responses. Distractions in the room should be eliminated, including small children or more than one or two observers. Questions should be reserved for test breaks. Be as familiar as possible with the programming software and the general steps for programming.

With respect to initial defaults for basic map parameters, a monopolar mode has proven useful (MP1 + 2 for Nucleus devices) along with 100 micro-second per phase pulse durations and the SPEAK (spectral maxima) processing strategy. This provides a good compromise of generally lower threshold and comfortable loudness levels, reasonable dynamic ranges, and minimizes nonauditory side effects. For the initial test electrodes, selecting an electrode in the middle of the array increases the likelihood of obtaining usable electrodes quickly.

Before electrical testing can begin, the location of the ABI receiver-stimulator antenna coil must be clearly identified. The surgeon hopefully will have placed the receiver-stimulator within about 1.5 to 2 inches of the pinna in an area of the skull where there is minimal curvature to allow the transmitter coil to sit as flat as possible over the implant. This will facilitate providing an optimal power signal to the implant, which of course is fundamental to all ABI testing.

In ABI recipients with NF2, typically there is no magnet in the implant receiver-stimulator to assist with aligning the transmitter coil over the implant antenna since the magnet is removed at the time of implantation. In lieu of the implant magnet, the telemetry feature of the Nucleus device can be used to indicate when the transmitter coil is in approximately the correct location. Then an elastic headband can be used to hold the transmitter coil over this location for initial threshold and comfortable loudness measurements on a few electrodes. When this is done, mark the location on the scalp of the center of the transmitter coil, shave a quarter-sized area around this mark, clean the area with alcohol, and carefully dry and apply a retainer disk. The retainer disk is a round piece of tape with a small metal disk inside that is used in lieu of the implant magnet to keep the transmitter coil attached to the patient's head. The retainer disk itself, which is not magnetic, should be placed about an eighth of an inch higher (toward the top of the head) than the marked location, because the transmitter coil will tend to sit toward the lower edge of the disk. Then verify that the initial T and C levels on the tested electrodes are similar. Proceed with obtaining T and C levels on the rest of the electrodes, skipping for the moment any electrodes with more than very mild nonauditory side effects. When there is time, go back and test those other electrodes.

Initial ABI recipient test responses can be quite variable and perhaps even confusing to new as well as more experienced clinicians. Patients should be informed that optimizing the programming of their sound processor is critically dependent on clear, definite descriptions of what they are experiencing, especially threshold and comfortable loudness judgments. New clinicians should be alert for indefinite or highly variable responses that indicate the patient may not actually be hearing or feeling anything related to the stimulation from the ABI electrodes. It is possible to complete most of a test session, program a sound processor, and then find out the patient doesn't report hearing anything at all. Over decades of testing, there have been several instances of variable and indefinite responses from individuals with NF2 who have been taking pain medications that affect the central nervous system (CNS). Obviously, the ABI stimulates part of the CNS, so it is not surprising that there can be an effect on test results. Patients should be encouraged to be as certain as they can of their responses and as consistent as possible in reporting them.

12.2.3 Nonauditory Side Effects

Normally, ABI recipients will report nonauditory side effects on at least some electrodes, often in conjunction with hearing sensations. Side effects often can be reduced or eliminated by using longer pulse durations. Generally, a minimum of four electrodes can result in a usable ABI sound processor program, although within certain limits, more options for stimulation are generally better.

If it appears that few if any electrodes are going to provide auditory sensations for a patient, try to prepare everyone for this outcome as early in the process as possible to help prevent sudden disappointment. If things continue to proceed negatively, it will be necessary at some stage to inform the patients that they do not have any usable electrodes, and that the ABI is not going to work for them. Unless a person hears on at least one electrode, this situation rarely if ever reverses itself. If the patients have had an ABI when their first vestibular schwannoma was removed, then of course an excellent option is to have another ABI when the second VS is removed. We have done this many times, and at least half of these patients eventually have become some of our best-performing ABI users. If the patients' ABI was implanted on their second side, then of course there is no easy option for a second ABI.

In cases where patients report mild side effects in conjunction with auditory sensations on some electrodes, then those electrodes often may be retained for use since the side effects typically are not problematic when actually listening with the sound processor. Some patients who initially have had even moderate side effects on essentially all of their electrodes (in conjunction with auditory percepts) often have been able to use their ABIs anyway because the side effects have decreased or disappeared over time. Patients often have decided that it was worth putting up with some side effects in the interest of having some hearing. Careful monitoring of status is important in these individuals.

12.2.4 Electrode-Specific Pitch Assessment

Since it is well-established that ABI recipients can experience electrode-specific pitch percepts, an approach needs to be used to test and assign electrodes appropriately to frequency analysis bands. Detailed testing can make a substantial difference in perceptual performance, especially for patients who have more marked pitch sensations. In our experience, even 2 pitch-ranked electrodes can provide better speech recognition than 10 or more electrodes in random pitch rank order. Some patients report little if any pitch differences across electrodes. About 60% of adult ABI recipients at our center have experienced a generally rising pattern of pitch from the lateral to medial end of the electrode array. So, in the absence of actual electrode pitch measurements, it has worked well simply to assign electrodes numerically to frequency analysis bandwidths (lowest electrode number to the lowest frequency analysis bandwidth and the highest number electrode to the highest analysis bandwidth). This usually allows new patients to begin using their sound processors by the end of the first morning. This approach also has been used effectively in instances where patients don't report any significant difference in pitch sensation across electrodes. Reports of pitch sensations can substantially change as ABI recipients get more experience listening to ABI sound. ABI recipients often report changes in electrode pitch percepts over time; therefore, they should be periodically re-tested with appropriate alterations made in ABI programs. At some stage, particularly if patients have developed very good or excellent sound-only speech recognition, making changes to their electrode assignments may be more disruptive than beneficial. Good clinical judgment and the patient's own preferences must be used in this and all phases of ABI programming.

12.2.5 Long-Term ABI Use, Performance Assessment, and Rehabilitation

ABI recipients will vary in their abilities to use and manage their sound processors and related equipment because of physical disabilities related to NF2, including partial or complete blindness. These issues will have to be managed as well as possible by creative clinicians. Experience has shown that blindness particularly is a difficult issue because about half of the blind ABI recipients at our Center have become nonusers. Most ABI recipients do not have significant issues of this kind, and preparing them to take home and use their ABI systems is generally straightforward. Patients should be reminded that improving with ABIs requires regular use, and that generally the more they use it the faster they will improve and the better they will do. Basically, this is reiterating what they should have been told preoperatively, including that ABI performance can improve for as long as 10 years or more. Patients should be informed that even modest amounts of regular experience can result in considerable improvement over the long term. Once patients get over the initial hump, they usually begin to see this for themselves. Many ABI recipients have remarked how surprised they were at how indispensable their ABI sound eventually became.

Before leaving for home, new ABI recipients should be scheduled for their 3-month follow-up visit. Follow-up programming usually can be accomplished in less than a half day allowing for appointments with surgeons to be scheduled during the rest of the day. As opposed to CI follow-ups, it may be necessary to repeat much of the initial ABI testing in order to accommodate normal changes that can occur over time in ABI recipients' electrical hearing. Therefore, ABI reprogramming sessions should start on time and not be interrupted. It works best for these sessions to be completely separated from the physician appointments. That way any delays do not cut into the time needed by other specialists.

With respect to long-term speech recognition assessment, a combination of tests was used initially, including environmental sounds recognition, to document ABI performance. Over the years, it has been necessary to streamline the process. Presently, a four-choice sound-only word test (NUCHIPS) is used, as well as a sentence test (City University of New York Sentences, sound, vision, and sound + vision modes). This has worked well as an efficient means of monitoring patient performance. Other newer tests may be as effective, but it is of course important to use the same tests over time. Since ABI performance abilities vary widely, the tests selected should allow for this. For example, sound-only word or sentence recognition tests may be inappropriate for a substantial number of ABI recipients initially.

With respect to aural/auditory rehabilitation for ABI recipients, this can be of considerable value for many by speeding progress and improving performance. It is best conducted by certified professionals experienced in working with ABI recipients, but a certain amount of effective listening practice can be achieved even at home. There is no space here for detailed coverage of rehabilitative techniques for ABI recipients, but some general guidelines can be offered. The general approach should be based on the fact that, for most recipients, ABI sound is most useful when combined with lipreading cues. Therefore, ABI auditory rehab should focus on the sound plus lipreading mode. This will help patients associate their new sounds with what they are accustomed to seeing on people's faces. Simple words of their own choosing can be used initially, followed by short phrases, simple sentences, and so on. What works well is to provide a short list of words, phrases, sentences, or even a short paragraph to both the listener and the talker. The initial step would be for the talker to repeat simply the words in the order they are written on the page with the listener repeating them back as they are said. The goal is for the listener to watch and listen so that the listener is receiving in combined modalities. With practice, it will be possible for the talker to mix the order of the words, and perhaps even eventually to remove the lipreading cues entirely. This approach may seem too simple, but it actually works well for ABI recipients, particularly early on. This general method can form the basis of efficient and effective listening practice for ABI recipients. More advanced rehab activities can be based around the Speech Tracking technique originally described by De Filippo.[38] The basic idea is to provide appropriate, efficient, and effective aural rehabilitation for ABI users, to give them a feeling of achievement, and to emphasize to them that short but regular listening practice over the long term can result in considerable improvements. It certainly also has been the case that many ABI recipients have developed outstanding perceptual skills without the benefit of formal rehab by just using their implants regularly in their normal communication environments. Perhaps the factor most associated with this has been having small children to monitor in the household. Because of this necessity, perhaps these patients have developed into our best-performing users of all.

References

[1] Hitselberger WE, House WF, Edgerton BJ, Whitaker S. Cochlear nucleus implants. Otolaryngol Head Neck Surg. 1984; 92(1):52–54

[2] Shannon RV. Auditory implant research at the House Ear Institute 1989–2013. Hear Res. 2015; 322:57–66

[3] Nakatomi H, Miyawaki S, Kin T, Saito N. Hearing restoration with auditory brainstem implant. Neurol Med Chir (Tokyo). 2016; 56(10):597–604

[4] Lenarz T, Moshrefi M, Matthies C, et al. Auditory brainstem implant: part I. Auditory performance and its evolution over time. Otol Neurotol. 2001; 22 (6):823–833

[5] Nevison B, Laszig R, Sollmann WP, et al. Results from a European clinical investigation of the Nucleus multichannel auditory brainstem implant. Ear Hear. 2002; 23(3):170–183

[6] Otto SR, Brackmann DE, Hitselberger WE, Shannon RV, Kuchta J. Multichannel auditory brainstem implant: update on performance in 61 patients. J Neurosurg. 2002; 96(6):1063–1071

[7] Siegbahn M, Lundin K, Olsson G-B, et al. Auditory brainstem implants (ABIs)—20 years of clinical experience in Uppsala, Sweden. Acta Otolaryngol. 2014; 134(10):1052–1061

[8] Matthies C, Brill S, Varallyay C, et al. Auditory brainstem implants in neurofibromatosis type 2: is open speech perception feasible? J Neurosurg. 2014; 120(2):546–558

[9] Brackmann DE, Hitselberger WE, Nelson RA, et al. Auditory brainstem implant: I. Issues in surgical implantation. Otolaryngol Head Neck Surg. 1993; 108(6):624–633

[10] Shannon RV, Fayad J, Moore J, et al. Auditory brainstem implant: II. Postsurgical issues and performance. Otolaryngol Head Neck Surg. 1993; 108 (6):634–642

[11] Matthies C, Brill S, Kaga K, et al. Auditory brainstem implantation improves speech recognition in neurofibromatosis type II patients. ORL J Otorhinolaryngol Relat Spec. 2013; 75(5):282–295

[12] Thong JF, Sung JK, Wong TK, Tong MC. Auditory brainstem implantation in Chinese patients with neurofibromatosis type II: the Hong Kong experience. Otol Neurotol. 2016; 37(7):956–962

[13] Colletti V, Shannon RV. Open set speech perception with auditory brainstem implant? Laryngoscope. 2005; 115(11):1974–1978

[14] Grayeli AB, Kalamarides M, Bouccara D, Ambert-Dahan E, Sterkers O. Auditory brainstem implant in neurofibromatosis type 2 and non-neurofibromatosis type 2 patients. Otol Neurotol. 2008; 29(8):1140–1146

[15] Roberts DS, Slattery WH, Chen BS, Otto SR, Schwartz MS, Lekovic GP. Compassionate use" protocol for auditory brainstem implantation in neurofibromatosis type 2: early House Ear Institute experience. Cochlear Implants Int. 2017; 18(1):57–62

[16] Puram SV, Herrmann B, Barker FG, II, Lee DJ. Retrosigmoid craniotomy for auditory brainstem implantation in adult patients with neurofibromatosis type 2. J Neurol Surg B Skull Base. 2015; 76(6):440–450

[17] Lundin K, Stillesjö F, Nyberg G, Rask-Andersen H. Self-reported benefit, sound perception, and quality-of-life in patients with auditory brainstem implants (ABIs). Acta Otolaryngol. 2016; 136(1):62–67

[18] McKay CM, Azadpour M, Jayewardene-Aston D, O'Driscoll M, El-Deredy W. Electrode selection and speech understanding in patients with auditory brainstem implants. Ear Hear. 2015; 36(4):454–463

[19] McSorley A, Freeman SR, Ramsden RT, et al. Subjective outcomes of auditory brainstem implantation. Otol Neurotol. 2015; 36(5):873–878

[20] Herrmann BS, Brown MC, Eddington DK, Hancock KE, Lee DJ. Auditory brainstem implant: electrophysiologic responses and subject perception. Ear Hear. 2015; 36(3):368–376

[21] Behr R, Colletti V, Matthies C, et al. New outcomes with auditory brainstem implants in NF2 patients. Otol Neurotol. 2014; 35(10):1844–1851

[22] Sanna M, Di Lella F, Guida M, Merkus P. Auditory brainstem implants in NF2 patients: results and review of the literature. Otol Neurotol. 2012; 33(2): 154–164

[23] Colletti V, Shannon R, Carner M, Veronese S, Colletti L. Outcomes in nontumor adults fitted with the auditory brainstem implant: 10 years' experience. Otol Neurotol. 2009; 30(5):614–618

[24] Maini S, Cohen MA, Hollow R, Briggs R. Update on long-term results with auditory brainstem implants in NF2 patients. Cochlear Implants Int. 2009; 10 Suppl 1:33–37

[25] Bento RF, Neto RVB, Tsuji RK, Gomes MQT, Goffi-Gomez MVS. Auditory brainstem implant: surgical technique and early audiological results in patients with neurofibromatosis type 2. Rev Bras Otorrinolaringol (Engl Ed). 2008; 74 (5):647–651

[26] Otto SR, Shannon RV, Wilkinson EP, et al. Audiologic outcomes with the penetrating electrode auditory brainstem implant. Otol Neurotol. 2008; 29(8): 1147–1154

[27] Colletti V. Auditory outcomes in tumor vs. nontumor patients fitted with auditory brainstem implants. Adv Otorhinolaryngol. 2006; 64: 167–185

[28] Kanowitz SJ, Shapiro WH, Golfinos JG, Cohen NL, Roland JT, Jr. Auditory brainstem implantation in patients with neurofibromatosis type 2. Laryngoscope. 2004; 114(12):2135–2146

[29] Lenarz M, Matthies C, Lesinski-Schiedat A, et al. Auditory brainstem implant part II: subjective assessment of functional outcome. Otol Neurotol. 2002; 23 (5):694–697

[30] Vincent C, Zini C, Gandolfi A, et al. Results of the MXM Digisonic auditory brainstem implant clinical trials in Europe. Otol Neurotol. 2002; 23(1):56–60

[31] Colletti L, Shannon R, Colletti V. Auditory brainstem implants for neurofibromatosis type 2. Curr Opin Otolaryngol Head Neck Surg. 2012; 20(5):353–357

[32] Otto SR, Shannon RV, Brackmann DE, Hitselberger WE, Staller S, Menapace C. The multichannel auditory brain stem implant: performance in twenty patients. Otolaryngol Head Neck Surg. 1998; 118(3 Pt 1):291–303

[33] Otto SR, House WF, Brackmann DE, Hitselberger WE, Nelson RA. Auditory brain stem implant: effect of tumor size and preoperative hearing level on function. Ann Otol Rhinol Laryngol. 1990; 99(10 Pt 1):789–790

[34] Mandalà M, Colletti L, Colletti G, Colletti V. Improved outcomes in auditory brainstem implantation with the use of near-field electrical compound action potentials. Otolaryngol Head Neck Surg. 2014; 151(6):1008–1013

[35] Colletti V, Sacchetto L, Giarbini N, Fiorino F, Carner M. Retrosigmoid approach for auditory brainstem implant. J Laryngol Otol Suppl. 2000(27):37–40

[36] Wong AY, Irwin MG. Large venous air embolism in the sitting position despite monitoring with transoesophageal echocardiography. Anaesthesia. 2005; 60(8): 811–813

[37] Otto SR, Moore J, Linthicum F, Hitselberger W, Brackmann D, Shannon RV. Histopathological analysis of a 15-year user of an auditory brainstem implant. Laryngoscope. 2012; 122(3):645–648

[38] de Filippo CL. Tracking for speechreading training. Volta Review. 1988; 90(5): 215–239

13 Programming, Rehabilitation, and Outcome Assessment for Adults: II

Cordula Matthies, Anja Kurz, and Wafaa Shehata-Dieler

Abstract

Programming of auditory brainstem implant (ABI) in adult patients aims for providing as many auditory electrodes as possible at most comfortable levels and preferably evoking a wide range of pitch sensation, through a standardized structured protocol. This includes repeat follow-up at defined intervals for checking of technical integrity, stable impedances, and re-arranging pitch sequence according to individual auditory development. First, nonauditory or partially auditory electrodes are checked repeatedly for acoustic input and may be selected for secondary activation.

Training is guided by specialized speech therapists, trained by the University Clinic, and comprises regular exercises with family, with mobile and computer-based programs, and repeated outpatient/inpatient training series.

Troubleshooting in case of absent sound perception or secondary failure has to consider technical defects as well as lost or displaced electrode contacts as well as degenerative processes and will lead to identification of those candidates with good prospects through revision surgery.

Outcome of patients' acoustic abilities considers detection, discrimination, and identification of sound qualities and is evaluated regularly by standardized investigations such as loudness scaling, vowel confusion test, syllable and pattern identification by Monosyllabic-Trochee-Polysyllabic (MTP) test and word and sentence recognition by Freiburg, and Matrix and Hochmair-Schulz-Moser (HSM) tests.

Long-term improvement is a never-ending process with speech discrimination developing over days to 6 months and continuous functional increase over 3 years, and further ultrasensitive abilities like perception of bird wings movements and of music melodies over one to several years.

Keywords: auditory brainstem implants, ABI in adults, auditory perception, stimulation strategy, neurofibromatosis type 2, stimulation side effects, Matrix test, Hochmair–Schulz–Moser test, evoked auditory brainstem response

13.1 First Implant Activation

13.1.1 Clinical Preparation

Timing

An early temporary activation of the auditory brainstem implant (ABI) may be planned within the first 7 to 10 days after surgery. This temporary activation gives the opportunity to control the integrity of the ABI system and the impedances of the electrodes, and it may provide an early chance to the patient of experiencing some sound perception.

Before permanent activation, after surgical implantation of the ABI, a minimum period of 4 weeks is calculated for the local integration of the ABI electrode carrier within the foramen of Luschka. The first 4 to 6 weeks are regarded as the most sensitive period for electrode dislocation, either "spontaneously" or secondarily to a fall. The start of ABI activation should be planned for *after* this period.[1,2] Routinely, at 6 weeks after surgery, the date for ABI activation is scheduled and the patient is admitted for 3 days to the Comprehensive Hearing Center (CHC).

Neurological–Neurosurgical Evaluation

At the time of admittance for activation, a general clinical and neurological–neurosurgical examination is performed. Specific attention is given to the recent history of special events reported by the patient such as constant or repetitive headaches, local discomfort at the scar and implant site, signs of local inflammation, balance disturbance, vertigo, and falls.

The region of the scar and of the implant are inspected for complete healing, closed surface over the implanted parts, and for exclusion of fluid accumulation, hydrocephalus, redness or other signs of inflammation. In neurological testing, special attention is paid to caudal cranial nerves, vestibular and cerebellar functions, and exclusion of hydrocephalus.

Radiological Investigations

During the first 6 months, radiological diagnostics should be limited to cranial computed tomography (CT), while magnetic resonance imaging (MRI) is not recommended.

A first postsurgical cranial CT is recommended within the first few days after surgery, before demission from the clinic. This should exclude local hemorrhage, pneumocephalus, and brainstem displacement, and it should outline the course of the ABI cable and the location of the ABI electrode carrier. These early images will serve as a baseline for future comparison.

After 6 months of surgery, with the MED-EL device a cranial MRI is allowed under specific circumstances (▶ Fig. 13.3 a, b). But within the 6-monthinterval after ABI implantation, MRI is to be avoided as it might cause a lead dislocation.

At re-admission for activation, in the usual case of an uneventful course during the healing period, no further cranial imaging is planned. In case of recent falls or suspicion of any inflammation or of development of a hydrocephalus, a cranial CT is indicated.

Audiological Preparations

Speech Processor

A precondition to ABI activation and programming is the selection of the adequate sound processor unit. This is done with the patient before the ABI surgery in order to arrange an activation session with it.

13.1.2 Setting at Intensive Treatment Unit (ITU) (▶ Fig. 13.1)

Patient Monitoring and Setting with Professional Personnel

For adequate patient monitoring, first activation of a new ABI is ideally performed at the ITU in the presence of a neurosurgeon, an otolaryngologist, or a neuro-anesthesiologist, as stand-by in case of cardio-pulmonary disturbances. The patient receives a venous cannula in the forearm and is connected to continuous electrocardiogram (ECG) monitoring and pO2 monitoring. Besides, an audiologist and an electrical engineer will be present.

Technical Setup

The chosen sound processor is assembled and the connecting head piece attached. A magnet is placed in the head piece and checked for magnetic attraction. A stronger magnet can be inserted easily by the audiologist if required. The sound processor is connected to the programming platform containing the most recent fitting software (▶ Fig. 13.1).

Instructions to the Patient before and during ABI Activation

Communication during all ABI fitting sessions is enhanced/supported by the use of a large computer screen with text editing the investigator's instructions and questions.

Before starting the ABI activation, the procedure is explained to the patient: At first, a test of the integrity of the ABI system ("reduced telemetry" setting) will be performed. The "reduced telemetry" protocol is predefined for ABI patients in the MAESTRO software. In this procedure, the integrity and coupling of the implant are assessed without stimulation at the electrode contacts.

Thereafter, each electrode will be tested, one by one, and the patient will be asked to report the perception of any sensation, be it

• Some auditory sensation,
• Some tinnitus or ringing sensation,
• Any other sensory perception such as paresthesias, vertigo, dizziness a.s.o., or
• Any combination of auditory and nonauditory effects.

These categories are noted in the activation protocol. The stimulus intensity will be increased to a comfortable loudness level and any discomfort is reported. Electrodes with some auditory impression shall be identified from nonauditory electrodes and marked in the ABI scheme (▶ Fig. 13.2). At any unpleasant or uncomfortable sensation, this will be stopped instantaneously.

Stimulation Parameters

Stimulation via the implanted ABI is dependent on the technical characteristics of the used implant. While ABI systems by Cochlear Company apply bipolar stimulation modes, all the MED-EL Company systems perform in a monopolar mode. The recommended order of stimulation in the MED-EL electrode carrier is to start stimulating opposite electrodes as follows: E4, E9; E1, E12; E2, E3; E5, E6; E7, E8, E10, E11 (▶ Fig. 13.2).

The subsequent stimulation parameters will be adjusted highly individually:

• Stimulation amplitude (current units, CU, or micro-ampere, μA),
• Stimulation duration (100 to 300 μs),
• Stimulation frequency (16 to 33 Hz),
• Stimulation mode/strategy (FSP, HDCIS for ABI).

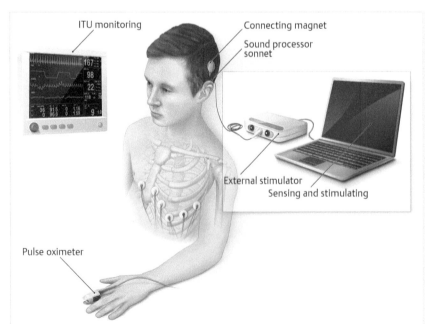

Fig. 13.1 Auditory brainstem implant (ABI) activation setup. The technical stimulation setup (used with permission from MED-EL, Innsbruck, Austria) for activation and programming of the ABI includes the external stimulator with connection cables and connecting magnetic head piece and the master computer platform, with the specialized software for sensing and stimulating the ABI. Intensive care unit monitoring of heart rate, blood pressure, oxygen saturation, and temperature are provided for the first programming session.

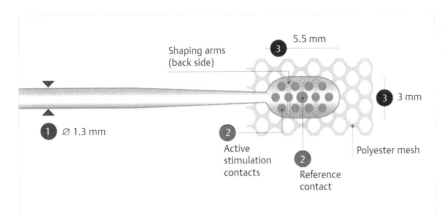

Fig. 13.2 Auditory brainstem implant (ABI) electrode carrier. The ABI electrode carrier (used with permission from MED-EL, Innsbruck, Austria) contains 12 electrode channels composed of platinum iridium, each being connected to independent current control sources and identified by its number. The central electrode is used as a reference. The electrodes are embedded in a silicone paddle-shaped carrier. The accompanying dacron net may be tailored with scissors depending on the extension of the lateral recess and the selected location for optimal lead placement. Before placing of the final electrode, a four-contact test electrode (embedded in a carrier of equivalent size) may be used for bipolar mapping.

13.2 Implant Programming

13.2.1 Activation Procedure

Control of Implant and Electrodes

At first activation, the control of the implant integrity and its connectivity to brain structures is essential and mandatory. Only after the proof of the system integrity, programming may be started. Whenever, in future adaptation procedures, a change of the stimulation program is attempted, this control has to be implemented as the basic first step. Depending on technical integrity and on the results of the electrode testing and produced effects, one can proceed further.

In the worst of cases, if all the channels are open, one needs to deactivate the system and consider revision surgery or explantation (see below). Also, in further programming procedures, the baseline control will serve as a reference to identify possible changes within the implant or in its relation with the brainstem.

Control of Implant Integrity and Viability

The electrode impedance is tested by applying a low intensity stimulation of 300 CU (phase duration of 24.2 µs) for most recent MED-EL implant types (Synchrony, Concerto, Sonata, Pulsar) that may be perceived by the patient. In ABI patients, not all electrode contacts might provide an auditory sensation. Hence, care should be taken in performing a "full impedance" check. It is recommended to proceed to the next step (see below, Perception Level of Single Electrodes). If all tested electrodes provide an auditory effect, no side effects, and a comfortable loudness level is achieved by stimulating with more than 7.2 CU, a "full impedance" measurement can be considered. The full impedance measurement evaluates the adequate contact of the electrodes with the brainstem surface and the integrity of the whole implant.

Perception Level of Single Electrodes

A step-by-step procedure is started with stimulation of one electrode at slowly increasing stimulation amplitude; here the patient will be asked to report the threshold level and any auditory or auditory-like sensations, and, thereafter, the comfort level and the level of discomfort as well as the level and type of side effects. The applied stimulation parameter and elicited effects are documented in the stimulation protocol for each electrode by the audiologist or the technical assistant.

Repeat Electrode Check

After a first testing of all the electrodes, a brief repeat testing is performed to control the sensation levels and which electrodes provide any acoustic sensation.

13.2.2 First Programming Procedure

After success in the first activation of the ABI, an individual program has to be designed and saved to the patient's sound processor. This program should largely exclude unpleasant side effects and enable some useful sound or noise perception.[2,3,4,5]

Designing the First Individual ABI Program

Electrode Selection

The electrodes causing unpleasant side effects are deactivated and marked in the protocol.[1] However, they should be re-tested in future procedures as they may produce sound sensations in some patients later on. Electrodes that repeatedly produce sound or noise sensations will be switched on. The stimulation intensity is adapted according to the patient's feedback at the most comfortable level.

Electrode Pitch

The next step involves a trial to put the electrodes in a sequence of tone heights. The patient is confronted with the sound produced by two electrodes and has to tell which gives a higher or lower pitch. Thereby, the investigator arranges the electrodes in a pitch sequence. This test is rather difficult and only a few patients will be able to complete it at first attempt.

First ABI Program

Once the auditory electrodes have been differentiated from the nonauditory ones, the latter are deactivated, and the auditory electrodes are switched on and are adjusted for their pitch and comfort levels. At the first programming, usually one ABI program is saved to the patient's sound processor.

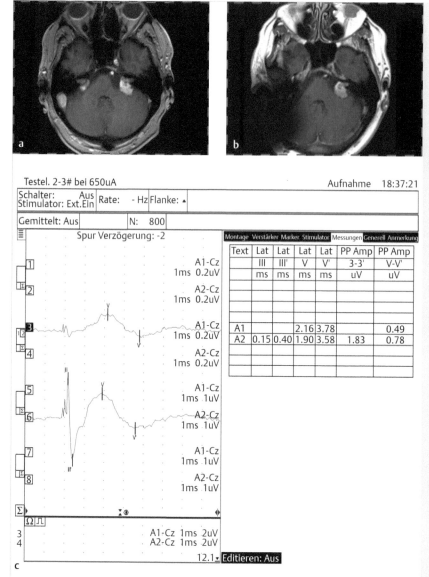

Fig. 13.3 **(a)** The presurgical magnetic resonance imaging (MRI) demonstrates the bilateral vestibular schwannomas, the right sided one 1 year after Cyberknife radio surgery. **(b)** The postsurgical MRI, 9 months after resection and ABI implantation, is free of any recurrence and with stable tumor extension on the left. **(c)** Intraoperative evoked auditory brainstem response (EABR). By test stimulation via the 4-pole-test electrode contralateral (trace A1, left side) and ipsilateral (trace A2, right surgical side) recording is positive with EABR components III, immediately after the stimulus artefact, III' and V/ V' well visible and reproducible.

For orientation, before starting the individual electrode configuration, an analysis of the intraoperative EABR and compound action potentials and their levels may indicate from which electrodes successful auditory sensations will be elicited (▶ Fig. 13.3 c).[6]

Instructions to the Patient after First Programming

Basic Instructions

The patient is instructed with regard to
- Handling the sound processor and the batteries,
- Using the remote control, and
- Increasing and decreasing the stimulation intensity.

Basic Tests

Simple tests are performed together with the patient in order to find out whether certain noises and sounds are perceived:
- Low frequency noise: drumming on the table
- High frequency noise: ringing of a door bell
- Identification of noise construction: twofold drumming, threefold drumming
- Identification of sound construction: twofold or threefold syllables: la-la, la-la-la

Then the next programming session is planned for the following day and the patient is encouraged to try out to listen to the sound processor for a couple of hours during the rest of the day.

13.2.3 Second Programming Procedure

The second ABI programming session is usually scheduled for the next morning when the patient is fit and not exhausted from other clinical investigation. This session serves for controlling whether the initial program is to be continued or needs to be changed and whether it is possible to leave the patient with it for a couple of weeks. Again, the exclusion of any unpleasant side effects and the identification of the comfortable stimulation intensity are two factors of great importance at this step and pre-conditions for the patient to be able to undergo hearing training during the coming weeks and months.

Adaptation of the First Individual ABI Program

First Patient Feedback

The patient reports on his/her first impressions with the activated ABI. Particularly, unpleasant sensations and the intensity of the perceived sensations are explored.

Electrode Selection

The previously selected electrodes are re-tested for sensation levels and comfort levels. If a minimum number of five electrodes are identified to give some auditory sensation, then no further electrode is tried currently.

Second ABI Program

Those electrodes that have been confirmed as auditory are kept switched on and are adjusted for sensation level and loudness. In the second programming session, live voice (produced by an audiologist) is used as reference for establishing a comfortable loudness level. It is not anticipated that the patient understands speech; it is rather the loudness perception of a periodically fluctuating stimuli such as speech which is tested. Then, the patient is prepared for expected and unexpected stimulation intensity. This can further be tested by applying very low and very high intensity noises.

One or Two ABI Programs

In some patients, early on, two different ABI programs are useful to be installed, one producing rather loud sensations and the other at lower intensity for noisy circumstances.

Instructions to the Patient at the End of the Second Programming Session

Basic Instructions

The patient is instructed for a second time with regard to
- Switching on and off of the sound processor,
- Increasing and decreasing stimulation intensity by using the remote control,
- Changing the ABI program,
- Handling the processor and the batteries,
- Duration of wearing the ABI, and
- Troubleshooting.

Early Tests

As on the first day, some simple tests are performed together with the patient to find out whether certain noises and sounds are perceived:
- Low frequency noise: drumming on the table
- High frequency noise: ringing of a door bell
- Identification of noise construction: twofold drumming, threefold drumming
- Identification of sound construction: twofold or threefold syllables: la-la, la-la-la
- Identification of vocals: dark (A, O, U) or light vocals (E, I)

Planning the Next Steps

If the patient feels confident to handle the ABI processor and does not report any discomfort, then demission from the clinic may be planned or a third programming session is scheduled and demission is planned for thereafter. (In case of a third programming session, its schedule is equivalent to the second one.)

At demission, the patient receives:
- A prescription for hearing training with a specialized speech therapist,
- A date for the next programming session at about 4 weeks later,
- An ABI identification card, and
- An ABI booklet for him/her and his/her family doctor and local otolaryngologist.

ABI Identification Card

Patients with an implanted ABI need to carry a special *implant identification card* with them all the time, preferably together with their personal identification card. The implant identification card provides the patient's identity parameters, implant type and serial number, and a phone number to be contacted in case of trauma or other emergencies.

The ABI booklet refers to the type of the patient's personal ABI system and specifies MRI compatibility and safety checklists with regard to medical diagnostic and interventions.

13.2.4 Standardized Follow-up Program

Timing and Elements of Sessions

At the Comprehensive Hearing Center Wuerzburg, CHC, for all patients with auditory implants (mostly cochlear implant [CI] patients),a standardized follow-up program has been implemented. In this program, regular fitting sessions at intervals of 3, 6, and 12 months after initial activation are combined with medical consultation, audiological assessment, and rehabilitation (if desired). Thereafter, follow-up fitting sessions are recommended twice per year. Most parts of this program (fitting, rehabilitation, consultation) are offered for ABI patients as well. However, in some cases more frequent additional appointments at shorter intervals are required.

Three standardized steps of control are to be performed before follow-up programming is started:
1. *Wuerzburg Loudness Scaling* (Wuerzburg Hörfeldskalierung WHF) (▶ Fig. 13.4): Each ABI patient performs this non-speech test which allows a first evaluation of perceived loudness at the different frequencies of the speech perception spectrum, namely at 500, 1000, 2000, and 4000 Hz (for further details, please refer to "Loudness Scaling").[1]
2. Individual patient feedback: The patient reports on his/her first impressions with the activated ABI. Unpleasant sensations and side effects are elicited.

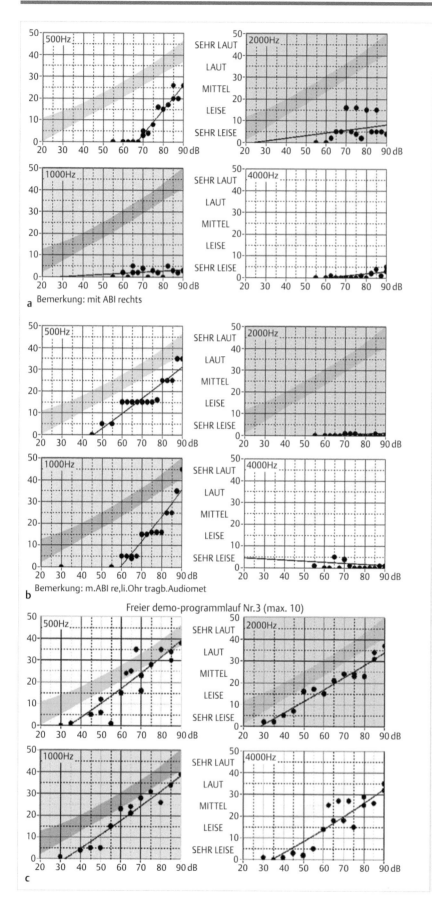

a Bemerkung: mit ABI rechts

b Bemerkung: m.ABI re,li.Ohr tragb.Audiomet

Freier demo-programmlauf Nr.3 (max. 10)

c

Fig. 13.4 The Wuerzburger loudness scaling (WALS) shows a significant improvement over time **(a–c)** from early to 3 to 6 months after activation. In September 2017, low loudness is perceived at 500 and 1000 Hz. In December 2017, low loudness is perceived at 500, 1000, and 2000 Hz.
In March 2018, intensity perception is markedly improved with good loudness perceived at 500 to 4000 Hz and approaching normal loudness levels. This development in perception of different frequencies is an important step toward speech perception. **(c)** WALS at 6 months.

3. This is followed by a technical checkup of the externally worn sound processor:
   - Check for broken cable
   - Assess microphones (listening check)
   - Visual inspection of contacts (battery compartment)
   - Cleaning/replacement of ear hook (if necessary)

Programming

As in "First Programming Procedure", *implant integrity and coupling* are determined. In the most preferred program, single-channel stimulation is administered for all active electrodes to determine the threshold of hearing and the most comfortable hearing level. Again, the overall loudness is defined using live voice.

Next, the *pitch sequence* is evaluated. An advantage of starting with the most preferred program of the previous programming session is that the previously installed pitch order is still in place. However, this order is likely to have changed and needs to be reassessed comparing two tones (balancing). Sometimes, two or more electrodes elicit the same pitch and cannot be placed in order. This needs testing, if either electrode should remain activated or one of them is deactivated for this session (can be reactivated at another programming session).

Further *fine-tuning* is possible using frequency-specific narrow band noise at moderate loudness that is presented via head-phones to the patient. The audiologist adjusts the most comfort-able level (MCL) until a comfortable loudness is achieved in *each* active electrode.

13.2.5 Assessment of Audiological Status

As described in previous sections, simple tests are performed to find out whether certain noises and sounds are perceived:
- Low frequency noise: drumming on the table
- High frequency noise: ringing of a door bell
- Identification of noise construction: twofold drumming, threefold drumming
- Identification of sound construction: twofold or threefold syllables: la-la, la-la-la
- Identification of vocals: dark (A, O, U) or light vocals (E, I)

In patients with some speech understanding, a small number of speech tests is administered (see "Speech Tests") and results are documented in the patient file.

13.3 Troubleshooting

13.3.1 ABI Activation without any Auditory Sensation

Lack of Auditory Sensation at First Activation

At first activation, electrode by electrode, the patient might report an absence of any auditory sensation.

A variety of causes need to be taken into consideration and some may be excluded:
- **1.1** A technical defect of the speech processor prevents adequate stimulation.

- **1.2** A technical defect of the magnet/the transduction system prevents adequate stimulation.
- **1.3** A technical defect of the implant leads to failure.
- **2.1** The implant electrode carrier has moved from the correct position.
- **2.2** The implant electrode carrier has lost its contact with the brainstem and is floating within the lateral recess.
- **3.1** The patient has some sensation, but cannot ascribe it to hearing due to very long-standing bilateral deafness and loss of memory of acoustic perception.
- **3.2** The cochlear nucleus is too degenerated to cause any auditory sensations, after long-standing brainstem compression or after radio-surgery.

Control of Implant and Electrodes in the Absence of Function

In order to elucidate the underlying cause of missing auditory sensation the following aspects need to be checked:

For **1.1** to **1.3**, *technical defects*:
- Check of the external parts (head pieces, sound processor, and external magnet) by exchanging them and re-measuring the impedances. *If impedances are normal, fitting is continued.*
- Check of impedance of each electrode by comparing the intraoperative impedances and the final surgical phase.
- If some electrodes provide measurable impedances and others are out of range, a lack of
  - contact of those electrodes or a defect of parts of the electrodes or cables must be assumed.
    The clinical effect at intact electrodes is tested.
- If all the electrode impedances are out of range, an implant failure or a lack of electrode contact with neural structures must be assumed.

For **2.1** to **2.2**, *dislocated electrode carrier*:
If electrode impedances are out of range, imaging by cranial CT is performed and compared to the early postoperative cranial CT:
- A change of site of the electrode tip and its depth within the lateral recess are highly can cause electrode dislocation.
- In case of high impedances/open channels, floating of the electrode carrier is likely.
- In case of preserved contacts and normal impedances, but no acoustic sensation, dislocation is to be assumed.

For **3.1** to **3.2**, *dysfunctional brainstem/auditory nucleus*:
A degeneration or dysfunction of the cochlear nucleus within the brainstem must be suspected under the following conditions:
- All external parts of the transducing and stimulating system are intact.
- All the electrodes of the ABI system show normal impedances.
- Impedances are similar or slightly lower than during implantation surgery.
- On stimulation with increasing stimulation intensities (up to maximum stimulation pattern), no auditory sensation is elicited.
- During stimulation, electric auditory brainstem responses may be recorded and compared to intra operative findings. Typically, stimulation artefact will be seen, and only a very small or no wave III and small or absent wave V. These

recordings may give proof of some conduction along the auditory relay stations, but the low amplitudes signify a very small number of active neurons, not sufficient to promote auditory sensations.

If intra operative EABR had been positive and had normal amplitudes, while postoperative EABR is low or absent, a displacement of the electrode carrier must be suspected. *This is a clear indication for revision.*

13.3.2 ABI Activation with Nonauditory Side Effects

Control of Implant and Electrodes in Dysfunction

Implant Dysfunction

A dysfunction of the implant can be ruled out by exchanging the external parts and controlling the electrode impedances to be within the normal range.

Implant with Broken Parts

Attention must be paid to extremely high impedances ("open channels" indicating disconnected/broken electrodes) or very low impedances indicating "leakage." In such a case, the patient might also describe some pain emanating near the scar and implant site during stimulation. Then an immediate discontinuation of the stimulation trial is mandatory and revision with complete explantation of the device, technical control, and re-implantation of a new device are necessary.

Intact Implant, but Clinical Dysfunction

If stimulation causes side effects and acoustic sensation is absent or acoustic sensation is found only on very few electrodes, the electrode carrier is most likely not at the precise location. A microsurgical revision may be indicated. If some electrodes give some useful auditory perception, these may be tried for a limited period. At re-evaluation, the development of any beneficial effects and acoustic results of the other electrodes will be investigated.

Implant Topography

Stimulation tests may be used to identify the functional anatomical position of the current electrode carrier:
- Upward displacement may be deduced from side effects such as facial twitching or severe vertigo (Vth, VIIth, and vestibular nerves/nuclei).
- Downward or lateral displacement may be deduced from side effects such as paresthesias in the throat or mouth (IXth nerve/nucleus).
- Medial displacement may be deduced from side effects such a paresthesias at the trunk, hips, or thighs (long sensory tracts).

Indication for Micro-surgical Revision

Depending on the proportion of number of useful auditory or dysfunctional electrodes, a decision for microsurgical revision is taken.

- *In case of 50% or more auditory electrodes*, a test phase with everyday application of the ABI stimulation program should be undertaken. At re-programming in 6 to 12 weeks intervals, testing of the achieved auditory benefit is to be tried early on for objective judgment besides the patient's subjective report. If clear benefit and improvement are documented, this concept should be continued.
- *In case of no auditory electrodes and no side effects on any electrodes*, the EABR should be repeated. In case of significant difference to the intraoperative recordings, a change of electrode carrier position must be suspected and revision is clearly indicated. If EABR are positive and similar to intraoperative testing, functional degeneration may be the cause. Degeneration may be a local problem at the brainstem or at higher brainstem or cortical levels.[7] A test phase with everyday application of the ABI stimulation program should be undertaken. At re-programming in 6 to 12 weeks intervals, testing of electrode effects and side effects and of EABR are to be tried. The question whether a microsurgical re-exploration and possible re-positioning of the ABI could be successful, needs to be discussed very individually, and any decision depends on the patient's attitude and general disease manifestation.
- *In case of few auditory electrodes (far below 50% of electrodes/channels) and* no side effects *on any electrodes*, these results should be analyzed in view of the intraoperative recording results.
  - *If intraoperative EABR had been positive* only on some electrodes and several electrodes had been mute, a limited auditory result at few electrodes corresponds to expectation.
  - *If intraoperative EABR had been positive* only on some electrodes and EABR components were deformed and small in amplitude, a limited auditory result at few electrodes corresponds to expectation.
- In case of few auditory electrodes (far below 50%) and reproducible side effects on many electrodes, these results should be analyzed in view of the intraoperative recording results.
  - If intraoperative EABR had been also positive on those contacts with current side effects, a microsurgical re-exploration is to be considered.

13.4 Rehabilitation Program

13.4.1 General Training Goals

In ABI patients, a successful outcome is aural, not tactile, sound perception enabling speech understanding. Open-set speech understanding is possible and has been reported previously.[3,4,5] However, unilateral or bilateral auditory nerve destruction is often accompanied by further disease-related side effects, for example, neurological deficits, so that aural rehabilitation may not be the sole concern. Ideally, a combined holistic approach of physical and aural rehabilitation is pursued.

In our center, we recommend, whenever possible, the same rehabilitation procedure as for CI recipients. Patients are seen at regular intervals of 1, 3, 6, and 12 months after initial activation. At each appointment, the programming aspect is the main objective accompanied by medical consultation and audiological assessment. However, special aural rehabilitation consultations are planned at all the visits in order to elaborate and support the ongoing progress.

13.4.2 General Auditory Training Strategy

The initial activation aims at establishing an auditory sensation that allows the recipient to perceive familiar and unfamiliar sounds in the surrounding. Auditory training with CI or ABI patients must train auditory abilities such as *detection, discrimination,* and *identification* of first sounds, later on speech-sounds.

- *Detection:* Firstly, awareness of everyday sounds is trained. The patient learns to be attentive to sounds and reacts to sounds. The detection process depends on loudness, frequency pattern, and familiarity of sounds. These factors shall be varied systematically to train detection ability.
- *Discrimination*: The aim of sound discrimination is the discovery of *differences* in loudness, frequency, rhythm, and quality. The training starts with large differences, for example, differentiating an octave for frequency discrimination, and then proceeds to smaller differences.
- *Identification*: Depending on the discriminative abilities of the patient, more capabilities for identification will evolve.

These auditory abilities can be trained by listening to everyday sounds and also by recording everyday noises such as telephone ringing, sounds of cutlery, voices of family members, and music instruments.

If this level of training is easily accomplished, the next aim is *to train speech perception*. The training for speech-perception follows a hierarchal manner of complexity and difficulty. Some of the first steps are:

- Discrimination of the number of syllables in words,
- Recognition of words with different syllables of a given (closed) set of words,
- Understanding words in an open set with very familiar words like numbers, and
- Understanding everyday sentences like "How are you?"

In the end,

- Discrimination of phonemes which are difficult to differentiate, such as o-u, e-i, is trained in monosyllable words or in Consonant-Vowel-Consonant syllables.

13.4.3 Training Materials

Everyday auditory experience and daily communication at home are hallmarks of continuous auditory training for the ABI patient. In addition, especially designed materials for auditory training in CI recipients can be purchased, for example, introduction books for family members and therapist, training CDs, and internet training material from CI manufacturers. Recently, smartphone applications (Apps) have been developed with different complexity levels for independent training at home, using a mobile phone or computer. Those training programs have been designed especially for CI recipients and might be suitable for ABI patients as well.

13.4.4 The Way to Train—Professional Training Support

Individual Home Training

There are several training and rehabilitation opportunities. The most convenient is the daily individual training at home. This represents the best foundation for achieving optimal auditory abilities. The patient may use the materials described above (see "Training materials") for his/her individual training.

Instruction Sheets

Instruction sheets contain training units gradually increasing in difficulty, instructions for the patient and her/his family members, recommendations, tips, and tricks. These are handed over to the patients and have proven to be quite helpful. The patient and her/his family members are made familiar with the instruction sheets during the rehabilitation session.

Online Programs for Hearing Rehabilitation

The patient receives an introduction to application and exercising of newly available computer programs for acoustic training.

Individual Speech Therapist

Besides the individual training at home, hearing exercises can be extended by a professional and specially trained speech therapist. Training of speech therapists for teaching and exercising with patients with auditory implants, especially cochlear and brainstem implants, is offered once to twice per year by the Comprehensive Hearing Centre of the ORL University Clinic and provides up-to-date knowledge on technical and functional technology development and the state-of-the-art hearing rehabilitation with implanted devices. Successful participation is being granted with a "Diploma of Advanced Auditory Rehabilitation in New Technologies." Thereby, a pool of qualified speech therapists has been built up and is continuously expanding.

The patient needs a prescription for this kind of aural rehabilitation that comprises a training session of at least once per week. This is the most preferred and recommended option in our center.

13.4.5 Residential Rehabilitation

ABI patients may be offered either semi-residential or full residential aural rehabilitation in addition to optional training with a specially trained speech therapist. There are a number of highly specialized aural rehabilitation centers in Germany. In order to be admitted, cost coverage must be confirmed via the health insurance prior to beginning.

An integral part of residential rehabilitation is the fine-tuning of the sound processor. It must be emphasized that programming of the sound processor must only be conducted by especially trained audiologists. The training for audiologists in this case is different from conventional CI programming and is not a part of a regular CI fitting course (in Germany). Therefore, ABI patients might participate in all offered therapies, but programming is conducted only by specially trained audiologist that must visit, if not on site.

A *semi-residential rehabilitation* concept involves not only the singular training for intense auditory perception training, but also group sessions where communication strategies (hearing in noise, coping strategies, communication tactics) and communication training for everyday situations are offered.

As in all chronic disease conditions, the opportunity to consult a trained psychologist is mandatory, and most centers offer psychology support.

In this semi-residential concept, the patient chooses to participate either half a day or a full day in a two-weekly term. Depending on the center, there might be other variations.

The full residential program lasts from 3 to 6 weeks. The concept is similar to that described for semi-residential program. Additionally, medical consultation by ENTs, tinnitus therapy, balance training, relaxation methods, physical exercises and sports, physiotherapy and physical therapy, music therapy, water gymnastics, and nutritional consulting may be offered.

13.5 Hearing Tests of ABI Function

13.5.1 General Considerations for ABI Hearing Tests in NF2

To evaluate the outcome of ABI rehabilitation, a number of tests assessing either nonspeech cues or speech cues can be conducted. In patients with no speech understanding, nonspeech tests are recommended that indicate loudness perception and ideally frequency discrimination.

In our center, the loudness scaling procedure is conducted prior to every programming session (starting after the basic programming session) in all ABI patients.

13.5.2 Nonspeech Tests

Non-speech tests provide information of the perceived sound level and frequency spectrum and permit to detect either threshold, the most comfortable level or the discomfort zone.

Loudness Scaling

The Wuerzburg Loudness Scaling (Würzburger Hörfeldskalierung WHF) (▶ Fig. 13.4) was developed in 1987 by Moser using a computer-based method to determine subjective loudness categories (© manufacturer Westra Electronic GmbH). Four fields representing four frequencies (500 Hz, 1 kHz, 2 kHz, and 4 kHz) at 16 different loudness levels from 20 to 90 dB sound pressure level (SPL) (total of 64 stimuli) are presented in a pseudorandomized order in the sound field. The patient is asked to judge the loudness perception via a sensitive touchpad with 50 loudness categories available.

Frequency Modulated Tones (FM)

Aided threshold can be determined with warble tones or FM in sound field. This is a behavioral threshold measurement method in which the patient is asked to indicate the softest sound that is audible. FM tones (warbles) are presented at octave and half-octave frequencies between 250 and 4000 Hz.

13.5.3 Speech Tests

The following speech tests are in most cases modified from the original speech test.

A female speaker conducts all speech tests at a level of 65±5 dB SPL. If possible, the patient's native language is presented and most frequently live voice is used. As usual, it begins with the easiest test and any test previously mastered with ease and at 100% may be skipped at the next test date, and the next more difficult step will be applied.

All tests are presented in three conditions:
- Visual only (lip reading only)
- Audio-visual (acoustic with lip reading)
- Sole acoustic input

The test sequence starts with the Freiburg bisyllabic number test, followed by the Monosyllabic-Trochee-Polysyllabic (MTP) test and a closed-set vowel confusion test. Finally, the Hochmair-Schulz-Moser (HSM) test as an everyday sentence test is administered and represents the most difficult level.

Vowel Confusion Test

A closed-set vowel confusion test has been adapted from Dorman et al.[8] In this test, eight tokens ("bib," "bab," "bub," "bob," "beb," "bäb," "büb," böb") are presented twice in a randomized sequence. They are written down on a list presented to the patient. The patient is asked to repeat or point on the token that he/she has understood.

Syllable and Pattern Identification

The MTP test, developed by Erber and Alencewicz,[9] is a closed-set word test consisting of 12 items measuring the ability to identify words and/or different syllable patterns. The patient is asked to point to a picture or verbally repeat the presented word. Word identification and pattern recognition scores are obtained.

Word Recognition

Freiburg bisyllabic number test, first described by K. Hahlbrock in 1953, is usually applied to determine the speech reception thresholds (SRT) at which 50% of words are correctly identified. The bisyllabic number test contains 10 lists in which a combination of two-syllabic and four-syllabic numbers (in total 10) are presented. In the modified ABI testing routine, a list of 10 numbers is presented via live voice at a level of 65±5 dB SPL. A correctly identified number corresponds then to 1 point and is further transformed to percentage.

Sentence Recognition

Matrix Test

The Oldenburg Matrix test (OLSA) uses an adaptive test procedure to estimate the signal-to-noise ratio required for 50% of word understanding. It consists of 40 lists of 30 test sentences each. Speech babble generated by superimposing all test items serves as the noise signal and is presented at a constant level of 65 dB SPL. The presentation level of the test sentences, consisting of five words each, is changed adaptively according to the number of correctly repeated words. Two training lists should be conducted prior to each run to compensate training effects. The target speech signal is usually presented from the front loudspeaker (S0) and noise either from the front (S0N0) or rear loudspeaker (S0N180).

In ABI subjects, the OLSA can be conducted with live voice (or recorded on CD) using speech only. For the majority of ABI patients, the classical noise component of the test is omitted.

HSM Test

The HSM[10] test is a sentence test that can be applied with or without background noise. It was developed specifically for the evaluation of hearing impaired and CI patients using everyday sentences. Its base consists of 30 German lists containing 20 sentences each. The speech signal can be presented at a fixed level, usually 65 dB SPL, combined with a Signal-to-Noise-Ratio (SNR) of 5 or 10.

Adapted for testing ABI patients, the sentences are read by a female speaker in live voice. The patient is asked to repeat all heard words. The quantity of correct words is scored. Meanwhile the test has been conducted in many languages.

13.6 Long-Term Programming and Adaptation

Long-term follow up:

As reported recently, in the abovementioned setting of rehabilitation, one-third to two-thirds of the ABI patients do develop open-set speech perception. For these special cases, long-term follow-up is now provided for about 13 years and allows a brief summary of upcoming developments.

13.6.1 Improvement

All patients with some positive acoustic electrodes in their ABI report some continuous improvement in their perception of environmental sounds, voices, and speech.

First 6 months: A first fast improvement phase is the first 6 months; during this period, most patients experience that they can identify different noises and they are able to differentiate male and female voices. If about 50% of electrodes/channels provide acoustic perception, in objective testing, they will show acoustic perception at various frequencies (▶ Fig. 13.4) and obtain some pure auditory (nonvisual) syllable discrimination (positive MTP test).

First 3 years: Over a period of 3 years, all patients notice further improvement, especially in word detection and identification. Patients with early positive MTP test will now develop toward some open-set speech discrimination (HSM test).

After 5 years: After 5 years, patients still observe new perceptions and better reliability in recognition of new sounds. Some patients are able to listen and to identify music pieces after 2 years, while others after 5 years.

13.6.2 Deterioration

Deterioration in perception may be avoided in most patients by regular controls of the system and fine-tuning of their stimulation programs.

If the previous auditory level cannot be reached again, an investigation of local changes in the vicinity of the electrode carrier have to be performed. Especially recurrent tumor with brainstem compression and compression of the cochlear nucleus, ipsilateral and also contralateral to the ABI electrode, may cause deterioration of hearing quality.

In case of compression, resection of the recurrent tumor with preservation of ABI electrode at the brainstem site will invariably lead to a recovery of the hearing function. The recovery process may take some weeks though.

13.6.3 Secondary Failure

Local infiltrative tumor growth invading the electrode to brainstem contact can lead to decreasing auditory function. Also, single or repeated falls, more often in children and juniors,[11] may lead to secondary implant failure.

In either case, local revision and, if necessary, tumor resection are indicated with a trial to preserve the ABI implant and re-position it. In some conditions, the integrity of the ABI system, the electrode contacts, wires, or the silicone isolation may be severed and the implantation of a completely new ABI device may become necessary.

Again, the auditory rehabilitation will work within weeks instead of the initial evolution over years.

13.7 Case Presentation

A clinical case of a patient with a family history of NF2 and auditory rehabilitation by ABI surgery is presented.

13.7.1 Patient History

At 44 years of age, this male patient was diagnosed with bilateral vestibular schwannomas, elsewhere. He belongs to a family with widespread NF2 manifestation with two female cousins and one female niece being diagnosed with NF2; one cousin has already been implanted with an ABI at our center.

After 10 years of observation, aged 55 years, with hearing decline on the left, he seeks treatment for his best hearing right side, and after intensive journeys and consultation with colleagues inside and outside the country, he finally decides for radiosurgery by Cyberknife on the right. Within 3 months thereafter, he experiences pain of the third trigeminal branch, otalgia, and fast auditory deterioration progressing to deafness despite dexamethasone medication. He has to give up his professional life as a craftsman and business man of his own company. Then he also experiences some further hearing decline on the other, previously less good left side and progression of the tumor on the left. With these conditions, he presents to our NF outpatient clinic for the first time. After discussing all the options such as Bevacizumab trial and tumor resection on the right deaf side with ABI placement, despite radiation, or tumor resection on the left side with some functional hearing preservation, we take a joint decision with him and his wife for the following sequence of steps:

• Tumor surgery on the right deaf side, ABI test, and ABI implantation

- Observation of hearing and tumor growth on the left, until auditory function by right ABI is sufficient
- Tumor resection on the left with the goal of subtotal removal and hearing preservation or Bevacizumab trial prior to this

13.7.2 ABI Rehabilitation

During the surgery in July 2017 (▶ Fig. 13.3a) along with monitoring of somato-sensory evoked potentials (SSEP), motor evoked potentials (MEP) of trigeminal and bilateral facial function, and electromyography (EMG) of motor cranial nerves, the right tumor was completely resected except for a circumscribed facial schwannoma at the meatus (▶ Fig. 13.3b). Exposure of the dorsal cochlear nucleus showed a wide lateral recess with arachnoid adhesion. By placing electrode and final electrode carrier, EABRs were obtained via two-thirds of the contacts; after more upward positioning, all electrodes gave EABR, some with perfect EABR and some at lower amplitudes ▶ Fig. 13.3c.

At first activation in September 2017, 11 electrodes provided pure acoustic sensations and pitch perception from 70 to 8,500 Hz. The Wuerzburg Loudness Scaling did not work at first trial (▶ Fig. 13.4a), but noise recognition and MTP syllable test were positive.

At re-programming in December 2017, the patient reported some improvement of his tinnitus during ABI hearing. Eleven electrodes were kept active with re-arranged pitch.

MTP test at December 2017 was positive, as follows:

visual only: 19/24 (79%); auditory only: 16/24 (67%); audio-visual: 24/24 (100%).

At re-programming in March 2018, the patient reported regular ABI training with computer programs and further subjective improvement.

MTP test in March 2018, 6 months after first activation, was positive at 100% at all settings:

visual only: 24/24 (100%); auditory only: 24/24 (100%); audio-visual: 24/24 (100%).

Vocal discriminations tests were positive at 9 to 11/14 test syllables (78%).

The Wuerzburg Loudness Scaling (WALS) showed an improvement over time (▶ Fig. 13.4 a–c) from early to 3 to 6 months:

- In September 2017, low loudness was perceived at 500 and 1,000 Hz.
- In December 2017, low loudness was perceived at 500, 1,000, and 2,000 Hz.

- In March 2018, intensity perception was markedly improved with good loudness perceived at 500 to 4,000 Hz.

13.8 Conclusion

These developments in Wuerzburg Loudness Scaling as well as in the MTP test indicate clearly the development to real speech perception. According to experiences with similar patients' data, besides some open understanding for syllables being present already now, patients are developing toward open speech understanding. This is very positive in view of the past history of fast hearing loss after Cyberknife radiosurgery.

References

[1] Goffi-Gomez MV, Magalhães AT, Brito Neto R, Tsuji RK, Gomes MdeQ, Bento RF. Auditory brainstem implant outcomes and MAP parameters: report of experiences in adults and children. Int J Pediatr Otorhinolaryngol. 2012; 76 (2):257–264

[2] Ramsden RT, Freeman SR, Lloyd SK, et al. Manchester Neurofibromatosis Type 2 Service. Auditory brainstem implantation in neurofibromatosis type 2: experience from the Manchester programme. Otol Neurotol. 2016; 37(9): 1267–1274

[3] Matthies C, Brill S, Kaga K, et al. Auditory brainstem implantation improves speech recognition in neurofibromatosis type II patients. ORL J Otorhinolaryngol Relat Spec. 2013; 75(5):282–295

[4] Matthies C, Brill S, Varallyay C, et al. Auditory brainstem implants in neurofibromatosis type 2: is open speech perception feasible? J Neurosurg. 2014; 120(2):546–558

[5] Behr R, Colletti V, Matthies C, et al. New outcomes with auditory brainstem implants in NF2 patients. Otol Neurotol. 2014; 35(10):1844–1851

[6] Mandalà M, Colletti L, Colletti G, Colletti V. Improved outcomes in auditory brainstem implantation with the use of near-field electrical compound action potentials. Otolaryngol Head Neck Surg. 2014; 151(6):1008–1013

[7] Rueckriegel SM, Homola GA, Hummel M, Willner N, Ernestus RI, Matthies C. Probabilistic fiber-tracking reveals degeneration of the contralateral auditory pathway in patients with vestibular schwannoma. AJNR Am J Neuroradiol. 2016; 37(9):1610–1616

[8] Dorman MF, Dankowski K, McCandless G, Smith L. Identification of synthetic vowels by patients using the Symbion multichannel cochlear implant. Ear Hear. 1989; 10(1):40–43

[9] Erber NP, Alencewicz CM. Audiologic evaluation of deaf children. J Speech Hear Disord. 1976; 41(2):256–267

[10] Hochmair-Desoyer I, Schulz E, Moser L, Schmidt M. The HSM sentence test as a tool for evaluating the speech understanding in noise of cochlear implant users. Am J Otol. 1997; 18(6) Suppl:S83

[11] Puram SV, Barber SR, Kozin ED, et al. Outcomes following pediatric auditory brainstem implant surgery: early experiences in a North American center. Otolaryngol Head Neck Surg. 2016; 155(1):133–138

14 Outcomes in Pediatric ABI: The Hacettepe University Experience

Levent Sennaroğlu, Gonca Sennaroğlu, Esra Yucel, and Burçak Bilginer

Abstract

This chapter reports the audiological outcome of pediatric auditory brainstem implantation (ABI) in Hacettepe University. Our preliminary ABI outcome was reported in 2009 and minimum patient age was 2.5 years at that time. In that report six children gained basic audiological functions. In 2016, we reported long-term ABI outcome where the minimum age was lowered to 1 year. Majority of the children had Categories of Auditory Performance (CAP) score of 5. Children with better thresholds were in categories 6, 7, and 8. Speech intelligibility scores were also better in children with lower thresholds. Children with common cavity performed better when compared to other inner ear malformation groups. In a most recent outcome of 84 pediatric ABI users who used their device for more than 1 year, 52% demonstrated 100% pattern recognition in words (closed-set condition), 24% demonstrated 100% word identification (closed-set condition), and 15% of them repeated more than half of the open-set sentences correctly in auditory-only condition.

Keywords: audiological outcome, cochlear nerve deficiency, cochleovestibular anomalies, inner ear malformation, pediatric auditory brainstem implantation, prelingual deafness

14.1 Brief History of ABI Experience in Hacettepe University

The first auditory brainstem implant (ABI) in Turkey was performed in Hacettepe University in 2002 after removal of a vestibular schwannoma in a postlingually deafened NF2 patient. In 2005, another NF2 patient received an ABI in our department. In 2006, we started ABI in prelingually deafened children. In July 2006, we performed three cases and our team waited to see initial audiological outcome before continuing the procedure. At the initial programming, all three children demonstrated response to sound. After observing their performance, our team continued with ABI surgery in children. Between June 2006 and January 2018, our team performed 116 primary and 5 revision pediatric ABIs.

14.2 Preliminary Results of Pediatric ABI

In 2009, our team published preliminary results of pediatric ABI cases.[1] This paper reported the results of the first 11 children who received an ABI between 2006 and 2008. They were all operated via retrosigmoid approach, always together with a neurosurgeon. Their ages were between 2.5 and 5 years. During initial programming, all patients demonstrated some nonauditory side effects. Some of the nonauditory stimulation were due to high stimulation level, besides acoustic stimulation. In these patients, current level was decreased until the patient could hear without any nonauditory side effect. The second group did not have any acoustical stimulation, but had only nonauditory side effects in some channels. In the latter group, the channel producing the side effects was turned off.

Six children achieved basic audiologic functions and were able to recognize and discriminate sounds, and many could identify environmental sounds such as a doorbell and telephone ring by the third month of ABI use.

Six of the patients demonstrated increase in the number of active channels between initial and follow-up programming. Their dynamic range also increased. Dynamic range increase is also related to better stimulability of the cochlear nuclei over time. This was interpreted as a kind of adaptation over time in the surrounding neural structures related to side effects.

Two children had additional handicaps. Additional handicaps slowed the progress of these children compared to other patients with cochlear implantation. The patients with attention deficit hyperactivity disorder were among the worst in terms of subjective auditory performances. Despite lack of open-set scores in children with additional disabilities, their parents reported that they feel much more confident in their educational settings and in their family.

14.3 Long-Term Results of ABI

In 2016, we published long-term results of pediatric ABI in Hacettepe University. Between 2006 and 2014, 60 children received ABI in Hacettepe University.[2] There were 35 children who had used ABI for at least 1 year. Among the radiological indications, complete labyrinthine aplasia, cochlear aplasia, common cavity, incomplete partition I, cochlear hypoplasia, and cochlear nerve aplasia were present.

Size of the ABI electrode was suitable for lateral recess. Only in two cases, foramen of Luschka had to be enlarged slightly. They were very young children operated at 1 year of age. There was no serious complication. Three children had transient facial paresis, which recovered completely in 2 weeks.

Categories of Auditory Performance (CAP) scores were assessed according to hearing thresholds. Children were separated into three groups according to their hearing thresholds: **Group I:** 25–40 dB, **Group II:** 41–50 dB, and **Group III:** ≥50 dB. Majority of the children had CAP score of 5. This means that they could understand common phrases without lipreading. In Group I, with better thresholds, certain patients were in categories 6, 7, and 8. Patients with such high scores were not present in groups with higher thresholds (Groups II and III). Similar finding was also present in Speech Intelligibility Rating (SIR) scores. Group I had better SIR scores than Groups II and III. Therefore, hearing thresholds are very important in auditory performance and speech intelligibility, where better CAP and SIR scores were observed with lower thresholds.

Functional auditory performance of cochlear implant (FAPCI) scores revealed that children with an ABI were in the lowest

10 percentile. This shows that language outcomes of ABI in children with severe inner ear malformations in general are not as good as cochlear implant (CI) users with normal anatomy.

Relationship of hearing threshold with language acquisition was also assessed. With lower thresholds, it is possible to obtain better language development.

The relationship of the number of active electrodes and the hearing thresholds was also investigated. For standardization, the number of active electrodes was defined as a percentage of the total number of electrodes. No relationship between the number of active electrodes and the hearing thresholds or language outcome was present.

Interesting findings were present in the type of inner ear malformation. Among the radiological classification, best performance was in the group "common cavity." In addition, the patients were separated into two groups according to the presence of cochlea vestibular nerve (CVN): "CVN present" (inner ear malformations such as common cavity) and "CVN absent" (complete labyrinthine aplasia etc.). Auditory performance was better in children with common cavity, or CVN present, and showed statistically significant difference. In common cavity, there is some cochlear neural tissue both in the cavity and in the CVN coming from the cavity. This may be the reason for better performance of this particular anomaly group in all test methods versus other etiologies.

When cognitive skills were taken into consideration, this also had a significant impact on the outcome. Group with impaired intelligence showed worse outcome in auditory performance, speech intelligibility, and language acquisition. As mentioned in preliminary results, attention deficit hyperactivity disorder, visual impairment, and mental retardation, combined as a group of handicap, negatively influenced SIR, CAP, and Manchester test scores.

Eighteen children had 100% pattern discrimination and the remaining 11 patients had scores between 33 and 96%. In multisyllabic words, 11 patients scored 100% and 8 patients scored between 25 and 92%. Among 35 children, 12 had open-set scores above 50%, 2 had 100%, and 10 patients scored above 50%. There was no correlation between number of active electrodes and closed- and open-set perception scores. On the other hand, hearing thresholds were inversely moderately correlated with closed- and open-set scores. In general, children demonstrated very good progress in the first 2 years but then the progress slowed down but continued at a slower pace.

14.3.1 Most Recent Audiological and Language Outcome of 84 Patients with ABI

Between June 2006 and January 2018, 116 children with complex inner ear malformations received an ABI by Hacettepe Implant team. Five of these were revision due to device failure. The results of 84 primary pediatric ABI patients who have been using their ABI for more than a year were analyzed and recently presented at European Pediatric Cochlear Implantation Meeting in Lisbon.[3] Of the total number of patients, 64% were female and 36% were male. Auditory verbal communication mode is used by 70% of these children and the rest have chosen total communication.

Auditory perception skills were evaluated by using Meaningful Auditory Integration Scale (MAIS)[4] and Categories of Auditory Performance (CAP-II).[5] Closed-set pattern perception subtest, closed-set word identification subtest, and open-set sentence recognition subtest were used from Children Auditory Perception Test Battery in Turkish.[6] Language performance was assessed with Test of Early Language Development (TELD-3)[7] and SIR.[8]

When we examined the relationship between duration of ABI use and progress of CAP scores, at the end of 6 months, it was observed that detection of environmental sounds obviously developed. By the first year of ABI use, they were able recognize most of the environmental sounds and their sources. One year later, most of the children were able to reach the "Discrimination of speech sounds without lipreading" (CAP-II) and "Understanding of common phrases without lipreading" (CAP-III) levels (▶ Fig. 14.1). It was noted that patients usually stayed at this level for a long period as it is more difficult to move to the next level. This is because the next level requires complex linguistic and cognitive skills, more than identifying daily words and sentences. By the end of third year of ABI use, they achieved their best performance on auditory perception skills. However, we should always keep in mind that their auditory perception skills continue to develop in different rates. It was also noted that in our study, children who were implanted at younger age (< 3 years old) showed faster progress and achieved higher scores in terms of auditory perception skills (▶ Fig. 14.2). As a final comment, substantial number of patients (25/30) were able to follow the conversation without lipreading or speech reading cues. Despite the small number of children (only 5/30 children) who could reach the final stage, it was promising that some of them were able to carry out conversation even by telephone.

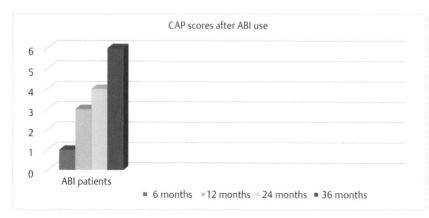

Fig. 14.1 Categories of Auditory Perception (CAP-II) scores in 3 years of follow-up.

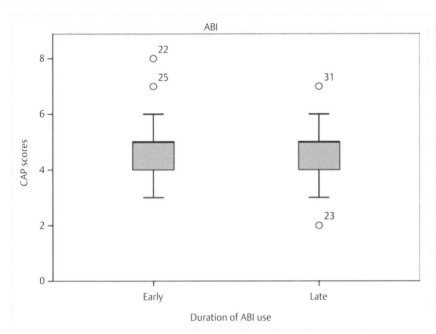

Fig. 14.2 Categories of Auditory Perception (CAP-II) scores and duration of auditory brainstem implant (ABI) use (between 5 and 10 years).

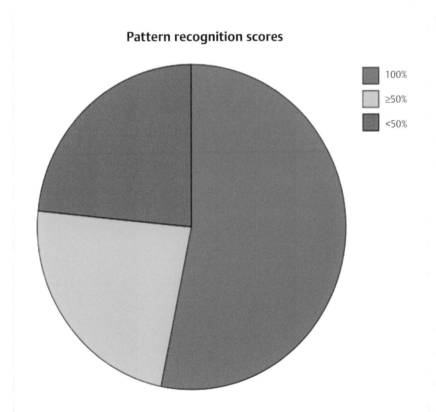

Fig. 14.3 Pattern perception scores of children.

We also used CIAT (Test for Auditory Perception Skills for Children in Turkish) battery in order to evaluate their speech perception skills.[2] In closed-set condition, 52% demonstrated 100% pattern recognition in words, while 24% showed pattern recognition of 50 to 100% (▶ Fig. 14.3). In word identification in closed-set condition using ABI only, 24% demonstrated 100% identification, while 36% identified 50 to 100% of the words presented

(▶ Fig. 14.4). Approximately 15% of them repeated more than half of the open-set sentences correctly in auditory-only condition. Sentence recognition of 20 to 50% was demonstrated by 21%.

We have also evaluated the language performance of the children by considering their receptive and expressive language skills. Although we collect the data by observing their communication performance in daily situations, we also rely

Word identification scores

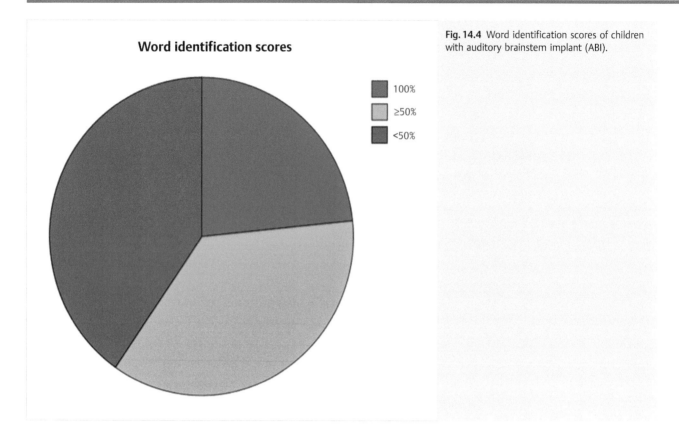

Fig. 14.4 Word identification scores of children with auditory brainstem implant (ABI).

Legend:
- 100%
- ≥50%
- <50%

on language performance test scores. However, comparing the gap between their chronological ages and language equivalent scores do not provide realistic scores as their hearing ages starts with ABI activation. So considering the gap only may not provide the correct results. Depending on the duration of the auditory deprivation, language development was estimated to be delayed. For this reason, we determined a linear increase considering the duration of implant use (▶ Fig. 14.5). We also encounter similar process in expressive language development (▶ Fig. 14.6). However, in expressive language development, the contents of the cues become more complicated and the words expected to be used are shifted to the plateau after a while due to the increase of the lengths of the speech sounds. Depending on the variables such as the enriched environmental stimulus surrounding the child, cognitive skills, educational status of the parents and/or caregiver, and the quality of rehabilitation program, the expressive language development may move to the next stage faster.

On the other hand, no statistical difference was obtained between the duration of ABI use and speech intelligibility according to the SIR classification.[8] However, as shown in ▶ Fig. 14.7, it can be observed that children who start using ABI at an early age were able to make faster progress and achieve higher scores in speech understanding than the ones who were implanted in older ages (< 3 years old). However, comprehension skills that also require the phonological resolution of vocalizations were observed as the most difficult task for children. Generally, they were in categories 2 and 3 in SIR. Their speech production can be defined as either "Connected speech is unintelligible" or "Connected speech is intelligible to a listener who concentrates and lip reads."

In our patient population, 24% had at least one additional difficulty such as CHARGE, cerebral palsy, Goldenhar, or mental motor retardation. When cognitive performance was taken into consideration, it was determined that there was a significant difference between their speech comprehension skills, auditory perception scores, and language skills. Children who were good performers in terms of cognitive skills were also able to use auditory perception skills in daily circumstances (FAPCI),[9] and develop better language skills (Manchester language test) with a more intelligible speech interaction (SIR) (▶ Table 14.1).

14.4 CI and ABI in Hypoplastic CN

As can be understood, results of pediatric ABI never reach the level of cochlear implantation in normal anatomy. Because of this, our team looked for options for bilateral stimulation in complex inner ear malformations (IEMs). We have a number of patients where CI was not sufficient and they received contralateral ABI. Their results are much better than ABI-only situation. Therefore, bimodal stimulation with CI on one side and an ABI on the contralateral side turned out to be an option for complex IEMs with severe cochlear nerve (CN) and CVN hypoplasia.

Decision-making is extremely important in this group of patients. Magnetic resonance imaging (MRI) may not be sufficient to determine the benefit of CI, if the CN or CVN is extremely hypoplastic. Results of audiological evaluation and MRI should be used together to make the decision. In the objective tests such as Auditory Brainstem Response (ABR) and Otoacoustic Emission (OAE), usually there is no response that supports the presence of hearing in majority of the cases. However, in ABR

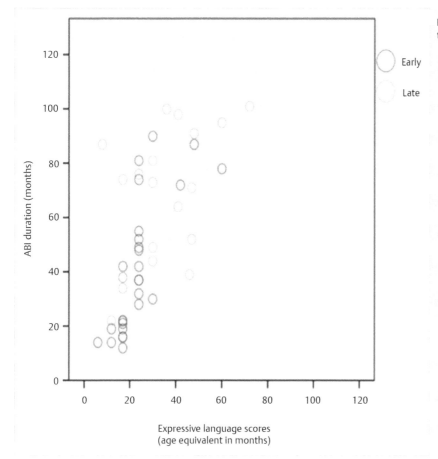

Fig. 14.5 Expressive language scores and duration of auditory brainstem implant (ABI) use.

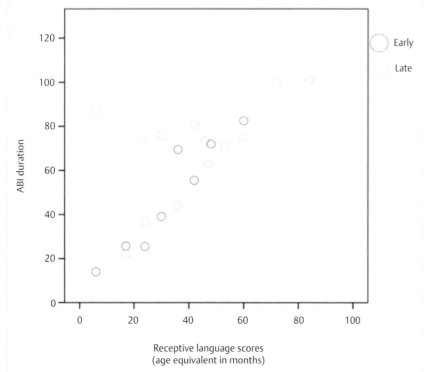

Fig. 14.6 Receptive language scores and duration of auditory brainstem implant (ABI) use.

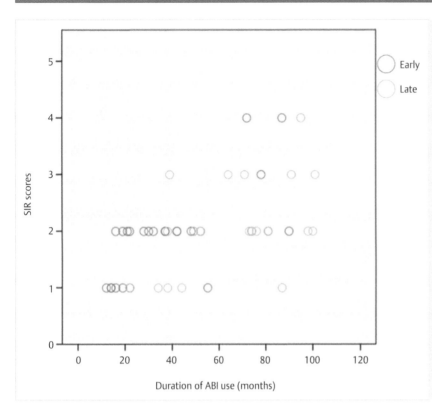

Fig. 14.7 Speech Intelligibility Rating (SIR) scores and duration of auditory brainstem implant (ABI) use.

Table 14.1 The relation between cognitive skills and auditory perception and speech language development

	FAPCI	SIR	CAP	Manchester	Receptive language	Expressive language
Normal	1,80	2,47	5,53	6,20	40,33	36,00
Dull	1,30	2,20	4,80	6,40	42,90	39,30
MR	*1,50*	*1,50*	*3,50*	*4,30*	*25,00*	*20,80*

results it is possible to observe cochlear microphonics (CM) in some inner ear malformations (especially in cases with CN hypoplasia/aplasia). We need to perform behavioral tests at the most comfortable time for the baby. Using the insert earphone, the responses of both ears are assessed separately. It is possible to determine which ear is better from the point of view of the audiologist. Thus, we have overcome the vibration problem caused by the speaker. Furthermore, in the hypoplastic cochlea, the basal part of the cochlea may be more intact than the apical part. This results in observing responses in high frequency region due to the stimulation of the basal part of the cochlea. For this reason, it is more efficient to start the test with 2,000 Hz instead of routine procedure of 500 Hz. In case of good response from one ear, accepted by both audiologists, CI is recommended for the better ear. If there is response on both sides, bilateral CI is planned in cases of CN hypoplasia. ABIs are recommended for the worse ear in which we cannot get any response in audiological tests in cases of CN aplasia or CN hypoplasia. Thus, bimodal stimulation is provided.

In Hacettepe University there are 14 patients who use CI and ABI together. These are patients with hypoplastic CN, hypoplastic or incomplete partition I cochleas, and common cavity

(CC). After their insufficient progress with CI for 1 to 1.5 years, decision for a contralateral ABI was made. Some of these children have thresholds of around 40 dB with CI, but because of the hypoplastic CN they show insufficient progress in language development. Therefore, it should be kept in mind that, even with CI for a year, it may be necessary to have ABI despite acceptable thresholds with CI. This also shows the difficulty of intracochlear test electrode to determine the appropriate modality of CI versus ABI intraoperatively during initial surgery. Even with actual CI it takes at least 1 year to make this decision. Inadequate cochlear nerve fibers, possibly not clearly visible with the MRI, may be sufficient to provide a meaningful stimulus to the auditory brainstem, but are not sufficient for neural activation at higher levels.

In 2014, there were six patients who used their ABI for more than a year and long-term results of CI and ABI of these six patients were presented at the 12th European Symposium on Pediatric Cochlear Implant, in Toulouse in 2015.[10] Average duration between CI and ABI was 1.5 to 2 years. This is due to the acceptable thresholds obtained after CI surgery. In the beginning, they demonstrated a progress, but after a certain period the language development came to a plateau. Therefore, there is a long period between CI and ABI surgery even though a careful follow-up is done. Their auditory performance and intelligibility scores were also presented. Although they had similar CAP scores in CI-only and ABI-only situations, auditory performance showed a dramatic increase when CI and ABI were used together. Average CAP score before ABI was 1, after ABI surgery it was 4.8. Same improvement was observed in SIR scores as well. Before and after ABI, average SIR scores were 1.2 and 3.3, respectively. This is now an acceptable method of treatment in cases of possible ABI indications.

Therefore, in complex IEMs with hypoplastic CN and CVN, it appears that the most acceptable treatment option is CI on the side with implantable cochlea, hypoplastic CN, or hearing response with insert ear phones and ABI on the contralateral side with worse anatomy and hearing. If there is response on both sides during audiological examination, bilateral CI is the best suggestion in spite of hypoplastic CN or CVN.

14.5 Simultaneous CI and ABI

Our team observed the important gap between CI and ABI in cases of insufficient progress in children with hypoplastic cochlear nerve. Therefore, the option of simultaneous CI and ABI was proposed in some selected cases. This is done in situations where the outcome with CI was presumed to be limited. The CI side has a CN, which is barely visible on 3 Tesla MRI and there is a very limited response with insert ear phones, while the other side has a definite ABI indication. Simultaneous CI and ABI surgery has two advantages. In children who are relatively late for surgery, between 2 and 3 years particularly with additional disabilities, waiting for the result of CI surgery may result in a late ABI surgery. Because of the disability, it is more difficult to decide whether the child is making progress with CI. As indicated before, it usually takes 1.5 to 2 years by the time the child receives contralateral ABI. Then the child becomes 3 to 3.5 years old and benefit from ABI decreases. In order to avoid delay, CI and ABI can be done in the same setting. If the child benefits from CI, then he or she will have bilateral stimulation from the start. In cases where CI is not beneficial, the child will not lose valuable time waiting for ABI. This approach was used in five patients so far in Hacettepe University and initial results were presented at the American Cochlear Implant Alliance Symposium in 2015 and were recently published.[11]

14.6 Bilateral ABI

As an implant team, our role has always been bilateral stimulation: we always give two hearing aids and two CIs to provide bilateral binaural hearing. The same must be valid for an ABI as well. As can be understood from the previous paragraphs, an ABI provides hearing and language in prelingually deafened children when used unilaterally. As the side effects and complications are minimal in experienced centers, it is advisable to perform the procedure bilaterally, because these are the children who definitely need bilateral hearing input more than children with normal anatomy.

We have two children with bilateral ABI.

References

[1] Sennaroglu L, Ziyal I, Atas A, et al. Preliminary results of auditory brainstem implantation in prelingually deaf children with inner ear malformations including severe stenosis of the cochlear aperture and aplasia of the cochlear nerve. Otol Neurotol. 2009; 30(6):708–715

[2] Sennaroğlu L, Sennaroğlu G, Yücel E, et al. Long-term results of ABI in children with severe inner ear malformations. Otol Neurotol. 2016; 37(7):865–872

[3] Sennaroğlu L, Sennaroğlu G, Yücel E, et al. Long-term Results of ABI in Children with Severe Inner Ear Malformations. Presented during 13th European Symposium on Pediatric Cochlear Implant. May 25–28, 2017. Lisbon, Portugal

[4] Robbins AM, Renshaw JJ, Berry SW. Evaluating meaningful auditory integration in profoundly hearing-impaired children. Am J Otol. 1991; 12 Suppl: 144–150

[5] Archbold S, Lutman ME, Nikolopoulos T. Categories of auditory performance: inter-user reliability. Br J Audiol. 1998; 32(1):7–12

[6] Yücel E, Sennaroglu G. Çocuklarİçinİşitsel Algı Testi. Advanced Bionics, 2011

[7] Guven S, Topbas S. Adaptation of the test of early language development (TELD-3) into Turkish: reliability and validity study. International Journal of Early Childhood Special Education(INT-JECSE). 2014; 6(2):151–176

[8] Allen C, Nikolopoulos TP, Dyar D, O'Donoghue GM. Reliability of a rating scale for measuring speech intelligibility after pediatric cochlear implantation. Otol Neurotol. 2001; 22(5):631–633

[9] Clark JH, Aggarwal P, Wang NY, Robinson R, Niparko JK, Lin FR. Measuring communicative performance with the FAPCI instrument: preliminary results from normal hearing and cochlear implanted children. Int J Pediatr Otorhinolaryngol. 2011; 75(4):549–553

[10] Sennaroglu GAF, Atay G, Bajin MD, et al. Bimodal Stimulation: One Side Cochlear Implant and Contralateral Auditory Brainstem Implant. In 12th European Symposium Pediatric Cochlear Implant. 2015. Toulouse, France

[11] Sennaroglu L, Yarali M, Sennaroglu G, et al. Simultaneous Cochlear and Auditory Brainstem Implantation in Children with Severe Inner Ear Malformations: Initial Surgical and Audiological Results. Otol Neurotol. 2020 Jun;41(5):625–630.

15 Auditory Brainstem Implantation in Tone Language Speakers

Michael C.F. Tong, John Ka Keung Sung, and Kathy Y.S. Lee

Abstract

Chinese language is based on 4 (Mandarin) to 6 (Cantonese) lexical tones to differentiate the meaning of a word with the same phonetic segment. Pitch perception transcribing into tone differentiation is therefore important in speech perception of adults and children undergone auditory brainstem implant. Assessment materials are designed for gross discrimination in fundamental frequency and lexical tone identification as well as the ability to tonal speech production in children. In a cohort of 13 adult NF2 implantees, 78% may differentiate environmental sound and 60% were able to have closed set word identification with lipreading. Only one patient was able to use the device alone without lipreading. In a second cohort of children who were pre-lingually deaf undergone ABI with a follow-up of up to 5 years, all children who had normal intelligence and functioning implants were able to use the device and be integrated into an integrated normal school environment using auditory-verbal means of communication. The mean vowel and consonant identification scores of this group were 59% and 63% respectively. When comparing to cochlear implant controls who often had their performance plateaued within 3 years, the ABI children showed slow but progressive improvement of up to even 5 years of usage. The mean tone imitation score was 53% and the mean tone production score was 63% with some children achieving over 90% performance. An observation that young implantees may achieve tone perception and production earlier and with better performance was made and case illustrations of children with different outcomes were made in this chapter. The observations of the slow progress, etiology of deafness and co-morbidities were discussed with reference to the outcomes. Successful methods of habilitation of these children include focusing on pitch and tone-pairs discrimination, nonsense syllables and meaningful word identification, and bilingualism with the use of sign language.

Keywords: tone language, Chinese, auditory brainstem implant, adults, children, speech perception outcomes

15.1 Introduction

Globally, the Chinese language or its dialects are the most commonly spoken first languages, with over 900 million native mandarin Chinese speakers (rank 1 in Wikipedia) and over 70 million Cantonese speakers (rank 17). The specific nature of the Chinese languages and other tone-based or tone languages allow speech and hearing scientists to explore the ability of different methods to rehabilitate the hearing impaired, from amplification to electrical stimulation of the cochlea. Difference in pitch patterns affects tone and these changes cannot be detected by lip reading alone. One of the challenges regarding the use of electrical stimulation to restore hearing is reduced ability with pitch perception, affecting notably the perception of tones in speech and music. Over the past 20 years, tests have been developed to assess the perception and production of tones in tone language speakers. We have shown that tones are generally recognized through pitch differentiation problem in younger cochlear implantees as well as better performing adults with difficulties,[31] and it is possible that the same problem may exist in auditory brainstem implant (ABI) users. In this chapter, we outline the characteristics, the assessment, and the outcome of ABI implantation in our series of Cantonese-speaking Chinese adults and children to compare with that available in the literature.

15.2 What is a Tone Language?

A tone language is a language in which the variation of the fundamental frequency contour of a syllable can change the meaning of the word. Mandarin and Cantonese are both lexical tone languages widely spoken by the Chinese population. While Mandarin is the official spoken language in China, Cantonese is the second-largest spoken language in terms of scope of use. Cantonese is widely spoken in the southern part of China including the Guangdong Province, Hong Kong, Macau, and other Asian countries such as Malaysia and Singapore, and the communities of residents in various parts of the world including Australia, United Kingdom, Canada, and the United States of America. It is estimated that 62 to 70 million people worldwide speak Cantonese.[20]

The use of pitch configurations to distinguish one lexical item from another is one important feature distinguishing tone languages from Western languages such as English. Lexical tones are identified from one another by the fundamental frequency (F0) according to the F0 height and contour.[12] There are six and four tones in Cantonese and Mandarin, respectively. A change in tone within a phonemic segment contributes to a change in lexical meaning.[21] ▶ Fig. 15.1 and ▶ Fig. 15.2 illustrate the different fundamental frequency patterns of the Cantonese and Mandarin tones. ▶ Table 15.1 shows sets of examples.

15.3 Speech Assessment Unique to Tone Languages

Due to the inherent different linguistic systems between tone and non-tone languages, it is essential to design specific clinical assessment tools gearing to the particular properties of the language system. For individuals with ABI, the progress in general is slower when compared with individuals with cochlear implants (CIs). Besides the stage of sound detection, areas of assessment need to be more detailed at the basic level of suprasegmental perception. In the validated standardized test of the Cantonese Basic Speech Perception Test (CBSPT),[17] test

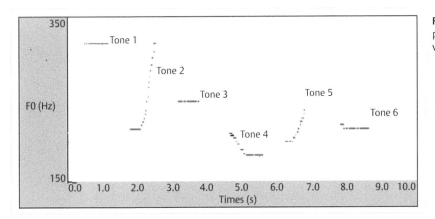

Fig. 15.1 The different fundamental frequency patterns of the six Cantonese tones for the vowel /a/.

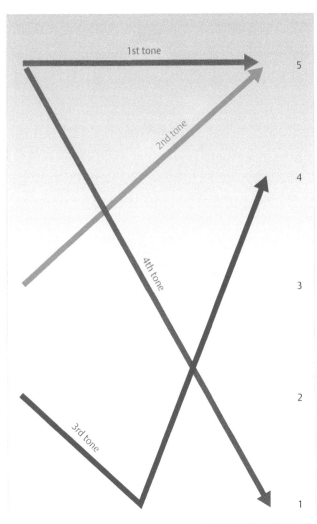

Fig. 15.2 Chart showing the relative changes in pitch for the four tones of Mandarin Chinese. On a scale of 1 to 5 with 5 being the highest pitch, the first tone remains constant at 5 (*high-level*), the second tone rises from 3 to 5 (*high-rising*), the third tone falls from 2 to 1 and then rises to 4 (*low-dipping*), and the fourth tone falls from 5 to 1 (*high-falling*). (https://en.wikipedia.org/wiki/Standard_Chinese_phonology#/media/File:Pinyin_Tone_Chart.svg)

facets include assessing suprasegmental features of pitch and stress perception, which are of paramount importance in tonelanguages.

15.3.1 Assessment of Pitch Perception

In tone language, pitch perception assessment could further be divided into
- Gross discrimination in fundamental frequency
- Basic lexical tone identification
- Lexical tone identification

Gross fundamental frequency discrimination testing is done by assessing the differentiation between a typical male speaker and female speaker producing the same sentence. The average fundamental frequency (F0) of a male and female is around 150 and 250 Hz, respectively. This is to test if one is able to make use of the great difference in pitch information for meaningful perception.

The next stage of basic lexical tone perception is to employ pairs of relatively easy-to-identify tone contrasts as test items. The earlier acquired tones and the tones with the greatest fundamental frequency pattern contrasts should be selected for discrimination in this basic test. In Cantonese, the high-level, high-rising, and low-falling tones are regarded as basic tones.[17] However, in Mandarin, research consistently shows that a high-falling tone is the earliest acquired tone and is the easiest to discriminate when paired with the other tones.[23]

The next level of evaluating pitch information is assessing the full set of lexical tone identification in the language. In Cantonese, there are six lexical tones. All possible combinations yield a total of 15 tone pair contrasts. The Cantonese Tone Identification Test (CanTIT)[16] is a validated and standardized assessment tool for measuring tone perception ability of the Cantonese-speaking population. Normed scores from age 3 to adults are provided. Reference scores of hearing-impaired children with various degrees of hearing loss are also included. With similar test construction principles, Mandarin speakers employ the Mandarin Tone Identification Test[33] as the assessment tool to assess the six tone pair contrasts.

15.3.2 Assessment on Stress Perception

The role of stress perception in English is very different from the tone languages of Cantonese and Mandarin. Depending on whether the two syllables receive equal or unequal stress, disyllabic words in English could further be divided into spondee and trochee. For example, "football" is a spondee with equal stress on the two syllables whereas "happy" is a trochee where

Table 15.1 Examples of lexical tone words in Cantonese and Mandarin

Lexical tones in Cantonese		
Tone	Transcription	Literal meaning
T1 (high-level)	/fu1/	Husband
T2 (high-rising)	/fu2/	Tiger
T3 (mid-level)	/fu3/	Trousers
T4 (low-falling)	/fu4/	Support
T5 (low-rising)	/fu5/	Wife
T6 (low-level)	/fu6/	Father
Lexical Tones in Mandarin		
Tone	Transcription	Literal meaning
T1 (high-level)	/ma1/	Mother
T2 (high-rising)	/ma2/	Hemp
T3 (low-dipping)	/ma3/	Horse
T4 (high-falling)	/ma4/	Scold

only the first syllable is stressed. Assessment on whether one could perceive the stress/unstressed pattern is important in English. Tone languages like Cantonese and Mandarin, however, do not have such a difference in stress pattern in disyllabic words. Both syllables receive equal stress. The rule of equal stress applies in all multisyllabic words, meaning every syllable in a word receives the same amount of stress. The more important aspect of stress in Cantonese and Mandarin, thus, lies in whether one could correctly identify the number of syllables so as to derive if the perceived word is a monosyllabic/disyllabic/trisyllabic or multisyllabic word. Assessment should include testing on identification of number of syllables.

15.3.3 Assessment of Segmental Aspects Involving Words

When moving up to the more advanced levels of speech perception involving use of meaningful words, linguistic characteristics including the phonological system, the grammar, and the syntactic structure must be considered. Frequency of occurrence of words used and sentence type should also be considered.

15.3.4 Assessment of Speech Production

Speech sound production assessment in tone languages should also include tone production accuracy in addition to segmental phonology of vowel and consonant production. Tone production skills maybe assessed at word level, phrase level, sentence level, or discourse level. The key is that all lexical tones in the concerned tone language should be included in the assessment items.

15.4 ABI in NF2 Chinese Speakers

The incidence and prevalence of neurofibromatosis type 2 (NF2)among Chinese has not been previously studied although it is estimated to be much lower than the quoted UK rate of 1:33,000.[11] The ABI poses further challenges for the tone

language speakers. First, postlingually deafened adults who need an ABI have bilateral vestibular schwannomas without their auditory nerves preserved as well as multiple comorbidities. Here we reviewed a series of Chinese adult patients with NF2 who underwent ABI surgery in the Chinese University of Hong Kong.

All patients underwent thorough audiovestibular, lipreading/oral communicative skills, and full radiological assessments before surgery. The implant used in all patients was the Nucleus ABI24 M and later ABI-5 series auditory brainstem device (Cochlear, Sydney, Australia) and one subject had a Combi-40 ABI (MED-EL, Innsbruck, Austria). The Nucleus SPEAK spectral peak speech coding strategy in monopolar mode was used in all patients except the patient using the MED-EL implant.

The extended trans labyrinthine approach for tumor removal and ABI insertion was used in all adults except for one revision surgery in which the retrosigmoid approach was employed. We use the facial nerve, cochlear nerve and other lower cranial nerves (glossopharyngeal and vagus nerves), and especially the choroid plexus as landmarks. The implant is inserted under direct vision and secured in position with a combination of adipose tissue, muscle grafts, and surgical tissue glue, before wound closure. In case the retrosigmoid approach was employed, direct access to the lateral recess was obtained posteriorly. Evoked auditory brainstem response (EABR) is used to confirm proper positioning of the implant electrode array during surgery. In two patients with functional hearing in the contralateral ear, ABI implanted during first-side surgery (as a "sleeper" device) was not switched on in one subject until hearing was lost in the contralateral ear, either from tumor progression or surgery. At the first switch-on session, threshold and maximum comfort levels were set, together with loudness balancing and pitch ranking of the electrodes. Electrodes were activated sequentially, and the intensity gradually increased to obtain thresholds while avoiding adverse effects under cardiovascular monitoring and with standby emergency resuscitation equipment. Nonauditory stimulated electrodes were disabled, and electrode array tonotopy was deduced by paired comparisons of pitch.

Remapping and re-evaluation were performed regularly over the first year. Speech and sound assessment measures, wherever possible, were performed and recorded at 6 months, 1 year, and 2 years, postoperatively. Open-set speech perception tests were conducted in Cantonese (Hong Kong Speech Perception Test Manual) except for the only Mandarin speaker in quiet listening conditions using live voice at normal conversational levels in three conditions: (1) use of ABI alone without the help of lipreading mode (A-mode), (2) lipreading alone without the use of ABI (visual or V-mode), and (3) lipreading together with use of ABI (audiovisual or AV-mode).

From 1997 to 2016, there were a total of 13 adult patients (12 Cantonese-speaking and 1 Mandarin-speaking patients) with NF2 who underwent surgery for removal of vestibular schwannoma and surgical placement of ABIs. Ten of these patients received ABIs after surgical excision of either their first-side vestibular schwannoma or second-side vestibular schwannoma. Two patients declined to have ABI implanted. One patient had consented for ABI but the surgery was abandoned intraoperatively because distorted anatomy prohibited access to the lateral recess. Two patients had their first-side vestibular schwannoma surgery done elsewhere. The bilateral implantee had implant migration and subsequent revision. The mean age of patients at presentation to our department was 28 years, ranging from 14 to 51 years. Ten (77%) patients were female. Most of the patients in the series were reported in Thong et al[28] and are being re-cited here.

The mean size of vestibular schwannoma at presentation for this group of patients was 27 mm (range, 15–41 mm) and the mean size at surgery was 30 mm (range, 15–55 mm). The mean age of patients at the time of ABI implantation was 25 years (range, 16–54 years). In all patients except one, ABI implantation was performed in conjunction with removal of the tumor. Only one patient had a second ABI at the time of removal of second-side tumor because of absence of responses on EABR testing postoperatively after the first surgery.

Device activations were performed between 5 and 9 weeks postoperatively for ABIs implanted during second-side surgery. In the two patients who had ABI implantation at first-side tumor removal, device activation was much later at 4 months (after removal of second-side tumor) and 23 months (after deterioration of hearing in the contralateral ear that had hearing-preservation tumor removal surgery done). The average number of active electrodes was 14 (range, 9–18). The patient who had bilateral sequential ABI implantation did not have EABR response on the second side postoperatively as well, although responses were present intraoperatively. A revision surgery had shown migration of the electrode, yet repositioning resulted in minimal auditory perception. Other surgical complications included: two (25%) patients had permanent facial palsy (House-Brackmann Grades II and III) and one (13%) patient had temporary facial palsy that resolved by 1 year. One patient had cerebrospinal fluid (CSF) leak postoperatively that was managed conservatively with bed rest and insertion of lumbar drain. One patient developed delayed postauricular wound infection at 2 months and this resolved with intravenous antibiotics and wound debridement and did not require implant removal.

15.4.1 Speech and Hearing Outcomes in NF2 Adults

Sound and speech assessment measures were performed for audiological outcomes at 6 months, 1 year, and 2 years,

postoperatively. Including the patient who had two sequential ABIs that did not have EABR postoperatively, environmental sounds could be differentiated by six (75%) patients (67% of implants) after 6 months of ABI use (mean score 46% [range, 28–60%]). One patient (Patient 5) stopped using the ABI after 6 months for reasons as mentioned later and therefore at the 1-year and 2-year postoperative assessments, only seven (78%) patients (56% of implants) continued to be able to differentiate between environmental sounds (1-year mean score 57% [range, 36–76%]; 2-year mean score 48% [range, 24–76%]). Closed-set word identification was possible in six (60%) patients (67% of implants) at 6 months (mean score 39% [range, 12–72%]), 1 year (mean score 68% [range, 48–92%]), and 2 years postoperatively (mean score 62% [range, 28–100%]). One patient demonstrated open-set sentence recognition in quiet in A-mode (use of ABI alone). However, sentence recognition was possible in AV-mode (lipreading together with use of ABI) in six (60%) patients (67% of implants) at 6 months postoperatively (mean score 49% [range, 27–67%]). At 6 months postoperatively, two patients had improvement with scores of 40 and 52% in AV-mode compared with V mode, whereas two patients had no improvement in AV-mode. After 1 and 2 years of ABI use, five (63%) patients (56% of implants) could recognize sentence in AV-mode (1-year mean score 31% [range, 12–79%]; 2-year mean score 35% [range, 12–67%]) and all scores were better than in V-mode (average improvement in scores of 25% at 1 year and 28% at 2 years).

At 2 years postoperatively, only five (50%) patients remained ABI users. In two patients, initial encouraging results with the ABI deteriorated over time and they stopped using the ABI. Patient 7 had the best results with the ABI but she unfortunately developed loud and persistent tinnitus after 2 years and this negatively affected her use of the ABI. In another patient, deterioration of vision soon after ABI implantation affected her ability to lip-read and the ABI was thereafter deemed unhelpful.

ABI users reported that there was improved environmental sound awareness and they were able to differentiate between everyday sounds such as the telephone and television. In one patient, the ABI was found to be helpful in improving understanding of speech and that there was less dependence on lipreading. In others, it was thought that the ABI helped lipreading and allowed them to communicate normally without writing.

In patients who were nonusers, the main complaint was that the ABI was too noisy, especially outdoors, and that it was difficult to tolerate for long periods. It was also thought that actual sound sensations were weak and of poor quality.

15.5 ABI in Non-NF2 Children with Tone Languages

It is an important step towards understanding the question of ABI in detecting tone changes in speech through the study of its development in children who are prelingually deafened. The introduction of ABIs in other non tumor inner ear diseases and deformities such as cochlear aplasia, labyrinthine aplasia (Michel deformity), and cochlear nerve aplasia[9] allows such opportunity for researchers to look into the issue. Following the pioneering work of Colletti and others, the indication for auditory brainstem implantation was extended to the treatment of pediatric prelingual deafness.[5,6]

The following are the data and findings from a published series of Cantonese-speaking children who underwent auditory brainstem implantations at our Center.[27] The audiological and tone language developmental outcomes of pediatric patients with ABIs followed-up for 1 to 5 years are compared with age-matched outcomes of a parallel group of CI users. This remains the only series presenting the outcomes of pediatric ABI users in a tone language setting.

15.5.1 Patient Demographics

ABI was performed in 11 Cantonese-speaking and 2 Mandarin-speaking prelingually deaf children who either failed or had contraindications for cochlear implantation between January 2009 and February 2015 in our unit. The age at implantation ranged from 1.7 to 3.8 years (mean 2.7 years). There were eight males and three females. Etiologies included cochlear nerve deficiency ($n=7$) and severe cochlear malformations ($n=2$) as shown radiologically. In the cochlear nerve deficiency group, two of the seven had coexisting auditory neuropathy spectrum disorder (ANSD) features in their auditory brainstem response (ABR) study.

15.5.2 Preoperative Assessment

All subjects were initially identified by the Hong Kong universal newborn hearing screening program and were referred to our unit for further assessment. Children who met the criteria for cochlear implantation would proceed to CI surgery. Children who showed limited or no benefit from hearing aids, and who had abnormalities on imaging such as cochlear aplasia or severe malformations would be further assessed for ABI candidacy. The decision to proceed with cochlear implantation was jointly made with the parents in view of the lack of benefit from hearing aids in speech and language development.

15.5.3 Audiological Perception Outcomes

Each subject's auditory perception ability was tested using the CBSPT. The following domains of auditory perception were tested:
- **Sound detection (seven-sound detection):** The ability to detect the Ling's seven sounds in a quiet environment
- **Suprasegmental (syllable identification):** The ability to identify the number of syllables in a sound string
- **Segmental:**
  - ○ **Vowel identification:** The ability to identify a word with an appropriate vowel in an array which is different from the vowel only
  - ○ **Consonant identification:** The ability to identify a word with an appropriate consonant in an array which is different from the consonant only

Raw scores of these domains were used to determine the subject's speech perception category (SPC) from 0 to 7 (see ▶ Table 15.2). The CBSPT only covers the test scope of up to

Table 15.2 Speech perception category from 0 to 7

Speech perception category	Definition
0	Minimal Sound Detection
1	Sound Detection
2	Suprasegmental Perception
3	Vowel Perception
4	Consonant Perception
5	10–20% Open-set Word Recognition
6	20–50% Open-set Word Recognition
7	>50% Open-set Word Recognition

consonant perception. For patients scoring over 75% in the consonant identification, open-set word recognition and sentence recognition tests were used to assess higher levels of speech perception ability. In addition, tone imitation and production tests were used on this specific group of Cantonese-speaking children. In tone imitation tests we test their ability to imitate words with different Cantonese tones while in tone production tests we assess their ability to correctly produce words with different Cantonese tones. Both were performed by experienced speech and language pathologists.

For comparison of CI outcomes with this group of ABI children, an age-matched group consisting of 17 children implanted between the ages of 1.1 and 3.1 years who had no significant developmental delay was selected. They were identified with severe to profound hearing loss with no indication of ANSD. Imaging including computed tomography (CT) and magnetic resonance imaging (MRI) suggested no significant abnormalities in the cochlear and internal auditory meatus.

Cochlear implantation was performed on 7 of the 11 Cantonese-speaking ABI subjects. One child had a hypoplastic middle ear with an unsuccessful electrode placement attempt. The remaining six subjects, who underwent uneventful surgery with satisfactory electrode position, did not show consistent sound detection nor benefit in speech and language development after 1 year of CI use with regular auditory programming attempts and speech training. Cochlear implantation was not considered for the other 4 of the 11 subjects as they all had severe cochlear malformations, or cochlear nerve deficiency. For the two subjects with cochlear nerve deficiency, the decision of not to implant them with a CI was made in conjunction with parental preference. Of the two Mandarin speakers, one had a prior intraoperative EABR showing no response in another center and one had complete cochlear aplasia. Both of them had no CI before ABI surgeries.

15.5.4 Speech and Language Outcomes of ABI in Tone Language-speaking Children

Results of the 11 Cantonese children are presented here. In the majority of subjects, seven-sound detection could be achieved at a relatively early stage postoperatively and this is comparable to age-matched CI users. Five subjects scored 100% with a mean score of 92.6% (range, 55.6–100%) at 1 year postoperatively. In Syllable Identification, four achieved 100% with a mean score of

77.8% (range, 0–100%), which happened more gradually over the first 2 to 3 years. In Vowel Identification, the average score was 59.1% (range, 16.7–87.5%). In Consonant Identification, the average score was 62.7% (range, 0–87.5%). Syllable Identification, Vowel Identification, and Consonant Identification were achieved by the majority of our subjects albeit at a relatively slower rate when compared to CI users. However, whereas outcomes of CI users plateaued after 2 to 3 years, ABI subjects appeared to continue to show improvement even 5 years after surgery. In Tone Imitation, the average score was 52.9% (range, 0–88.9%). In Tone Production, the average score was 63.6% (range, 0–96%). The Tone Imitation and Production scores are closer to CI users, with good results achieved by some of the subjects that had less impressive outcomes in other parameters such as the SPC.[17]

At the time of data collection, two subjects achieved categories 5 to 7 in the SPC[17] assessment which is equivalent to open-set word recognition. Two subjects achieved category 4, and the remaining two subjects categories 1 to 3. Similar to the other outcome measurement parameters, speech perception represented by the SPC showed a slow but steadily improving trend during the follow-up period. SPC 4 or better was achieved by 4 of the 11 subjects. With the current trend, we expect some of the subjects to achieve higher categories at the end of the 5-year postoperative follow-up period.

Three children did not perform well enough to complete our outcome assessment. Of note, these subjects have coexisting nonauditory developmental disabilities. Nevertheless, parents reported good compliance to ABI usage by their children who demonstrated improved awareness to environmental sounds.

15.6 Case Studies

15.6.1 Case 1: KC

KC was born full-term failing neonatal hearing screening while in the hospital soon after birth. Evoked response audiometry repeatedly showed bilateral profound hearing loss and auditory neruopathy. MRI and CT of the temporal bone had indicated absence of right eight nerve complexes in the internal auditory meatus. Both vestibulocochlear apparatuses were normal in configuration. Left cochlear implantation was performed at the age of 15 month after discussion with the parents and intraoperative EABRs were negative for electrical stimulation through the implant. He was subsequently switched on without any auditory responses and there was significant speech and development delay. At the age of 25months, left ABI through retrosigmoid approach with removal of the CI was performed and he was subsequently switched on a month after with 14 active usable electrodes. ▶ Fig. 15.3 shows the speech and language outcomes with comparison to the CI group data. The data show a delay of 2 to 3 years in vowel, consonant, and tone identifications; yet tone imitation and production had caught up with the CI group 1 year after surgery. The latter was more dependent on a good speech and language training program. KC is currently 12 years of age and integrated into a similar-age class of a mainstream school. He is a trilingual, Cantonese, English, and sign language speaker, and uses mostly oral communication mode in school and at home.

15.6.2 Case 2: MY

MY was born prematurely at 32 weeks of gestation and was noted to have "global developmental delay" before referring to us at the age of 26 months. He failed newborn ABR screening but passed the neonatal otoacoustic emissions (OAE) screening at the age of 2 months. There was also a history of seizure and limited benefit from bilateral hearing aids. ABR showed bilateral auditory neuropathy with presence of wave I but absence of brainstem responses at 100 decibel above normal hearing level (dBnHL) of acoustic stimulation. CT and MRI had indicated left Mondini deformity, hypoplastic right internal auditory canal (IAC) with one single nerve identified, and a high riding jugular bulb on the left and grossly normal anatomy and nerves in the left IAC. Left cochlear implantation was performed at 35 months of age and postoperatively, there was absence of EABR and behavioral responses. At the age of 40 months, left CI explantation and ABI were performed. He was successfully switched on with 15 active usable electrodes. He was in an integrated hearing impaired–normal kindergarten and was integrated into mainstream education in primary school. The speech and language outcomes are charted in ▶ Fig. 15.4. He has good consonant detection but is unable to correctly identify tones. He is currently 12 years old with a fair speech production and tone imitation with minimal auditory input and speech training.

15.6.3 Case 3: LC

LC failed neonatal hearing screening and was identified with global developmental delay soon after birth. Genetic screening confirmed labyrinthine aplasia, microtia, and microdontia (LAMM) syndrome and radiologically there was aplasia of the cochleovestibular apparatus bilaterally. After discussing with the parents, ABI was performed on the right side at the age of 20 months. Switch on 1 month after the surgery was successful in 11 electrodes which remained usable todate. Despite the mild developmental delay, he was integrated into mainstream education in primary school. Regarding the speech and language outcomes which are shown in ▶ Fig. 15.5, he is our star patient who could perform as good as our CI control group, including tone identification tests. At the moment we are planning for a second-side implant and he is now 9 years of age. LC is our youngest ABI patient, and this may be an important factor for the excellent speech and language outcomes despite the presence of comorbidities.

15.7 Interpretation of Speech and Language Outcomes of NF2 Adults

15.7.1 Detection of Environmental Sounds

As the only hearing rehabilitation option available for these patients, the main goal of the ABI is to help patients detect environmental sounds and provide auditory sensations to enhance their lipreading ability such that oral communication can still be possible.

In this small group of patients, 75%could detect and differentiate between environmental sounds. This is in concordance

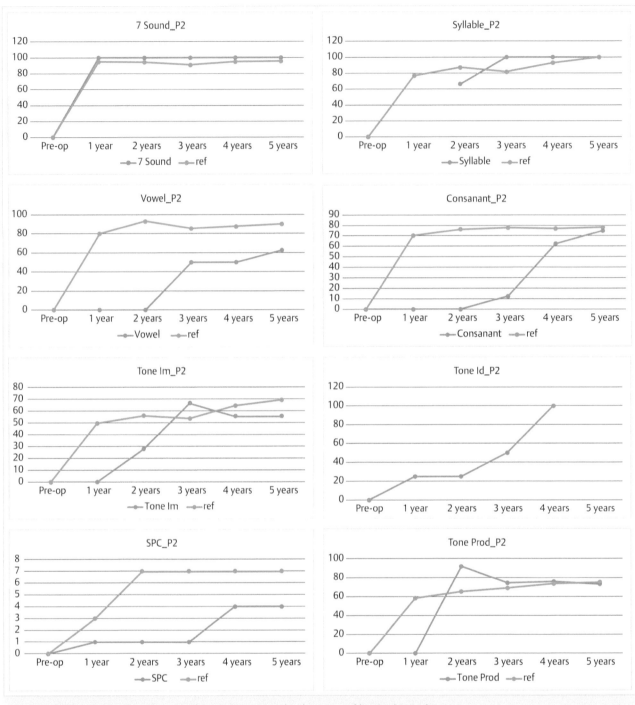

Fig. 15.3 Speech and language outcomes of Case 1 KC compared with group cochlear implantee data.

with Lenarz et al[19] who found that 82% of their patients found the ABI most useful for differentiating between the various environmental sounds.

15.7.2 Limitations in Speech Recognition without Lipreading

ABI implantation in NF2 patients has been observed to have significantly worse outcomes in general, compared with the high levels of speech recognition observed in non-NF2 adults[9,13] and

congenitally deaf children).[5,7,26] Although recent studies have shown excellent speech recognition in some NF2 patients such that telephone use is even possible (Sanna, 2012),[13] outcomes with the ABI are highly unpredictable and open-set speech perception in NF2 patients using the ABI alone is rarely possible.[14] In the series published by Sanna et al,[25]15 (65%) of 23 patients had no speech recognition with ABI alone although of the 8 patients who did, 4 were able to use the telephone. Vincent et al found that only 3 (21%) of their 14 patients had speech perception, of whom one could use the telephone (Vincent, 2001).

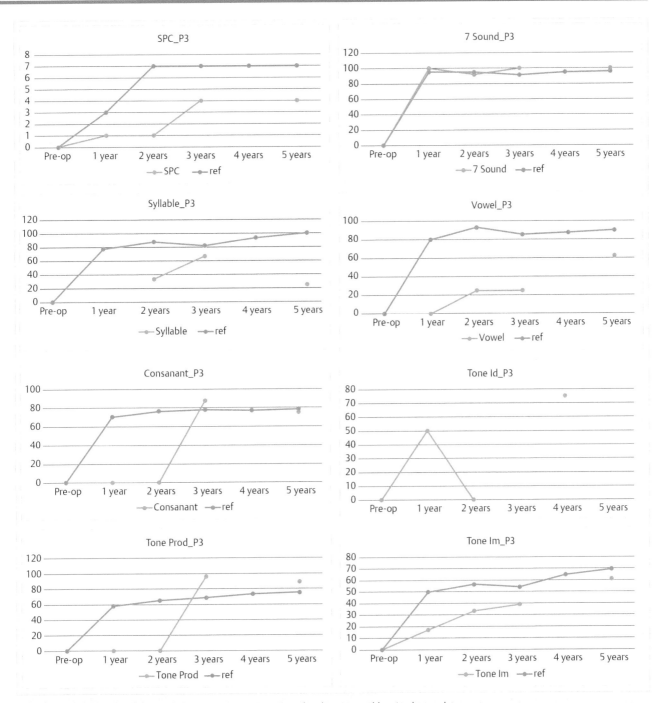

Fig. 15.4 Speech and language outcomes of Case 2 MY compared with group cochlear implantee data.

Outcomes across ABI surgical centers were recently compared at a meeting of surgeons in 2012 in an attempt to explain the variability observed in NF2 patients.[2,8] Patient, surgical, and device factors were compared and age at implantation and tumor size before surgery were not found to be significant factors. Factors that showed significant correlation were length of deafness, surgical position, number of distinct pitch electrodes, perceptual levels, and stimulation pulse rate. These factors are thought to be related to the health of the auditory brainstem tissue to be stimulated and the consensus opinion was that the most likely cause of poor ABI performance in NF2 patients is

mechanical or vascular damage to the cochlear nucleus during tumor removal or systemic damage to the brainstem from NF2 disease progression. We have been following the practice of utmost care during surgery to minimize physical and venous trauma to the surface of the brainstem in an attempt to improve hearing outcomes.

Tone language recognition requires more pitch perception information for language understanding, and we have already predicted that the outcomes of ABIs in our group of subjects may not be excellent in terms of open-set speech recognition. Just one of the patients in our series managed to achieve

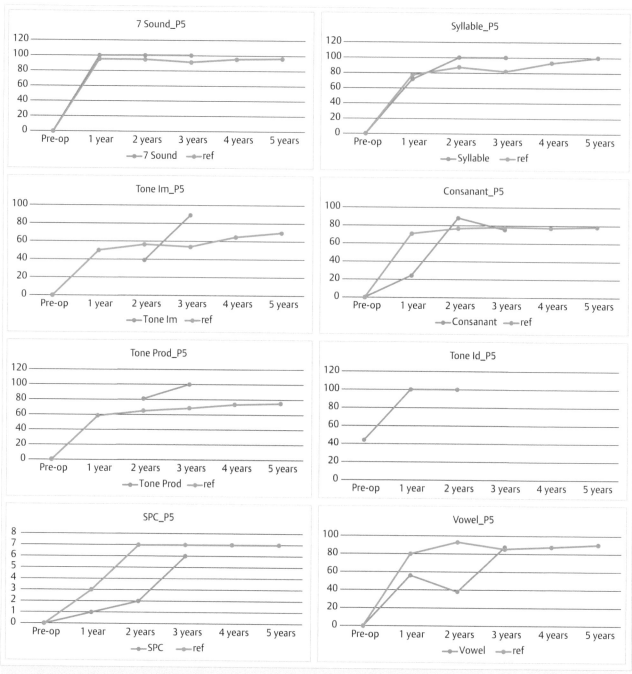

Fig. 15.5 Speech and language outcomes of Case 3 LC compared with group cochlear implantee data.

open-set speech understanding in A-mode. Difference in pitch distinguishes one word from another and hence changes the lexical meaning. Differentiating between the tones is essential for speech understanding. Current speech-processing strategies of the ABI may not be adequate for tone languages. This may be inferred from studies on CI patients whereby adjustments to speech processing parameters have been found to improve tone recognition and speech perception in Cantonese and other tone languages.[15,29] More research is needed to investigate optimal speech-processing strategies for tone language perception in ABI patients.

15.7.3 Expectation Management in NF2 Patients for ABI Surgery

With regards to improvement in lipreading for speech understanding, the results are far more encouraging. Our series showed an average of 28% improvement in speech recognition scores in AV-mode over V-mode at 2 years. This is comparable to reports that showed that the ABI provided auditory sensations that improved lipreading by an average of 30% points.[8] As an adjuvant to lipreading, ABI has been considered the most useful for understanding speech in quiet surroundings.[18] Noisy environment has been found to be the biggest cause of disturbance for ABI users and in Hong Kong or other Asian cities, this poses a real problem for our listeners. In two of our patients, speech recognition was worse in AV-mode compared with V-mode at 6 months and this subsequently improved at the 1-year assessment. This phenomenon was attributed to device-activation lipreading distraction whereby auditory sensations from the ABI distract the patient's concentration during lipreading in those who have not yet adapted.[19]

Improvement in auditory performance has been observed to occur over the first 6 to 9 months in general and in our series of patients, results were variable with some showing improvement in lipreading enhancement with time, and others showing deterioration.

At 2 years, there was only a 37% ABI user rate. The lack of perceived benefit experienced by the patients as well as progression of NF2 both contribute to non-use; for instance, deterioration of vision from commonly coexisting optic tumors affects lipreading ability. Development of multiple handicaps and deterioration in the patient's general condition can also interfere with hearing training and motivation to use the ABI. All our patients had the magnet removed from their ABI receiver-stimulator and less convenient adhesive retention disks were used to attach the external transmitter coil. It is therefore important to manage patient's expectations preoperatively as multiple factors, related and unrelated to the ABI itself, can affect hearing rehabilitation outcomes.

With regards to surgical-related failures, one of our patients who had bilateral sequential ABI done had no auditory responses subjectively and on EABR testing postoperatively on either side although responses were present intraoperatively. This patient was 54 and 55 years old at the first- and second-side ABI implantation, respectively, and was the oldest patient in our series. His tumor was not the largest in our series (24 × 25 mm) and postoperative imaging did not show obvious migration or displacement of the electrodes. Nevertheless, it is recognized that even a slight displacement of the electrode array can affect outcomes.

15.8 Interpretation in Prelingually Deafened Cantonese-Speaking Children

15.8.1 Prolonged Time Frame of Auditory Development in ABI Children

Good sound detection could be achieved in the first year for ABI users and this is comparable to age-matched CI users and published case series data.[3] CI users can typically achieve good outcomes within 2 years of surgery.[22] Our current data show a slower progress; yet there is continued improvement in all parameters during the 5-year follow-up period, consistent with findings from others whereas additional comorbidities may slow down progression.[32]

15.8.2 Poor (Slower) Speech Perception and Tone Production Outcomes in Subjects with Relatively Well-developed Environmental Sound Detection

Most of the subjects were able to detect sounds and did well in environmental sound detection tasks. The overall performance in speech perception was poorer in ABI than that of the CI children. The different location of electrodes between CI and ABI and tonotopic arrangement of the ABI electrode might have contributed to the difference in the ability to perceive the temporal and spectral information necessary for speech perception.[1,6] In some subjects, they were able to identify tones as good as the CI children, which indicated that there is indeed tonotopic arrangement in the brainstem with contribution to tone language speech understanding.

15.8.3 Comorbid Nonauditory and Cognitive Conditions

Pediatric performance might be strongly dependent on etiology of deafness, cognitive ability, and the integrity of the auditory pathways showing greater variability. Subjects with an auditory nerve and a cochlear malformation performed better than subjects with either a cochlear nerve deficiency or an ANSD. Similar to the pediatric CI population, subjects with multiple disabilities showed slower progress and limited benefit from an ABI. The poor open-set speech recognition and speech production associated with cognitive comorbidity suggests that disorders of central auditory signaling or speech and language processing are an important factor in ABI outcome.[4,24] Good family support, an indispensable indication for surgery in this group of children, guarantees good compliance and noticeable benefits of device use in training and daily activities.

15.8.4 Neural Plasticity

Despite the high variability of ABI outcomes and the associated time-frame, an early decision to convert from a CI to an ABI is advocated. ABI should be considered for optimal auditory perception and speech and language development when a lack of progress with a CI is evident.[4] Age may still be the most important factor as shown in our patient LC (see above).

15.8.5 Etiologies and Outcomes

The etiology of deafness is the main determining factor of outcome. In our series, the two outstanding performers (including LC) had major middle ear and inner ear deformities. The structural and functional integrity of the cochlear nerve and cochlear nucleus is an important prognostic factor for successful auditory rehabilitation, especially for open-set word recognition. The other subjects in our series with ANSD with cochlear nerve deficiency and retrocochlear deafness had less satisfactory outcomes.

A review of outcomes from different international centers[10,26] and ours shows the presence of a functional cochlear nerve (e.g., hearing loss due to inner ear malformations or meningitis) and the implied presence of cochlear nuclei in some children contributed to successful outcomes. Whereas in those children with cochlear nerve abnormalities, the nerve might be dysfunctional, preventing good signal transmission to the central auditory pathways, resulting in a poor clinical outcome with ABI.

15.8.6 Use of Adjuncts Sign Language and Lipreading

The group of children that we have been describing are usually implanted with an ABI at an older age than children who receive CIs. With a later starting point and slower progress, as we have reported in this study, auditory stimulation alone appears to be insufficient for development. We strongly recommend additional modes of communication to facilitate the overall development of children who find themselves in this group. Extensive counseling of parents emphasizing the importance of additional modalities of communication is essential. Bilingual programs and lipreading are two major adjuncts advocated for the children in our study. ABI is an important adjunct to the child's cognitive and language development, where lipreading and sign language are incorporated and in a few subjects who had been diagnosed with developmental delay, enhanced cognitive development after ABI had resulted in mainstream education.

15.9 Habilitation of ABI Users in Tone Languages

Our experiences so far have stressed the importance of a structured habilitation program as well as an integrated pathway to mainstream education. The greatest challenge of habilitating ABI users lies in the group of prelingually deaf individuals who do not have sufficient linguistic knowledge to assist their speech perception. On the one hand, intensive auditory training has to be provided to develop the speech perception ability. On the other hand, the linguistic competency needs to be built up via alternate means when the auditory route is not found to be the most efficient and effective approach.

While many children remain at the stage of sound detection and suprasegmental perception, about 20% of the children are able to attain open-set word recognition levels. The duration of ABI use for children to achieve open-set word recognition is 4 to 5 years, which is relatively longer when compared with children with CI. Instead of moving up the speech perception hierarchy hastily, the basic foundation has to be very solid and speech perception training has to be performed in a much refined and meticulous manner. Children need time to develop those basic skills before moving up the hierarchy. Discrimination tasks in the format of judging whether two speech sounds are the same or different have to be well practiced. The focus of habilitation could be summarized as the following four areas:

1. Suprasegmental perception of pitch
   - Gross pitch discrimination: Discriminate and identify male versus female voice
   - Discriminate and identify tone pairs with high contrasts
   - Discriminate and identify tone pairs with low contrasts
   - Identify all lexical tones
2. Suprasegmental perception of stress
   - Discriminate and identify number of nonsense syllables
3. Transition from suprasegmental to segmental word identification
   - High contrast word identification using meaningful words with different number of syllables, different vowels, and different consonants
4. Develop the linguistic system via alternative means such as sign language if needed

It is hoped that the information highlighted the essential elements when performing speech assessment and habilitation on ABI users who are speakers of tone languages.

15.10 Conclusion

As NF2 is rare in Hong Kong, our experience of ABI implantation in this group of patients is limited. However, the data seem to show poorer outcomes compared with English-speaking and other non-tone language-speaking NF2 patients. Environmental sound awareness and lipreading enhancement are the main benefits observed in our patients. The latter fortunately was achievable in our patients as Chinese languages seem to be a more visually provoking languages as found in our unpublished studies. More work is needed to improve auditory implant speech processing strategies for tone languages and these advancements may yield better speech perception outcomes in the future.

Regarding prelingually deafened children, our results show that with persistent device use, meaningful auditory perception can develop in most subjects. For children who fail to show benefit from a CI, early implantation and activation of ABI is important to maximize their speech development. While the cause of deafness is the main determining factor for outcome, the presence of additional nonauditory and cognitive disabilities are associated with poorer performance.

References

[1] Bayazit YA, Kosaner J, Cinar BC, et al. Methods and preliminary outcomes of pediatric auditory brainstem implantation. Ann Otol Rhinol Laryngol. 2014; 123(8):529–536

[2] Behr R, Colletti V, Matthies C, et al. New outcomes with auditory brainstem implants in NF2 patients. Otol Neurotol. 2014; 35(10):1844–1851

[3] Colletti L, Colletti G, Mandalà M, Colletti V. The therapeutic dilemma of cochlear nerve deficiency: cochlear or brainstem implantation? Otolaryngol Head Neck Surg. 2014; 151(2):308–314

[4] Colletti L, Shannon RV, Colletti V. The development of auditory perception in children after auditory brainstem implantation. Audiol Neurotol. 2014; 19 (6):386–394

[5] Colletti V, Carner M, Fiorino F, et al. Hearing restoration with auditory brainstem implant in three children with cochlear nerve aplasia. Otol Neurotol. 2002; 23(5):682–693

[6] Colletti V, Carner M, Miorelli V, Guida M, Colletti L, Fiorino F. Auditory brainstem implant (ABI): new frontiers in adults and children. Otolaryngol Head Neck Surg. 2005; 133(1):126–138

[7] Colletti V, Shannon RV. Open set speech perception with auditory brainstem implant? Laryngoscope. 2005; 115(11):1974–1978

[8] Colletti L, Shannon R, Colletti V. Auditory brainstem implants for neurofibromatosis type 2. Curr Opin Otolaryngol Head Neck Surg. 2012; 20(5):353–357

[9] Colletti V, Shannon R, Carner M, Veronese S, Colletti L. Outcomes in nontumor adults fitted with the auditory brainstem implant: 10 years' experience. Otol Neurotol. 2009; 30(5):614–618

[10] Couloigner V, Gratacap M, Ambert-Dahan E, et al. [A report of three cases and review of auditory brainstem implants in children]. Neurochirurgie. 2014; 60 (1–2):17–26

[11] Evans DG, Howard E, Giblin C, et al. Birth incidence and prevalence of tumor-prone syndromes: estimates from a UK family genetic register service. Am J Med Genet A. 2010; 152A(2):327–332

[12] Gandour J. Perceptual dimensions of tone: evidence from Cantonese. J Chin Linguist. 1981; 9:20–36

[13] Grayeli AB, Kalamarides M, Bouccara D, Ambert-Dahan E, Sterkers O. Auditory brainstem implant in neurofibromatosis type 2 and non-neurofibromatosis type 2 patients. Otol Neurotol. 2008; 29(8):1140–1146

[14] Kanowitz SJ, Shapiro WH, Golfinos JG, Cohen NL, Roland JT, Jr. Auditory brainstem implantation in patients with neurofibromatosis type 2. Laryngoscope. 2004; 114(12):2135–2146

[15] Lee T, Yu S, Yuan M, Wong TK, Kong YY. The effect of enhancing temporal periodicity cues on Cantonese tone recognition by cochlear implantees. Int J Audiol. 2014; 53(8):546–557

[16] Lee KYS. The Cantonese Tone Identification Test (CANTIT). Hong Kong: Department of Otorhinolaryngology, Head & Neck Surgery, the Chinese University of Hong Kong; 2012

[17] Lee KYS. The Cantonese Basic Speech Perception Test (CBSPT). Hong Kong: Department of Surgery, the Chinese University of Hong Kong; 2006

[18] Lenarz M, Matthies C, Lesinski-Schiedat A, et al. Auditory brainstem implant part II: subjective assessment of functional outcome. Otol Neurotol. 2002; 23 (5):694–697

[19] Lenarz T, Moshrefi M, Matthies C, et al. Auditory brainstem implant: part I. Auditory performance and its evolution over time. Otol Neurotol. 2001; 22 (6):823–833

[20] Lewis MP, Simons GF, Fennig CD, eds. Ethnologue: Languages of the World. 17th ed. Dallas, TX: SILInternational; 2013. Online version: http://www.ethnologue.com

[21] Matthews S, Yip V. Cantonese: A Comprehensive Grammar. London: Routledge; 1994

[22] Niparko JK, Tobey EA, Thal DJ, et al. CDaCI Investigative Team. Spoken language development in children following cochlear implantation. JAMA. 2010; 303(15):1498–1506

[23] Peng SC, Tomblin JB, Cheung H, Lin YS, Wang LS. Perception and production of mandarin tones in prelingually deaf children with cochlear implants. Ear Hear. 2004; 25(3):251–264

[24] Pisoni DB. Cognitive factors and cochlear implants: some thoughts on perception, learning, and memory in speech perception. Ear Hear. 2000; 21 (1):70–78

[25] Sanna M, Di Lella F, Guida M, Merkus P. Auditory brainstem implants in NF2 patients: results and review of the literature. Otol Neurotol. 2012; 33(2):154–164

[26] Sennaroglu L, Ziyal I, Atas A, et al. Preliminary results of auditory brainstem implantation in prelingually deaf children with inner ear malformations including severe stenosis of the cochlear aperture and aplasia of the cochlear nerve. Otol Neurotol. 2009; 30(6):708–715

[27] Sung JKK, Luk BPK, Wong TKC, Thong JF, Wong HT, Tong MCF. Pediatric auditory brainstem implantation: impact on audiological rehabilitation and tonal language development. Audiol Neurotol. 2018; 23(2):126–134

[28] Thong JF, Sung JK, Wong TK, Tong MC. Auditory brainstem implantation in Chinese patients with neurofibromatosis type II: the Hong Kong experience. Otol Neurotol. 2016; 37(7):956–962

[29] Tong MC, Lee KY. Do Chinese speakers need a specialized cochlear implant system? ORL J Otorhinolaryngol Relat Spec. 2009; 71(4):184–186

[30] Vincent C, Zini C, Gandolfi A, et al. Results of the MXM Digisonic auditory brainstem implant clinical trials in Europe. Otol Neurotol. 2002; 23(1):56–60

[31] Xu L, Chen X, Lu H, et al. Tone perception and production in pediatric cochlear implants users. Acta Otolaryngol. 2011; 131(4):395–398

[32] Yücel E, Aslan F, Özkan HB, Sennaroğlu L. Recent rehabilitation experience with pediatric ABI users. J Int Adv Otol. 2015; 11(2):110–113

[33] Zhu S, Wong LLN, Chen F. Development and validation of a new Mandarin tone identification test. Int J Pediatr Otorhinolaryngol. 2014; 78(12):2174–2182

16 Variability in Performance of Auditory Brainstem Implants

Kathryn Y. Noonan, Gregory P. Lekovic, and Eric P. Wilkinson

Abstract

Many patient, device, and surgical factors contribute to patient success with auditory brainstem implants. This chapter examines device positioning, duration of deafness, choice of device, intelligence or motivation of patient, etiology of deafness, tumor size, age of patient, surgical technique, programming, and rehabilitation. Significant variability in techniques are discussed however the ideal approach to implantation is not fully understood.

Keywords: variability, performance, surgical factors, auditory brainstem implant, neurofibromatosis, outcomes

16.1 Background

All auditory implants are subject to a multitude of variables that affect their performance outcomes. Understanding this variability allows for continuous adjustments and improvements to achieve optimal audiometric results. Cochlear implants (CIs), for example, are subject to some variability in positioning and from the types of electrodes used. However, in the absence of a malformation, the CI will generally occupy the same position due to the anatomic confines of the structure. Techniques such as "soft surgery" and hearing preservation, designed to prevent trauma in the cochlea with subsequent postoperative hydrops and performance variabilities, have been developed. Preservation of low frequency hearing is possible and patients may use a combination of electric and acoustic hearing (EAS) to take advantage of low frequency pitch cues along with the speech signal reproduced by the CI. In part due to the tonotopic layout of frequency information in the cochlea, the information provided by a CI will result in a signal more readily decipherable by the higher auditory system, when compared with an auditory brainstem implant (ABI).

The higher auditory pathways and their variabilities certainly affect CI performance. Auditory neuropathy, caliber variations in the VIIIth cranial nerve in certain types of malformations, and cochlear malformations may result in decreased information from the periphery entering the auditory system, but the higher auditory pathways, including the brainstem nuclei, ascending pathways, and ultimately the auditory cortex, have inherent variability and play a role in outcomes. Older patients, for example, often take longer to gain benefit from CI due to temporal processing issues in the auditory cortex.

In ABI patients, the information coming from the peripheral auditory system is not as tonotopically organized as information coming from the cochlea. This information is degraded when compared to stimuli from a CI. However, outcomes in adults and children implanted with ABI show a wide variability, from no benefit, to benefits with lipreading, to closed-set speech perception, to open-set speech perception with relatively normal development of the auditory system.[1] What factors enter into such variability? In this chapter, we examine

multiple factors that play a role in the wide range of outcomes seen with ABI.[2] Known variables in the CI literature are explored as well as additional factors specific to the ABI. Device positioning, duration of deafness, choice of device, intelligence/motivation of patient, etiology of deafness, tumor size, age of patient, surgical technique, programming, and rehabilitation will be discussed in detail.

16.2 Potential Factors Involved in Variability

16.2.1 Surgical Factors

Device Positioning

Device positioning is an important variable impacting ABI audiometric outcomes. Due to the anatomy of the lateral recess there is significantly more variability allowed in the positioning of devices when compared to CIs. Ideally, the device is to be positioned within the lateral recess of the foramen of Luschka with the paddle in contact with the cochlear nucleus. The surgical landmarks for identification of the foramen of Luschka include the origin of the lower cranial nerves and the choroid plexus, a tuft of which reliably projects into the cerebellopontine angle from within the lateral recess. However, these landmarks may be absent or difficult to identify in some cases (e.g., if the lower cranial nerves are involved with tumor). Large schwannomas may dilate the lateral recess such that the electrode may not maintain its ideal position within a patulous foramen of Luschka. In other cases, the lateral recess may be obscured by the presence of tumor involving the lower cranial nerves; these are typically not removed when removing a vestibular schwannoma due to fear of lower cranial nerve complications. Rarely, the lateral recess may be imperforate, or its entrance blocked by arachnoid septations.

The cochlear nucleus has a three-dimensional tonotopic organization that runs orthogonal to the surface.[3] Therefore, flat paddle electrode arrays are suboptimal for taking advantage of this anatomic orientation. Some authors have sought to optimize implants to better correlate with the anatomy of the region. Otto et al investigated the use of a penetrating implant to capitalize on the three-dimensional organization of the cochlear nucleus. In their study, they were not able to show improved audiometric outcomes with the penetrating electrode; however, they did report consistently lower thresholds in the penetrating ABI recipients.[4] Although some patients showed promising results, eventually penetrating electrodes were abandoned in favor of devices with more straightforward placement strategies due to the technical difficulty of implantation.

Other authors have investigated the variability that stems from device location and angle of placement. Barber et al reported on the existence of a surface "sweet spot" that resulted in lower thresholds and less nonaudiometric side effects by

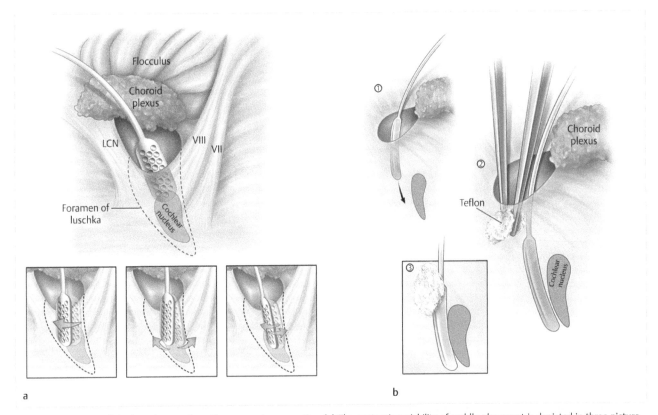

Fig. 16.1 Anatomy of the lateral recess from the surgeon's perspective. **(a)** The anatomic variability of paddle placement is depicted in three picture inserts. **(b)** Teflon placement for ideal positioning and contact between the electrode paddle and the cochlear nucleus.

achieving an optimal angle of the device.[5] Additionally, they reported a wide range of angle variability among their study population with a weak correlation between angle and audiometric outcomes. See ▸ Fig. 16.1 for details on ABI placement and the associated angle placement variability.

Anatomic variability between patients contributes to the difficulty of electrode placement. Intraoperative testing can facilitate device placement. Matthies et al discussed the use of a quadripolar test electrode and evoked auditory brainstem response (EABR) mapping to precisely localize the cochlear nucleus or placement "sweetspot" prior to device implantation.[6] Mandalà et al found a significant improvement in audiometric outcomes when they used near-field compound action potentials (CAP) to position the device compared to EABRs (p=0.0051).[7] In their study of 18 patients they report 78.9% correct on open-set testing in the CAP group compared with 56.7% speech perception in the traditional EABR cohort.[7] These studies show that significant variability in ABI performance can be explained by device placement making it a critical factor for success.

Anatomic Variability

Brainstem trauma from tumor removal or anatomic distortion may impact audiometric outcomes; however, there is limited date available on this topic. See ▸ Fig. 16.2 for an example of brainstem distortion noted on preoperative ABI scan. This hypothesis is supported by the fact that audiometric outcomes in nontumor patients generally are superior to patients with

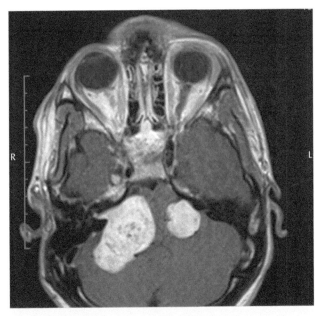

Fig. 16.2 Neurofibromatosis 2 patient with brainstem compression from bilateral vestibular schwannomas.

tumors.[1] Behr et al specifically investigated the impact of anatomic distortion by looking at the correlation between speech discrimination and tumor stage.[8] Their study focused on stage 3 (touching brainstem) and stage 4 (brainstem compression) vestibular schwannoma patients. Interestingly, their data found that there was no correlation between the tumor stage and word recognition, arguing against brainstem distortion as a significant factor impacting outcomes.[8] Goyal et al investigated the impact of anatomic variations in nontumor patients.[9] They studied cerebellar flocculus size in pediatric patients and corresponding audiometric outcomes. This study reported more difficulty with electrode placement in patients with high grade flocculus size. More data is needed to fully understand the impact of anatomic distortion.

Brainstem Trauma

It is also theorized that trauma from excitotoxicity or cautery injury may negatively impact on outcomes. Iseli et al conducted a study in gerbils where they compared cold-steel cutting of the cochlear nerve versus cauterizing and cutting the cochlear nerve.[10] They found no difference between the two approaches when the site was sufficiently far from the cochlear nucleus. However, more proximal bipolar cautery caused significant changes in the cochlear nucleus and likely impacts outcomes in ABI recipients. The House Clinic group investigated this parameter and reports improved outcomes with modified surgical techniques using conservative cautery, thus minimizing vascular damage.[11] Surgical technique and cautery use are important contributors to audiometric outcomes. Open-set speech outcomes are typically found at high volume centers only, underscoring the importance of surgeon's experience and surgical volume.[12]

Surgical Positioning

Surgical positioning may potentially contribute to ABI outcomes. Patient positioning affects brain relaxation, bleeding, and the amount of cautery needed for hemostasis. Two main surgical positions are employed for ABI surgery. In Europe, a semi-sitting position is used whereas in the United States a supine position is more popular. When comparing the European and US literature, there is statically significant better results with the semi-sitting position (p=0.041).[8] However, there are several other surgical differences including the surgeon, the device used, and the impact on hydrostatic that contribute to the figures in this study. Many surgeons in the United States avoid a semi-sitting position due to the perceived risk of air embolism. There are no controlled studies to specifically compare this variable.[13] It is therefore difficult to determine if surgical positioning has any significant impact on audiometric outcomes.

16.2.2 Patient Factors

Duration of Deafness

The patient's duration of deafness is another crucial variable impacting ABI performance. From the CI literature, we know this is an important factor for implantable audiometric outcomes. Multiple authors have demonstrated this axiom likely holds true with ABI users. Behr et al reviewed 26 patients with open-set scores greater than 30% and found an inverse relationship between duration of deafness and word recognition scores. Patients who were deafened for less than a year had better speech recognition outcomes than those who were deaf for

longer period. Matthies et al demonstrated similar findings in a prospective study of 18 patients receiving ABIs.[14] They looked at the cumulative duration of deafness between both ears and found it was one of the strongest predictors of sentence scores among their patients. These findings suggest duration of deafness is an important factor and advise implantation of surgical candidates as early as possible.

Intelligence/Motivation

When compared to CIs, ABIs require significantly more auditory rehabilitation and motivation to achieve optimal outcomes. Patients with multiple disabilities and other comorbid conditions have worse performance outcomes.[15]

Noij et al conducted a systematic review of 162 nontumor children who underwent ABI placement.[16] They found nonauditory disabilities correlated with worse audiometric outcomes. Additionally, they demonstrated that audiometric outcomes correlated with duration of use. Patients continued to improve for about 24 months before reaching a plateau. Similarly, Otto et al reported initial disappointment at activation but significant improvement after a period of adaptation and learning.[17] Their study showed continued gains for up to 8 years with device use and some patients with initial poor performance were able to achieve open-set after a few years of use.[17]

Age

Although there is still a relatively small body of ABI literature available, thus far age of implantation has not been shown to be a significant factor in predicting audiometric outcomes. Several studies have examined this parameter but did not find an age trend that reaches statistical significance.[16,18,19] A systematic review by Noij et al of 162 children found age was not correlated with audiometric outcomes.[16] Jung et al reviewed nontumor ABI patients and found postlingually deafened adults had higher CAP scores than the pediatric population; however, this finding was not statistically significant.[19] In the current literature, age does not appear to play a significant role in audiometric outcomes.

Etiology of Deafness

The etiology of deafness significantly contributes to audiometric outcomes. Originally the only indication for an ABI was neurofibromatosis type 2 (NF2) and therefore this patient population comprises the majority of the literature. Increasingly indications for implantation have expanded and new performance outcomes in non-NF2 patients are now available. Overall, patients without cerebellopontine angle tumors have better outcomes than patients with tumors.[1,20] Additionally, within the tumor group, size of the tumor does not predict audiometric outcomes.[4,8,14,17,18,20]

Indications for ABI now include trauma, altered cochlear patency, auditory neuropathy, and cochlear nerve aplasia. Some of the variability in patient outcomes may stem from disruption of central auditory pattern recognition. Colletti et al reviewed a large series of nontumor patients and found patients with more distal lesions had better audiometric outcomes than patients with proximal auditory pathway lesions.[1] Patients with neuropathy and other neurologic disorders were poor performers, while cochlear malformations were typically intermediate performers, and the best results were reported in patients with cochlear trauma or severely altered cochlear patency. Similar results of poor performance with absent cochlear nerves have been reported by other authors.[11,19,20,21,22] However, this is still an area of active research. Sennaroglu and others have reported on some rare patients with open-set speech understanding with an absent cochlear nerve.[21,22] They hypothesize there is a degree of cochlear nucleus development independent of the cochlear nerve but overall patients with cochlear nerves fibers tend to do better than those with complete nerve agenesis.

16.2.3 Device Factors

Choice of Device

Cochlear and MED-EL devices are the two main ABI options but there are no controlled studies to determine if one is superior to the other. Overall, better outcomes are reported in the literature with use of the MED-EL device.[23] The MED-EL implant has an 8×3 mm electrode array with 12 electrodes, while Cochlear offers a 5×3 mm electrode array with 21 electrodes.[11,23] The MED-EL is more flexible which may aid in placement.[10] Shannon et al compared devices between centers in the 2012 expert consensus statement and found 31% of patients with the MED-EL device had good speech recognition compared to 5% with the Cochlear Corporation ABI.[11] There were many confounding variables including surgical positioning, surgical approach, and operative technique in this analysis making it impossible to truly equate outcomes. In the United States, Cochlear has FDA approval and is therefore widely used whereas many European studies report use of the MED-EL ABI.

Programming

ABIs require more complex programming when compared to CIs. During programming, each electrode on the array is assessed for auditory and nonauditory stimulation. Electrodes that provide auditory sensations are then tested for thresholds, comfort level, and pitch and that information is incorporated into the programming strategy. Electrodes with significant nonauditory side effects can have the stimulation strategy adjusted or if necessary can be deactivated. Intraoperative EABR can be used as a reference point for programming and has been found to correspond with auditory sensations.[24] Although many authors report no correlation between the number of active electrodes and hearing outcomes there is a minimum amount of active spectral channels required for adequate speech regonition.[6,8,17,22,25,26] Studies from the older eight-electrode array and the newer arrays have similar conclusions that a minimum percentage is required for optimal audiometric results.[14]

Spectral processing is also thought to contribute to ABI audiometric outcomes. One recent study attempted to further investigate the importance of spectral information by reducing the number of active electrodes to create a definitive pitch-ranked mapping. However, the authors found no benefit to this programming strategy and in fact the patients tended to have decreased performance when this strategy was employed.[27] Otto et al found a general trend in their series with pitch increasing in a lateral to medial direction, and subsequently

used this information for pitch ranking when necessary.[17] Optimization of programming strategies is a complex process but is essential for ideal audiometric outcomes.

16.3 Historical and Future Efforts to Develop Novel Strategies

As has been mentioned briefly, the placement of surface electrodes on the cochlear nucleus leaves deeper neuronal populations unstimulated, or through current spread, results in several neuronal populations being stimulated simultaneously. This nonselective, surface stimulation, particularly with a flat paddle electrode that does not conform, has led to interest in the development of newer electrodes. The penetrating ABI project, or PABI,[4] was instituted with the goal of recruiting deeper neuronal populations in the cochlear nucleus to include in an ABI program, as well as to provide more selective stimulation that might result in more discrete pitch perception and thus improve speech discrimination. Patients with the PABI used both a penetrating array and a surface array. Although the PABI did result in the more selective stimulation of neuronal populations and reduced charge density requirements for their stimulation, outcomes were not superior to surface ABI.[4]

Penetrating ABI research continues. Newer penetrating electrode technologies with multiple contacts and with the ability to provide more contacts, as well as continued research into the effects of selective stimulation on the higher auditory pathways may provide future penetrating arrays for clinical use.[28,29]

The outcome variability with ABIs has led to the convening of several meetings to discuss ideas and options for improving ABI performance.[8,22] Both MED-EL and Cochlear Corporation have convened such meetings with subject experts from the medical, radiological, audiological, and engineering present to discuss the literature and postulate on areas of potential improvement.

A separate chapter in this textbook will address alternative stimulation methods to electrical stimulation.[30]

References

[1] Colletti V, Shannon R, Carner M, Veronese S. Outcomes in nontumor adults fitted with the auditory brainstem implant: 10 years' experience. 2009;30(5):614–618

[2] Shannon RV. Advances in auditory prostheses. Curr Opin Neurol. 2012; 25(1):61–66

[3] Moore JK, Osen KK. The cochlear nuclei in man. Am J Anat. 1979; 154(3):393–418

[4] Otto SR, Shannon RV, Wilkinson EP, et al. Audiologic outcomes with the penetrating electrode auditory brainstem implant. Otol Neurotol. 2008; 29(8):1147–1154

[5] Barber SR, Kozin ED, Remenschneider AK, et al. Auditory brainstem implant array position varies widely among adult and pediatric patients and is associated with perception. Ear Hear. 2017; 38(6):e343–e351

[6] Matthies C, Brill S, Varallyay C, et al. Auditory brainstem implants in neurofibromatosis type 2: is open speech perception feasible? J Neurosurg. 2014; 120(2):546–558

[7] Mandal, à M, Colletti L, Colletti G, Colletti V. Improved outcomes in auditory brainstem implantation with the use of near-field electrical compound action potentials. Otolaryngol Head Neck Surg. 2014; 151(6):1008–1013

[8] Behr R, Colletti V, Matthies C, et al. New outcomes with auditory brainstem implants in NF2 patients. Otol Neurotol. 2014; 35(10):1844–1851

[9] Goyal S, Krishnan SS, Kameswaran M, Vasudevan MC, Ranjith, Natarajan K. Does cerebellar flocculus size affect subjective outcomes in pediatric auditory brainstem implantation. Int J Pediatr Otorhinolaryngol. 2017; 97:30–34

[10] Iseli CE, Merwin WH, III, Klatt-Cromwell C, et al. Effect of cochlear nerve electrocautery on the adult cochlear nucleus. Otol Neurotol. 2015; 36(4): 670–677

[11] Shannon RV, Behr R, Colletti V, et al. New Outcomes with Auditory Brainstem Implants in NF2 Patients. In: Munich ABI Consensus.; 2012

[12] Schwartz MS, Wilkinson EP. Auditory brainstem implant program development. Laryngoscope. 2017; 127(8):1909–1915

[13] Schwartz MS. Auditory brainstem implants in neurofibromatosis type 2. J Neurosurg. 2014; 121(3):760–761

[14] Matthies C, Brill S, Kaga K, et al. Auditory brainstem implantation improves speech recognition in neurofibromatosis type II patients. ORL J Otorhinolaryngol Relat Spec. 2013; 75(5):282–295

[15] Sung JKK, Luk BPK, Wong TKC, Thong JF, Wong HT, Tong MCF. Pediatric auditory brainstem implantation: impact on audiological rehabilitation and tonal language development. Audiol Neurotol. 2018; 23(2):126–134

[16] Noij KS, Kozin ED, Sethi R, et al. Systematic review of nontumor pediatric auditory brainstem implant outcomes. Otolaryngol Head Neck Surg. 2015; 153(5):739–750

[17] Otto SR, Brackmann DE, Hitselberger WE, Shannon RV, Kuchta J. Multichannel auditory brainstem implant: update on performance in 61 patients. J Neurosurg. 2002; 96(6):1063–1071

[18] Sanna M, Di Lella F, Guida M, Merkus P. Auditory brainstem implants in NF2 patients: results and review of the literature. Otol Neurotol. 2012; 33(2): 154–164

[19] Jung NY, Kim M, Chang WS, Jung HH, Choi JY, Chang JW. Favorable long-term functional outcomes and safety of auditory brainstem implants in nontumor patients. Oper Neurosurg (Hagerstown). 2017; 13(6):653–660

[20] Colletti V, Carner M, Miorelli V, Guida M, Colletti L, Fiorino F. Auditory brainstem implant (ABI): new frontiers in adults and children. Otolaryngol Head Neck Surg. 2005; 133(1):126–138

[21] Sennaroglu L, Ziyal I, Atas A, et al. Preliminary results of auditory brainstem implantation in prelingually deaf children with inner ear malformations including severe stenosis of the cochlear aperture and aplasia of the cochlear nerve. Otol Neurotol. 2009; 30(6):708–715

[22] Sennaroğlu L, Sennaroğlu G, Yücel E, et al. Long-term results of ABI in children with severe inner ear malformations. Otol Neurotol. 2016; 37(7):865–872

[23] Colletti L, Shannon R, Colletti V. Auditory brainstem implants for neurofibromatosis type 2. Curr Opin Otolaryngol Head Neck Surg. 2012; 20(5):353–357

[24] Herrmann BS, Brown MC, Eddington DK, Hancock KE, Lee DJ. Auditory brainstem implant: electrophysiologic responses and subject perception. Ear Hear. 2015; 36(3):368–376

[25] Kuchta J, Otto SR, Shannon RV, Hitselberger WE, Brackmann DE. The multichannel auditory brainstem implant: how many electrodes make sense? J Neurosurg. 2004; 100(1):16–23

[26] Otto SR, House W, Brackmann DE, Hitselberger WE, Nelson RA. Auditory brain stem implant: effect of tumor size and preoperative hearing level on function. Ann Otol Rhinol Laryngol. 1990; 99(10 Pt 1):789–790

[27] McKay CM, Azadpour M, Jayewardene-Aston D, O'Driscoll M, El-Deredy W. Electrode selection and speech understanding in patients with auditory brainstem implants. Ear Hear. 2015; 36(4):454–463

[28] Han M, Manoonkitiwongsa PS, Wang CX, McCreery DB. In vivo validation of custom-designed silicon-based microelectrode arrays for long-term neural recording and stimulation. IEEE Trans Biomed Eng. 2012; 59(2):346–354

[29] McCreery D, Yadev K, Han M. Responses of neurons in the feline inferior colliculus to modulated electrical stimuli applied on and within the ventral cochlear nucleus; Implications for an advanced auditory brainstem implant. Hear Res. 2018; 363:85–97

[30] Hight AE, Kozin ED, Darrow K, et al. Superior temporal resolution of Chronos versus channelrhodopsin-2 in an optogenetic model of the auditory brainstem implant. Hear Res. 2015; 322(322):235–241

17 ABI Program Development

Marc S. Schwartz and Eric P. Wilkinson

Abstract

The purpose of this monograph is to outline the current state of the art regarding the field of auditory brainstem implantation. Readers will include auditory brainstem implant (ABI)-experienced surgeons and audiologists and also practitioners without first-hand knowledge but who are curious about utilization of this device. This second group may perhaps have patients for whom ABI placement is a possibility or may have the intention of performing ABI surgery. The purpose of this chapter is to outline the considerations necessary for successfully entering this field. In order to accomplish this goal, it is important to understand the benefits and risks of the ABI. This is true for each of the various classes of potential ABI recipients.

Keywords: auditory brainstem implant, cochlear implant, medical device industry, surgical volume, comprehensive care

17.1 Risk–Benefit Analysis of the Auditory Brainstem Implant

Since the benefits of the ABI are audiological and its risks are primarily those of surgical complications, it is impossible to quantitatively compare one to the other. Any assessment of risk–benefit inherently involves value judgments. By definition, these judgments are subjective. Nevertheless, it is possible to describe these risks and benefits as well as to indicate how they may vary among not only different classes of patients but also between different surgeons and centers as well.

17.2 Audiologic Benefit

17.2.1 NF2 Patients

Most deaf patients with neurofibromatosis type 2 (NF2) who have been implanted with ABIs utilize them on a daily basis.[4] This signifies that these patients obtain benefit from their devices, at least in forming an auditory connection to their environments. It is important to understand, however, that, at least with NF2, auditory results are generally modest and are highly variable. ABIs do not restore normal hearing, and only a small percentage of patients obtain any significant understanding of conversational speech.

The auditory benefit obtained by NF2 patients with ABIs was initially described in detail by Otto, et al, in 2002.[5] A battery of tests were conducted on 61 patients who had been implanted with the 21-electrode Nucleus ABI24 designed to measure the comprehension of environmental sounds, consonant and vowels sounds, words, and sentences. The battery included both closed-set and open-set testing as well as testing of both sound only and sound in combination with vision (lipreading). On closed-set tests of environmental sounds, consonant and vowel sounds, and words, patients with ABIs scored significantly

higher than random chance. However, on open-set sentence tests, only a small percentage of patients achieved significant comprehension. In terms of speech understanding, the major benefit of ABIs for most patients is significant improvement when tested together with lipreading when compared to lipreading alone.

More recently, improved audiological results with ABIs in NF2 patients have been reported by two centers in Europe.[7,8] These centers use the MED-EL ABI and perform implantation using the retrosigmoid approach in the sitting position. The MED-EL device is not approved by the FDA for use in the United States. In these centers, results continue to vary among patients, but up to 30% of patients achieve significant open-set speech comprehension with sound alone. It should be noted that a PubMed search using the terms "auditory brainstem implant" and "neurofibromatosis type 2" yields 14 reports, with none of the other 12 reporting significant open-set speech comprehension in a similar percentage of patients.[5,7,8,9,10,11,12,13,14,15,16,17,18,19]

17.2.2 Adult Non-NF2 Patients

More recently, ABIs have been implanted in adult patients without NF2. These patients undergo craniotomy for the express purpose of ABI implantation. A small number of adults who were deafened postlingually by causes not amenable to cochlear implantation, such as traumatic transection of the cochlear nerves and post-infectious ossification of the cochlea, have received ABIs with results reported to be better than for patients with NF2.[20] The indications for the implantation of ABIs in non-NF2 adults are very rare, and the small numbers of such patients make clear determination of the audiological benefits difficult.

17.2.3 Pediatric Patients

ABIs have also been used in congenitally deaf children unable to benefit from cochlear implantation due to cochlear malformations or absence of the cochlear nerve.[21,22] Again, reports are guardedly encouraging that results are considerably better than those for patients with NF2. It is important to understand, however, that the evaluation of pediatric patients is considerably more complicated than that of adults.[23,24] Although there is clear evidence of the development of speech understanding in a subset of these patients, it remains unclear what percentage or how many pediatric patients will benefit significantly. There are currently four ongoing studies of ABI implantation in the pediatric population in the United States. One of these is supported by the NIH.

17.3 Surgical Risk

Reports in the literature of ABI implantation universally show that ABIs can be placed with acceptable risk.[25] However, not all ABI implantations are reported, especially from low-volume centers. The overall risk of ABI implantation across all centers is unknown, and within the ABI community, although it is hearsay, it is strongly suspected that there have been several serious

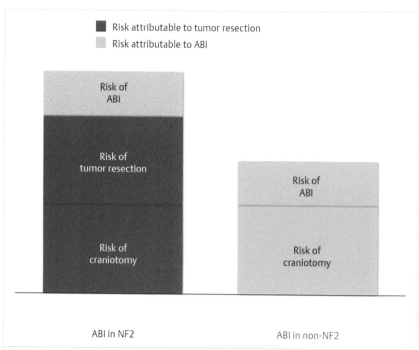

Risk attributable to tumor resection

Risk attributable to ABI

Risk of
ABI

Risk of
tumor resection

Risk of
craniotomy

Risk of
ABI

Risk of
craniotomy

ABI in NF2

ABI in non-NF2

Fig. 17.1 Stratification of risk of ABI placement both at the same sitting as tumor resection and as a stand-alone procedure.

adverse events. It should be accepted as tenet by all reasonable surgeons that no craniotomy can be carried out without risk.

The critical point is that the marginal risk of ABI implantation in patients with NF2, who are undergoing craniotomy for the primary purpose of tumor resection, is much less than the risk of ABI implantation in patients without NF2. This is because in NF2 the risk of craniotomy and approach to the cerebellopontine angle is assignable to the tumor resection, while, in the absence of NF2, all the risk of craniotomy must be assigned to the ABI placement itself (▶ Fig. 17.1).

Comprehension of this point leads directly to two conclusions. First, surgeons implanting ABIs in the absence of NF2 are assuming a much higher risk than are surgeons who implant ABIs in the course of tumor resection. This is true even if the overall risk of surgery in NF2 is higher than the risk of ABI placement alone. Second, the audiological results of ABI placement without NF2 must be significantly higher than results in NF2 to justify the procedure in the first place. That is, while environmental sound awareness without open-set speech discrimination has clearly been shown to be a worthwhile result for NF2 patients, this level of audiological benefit may not justify craniotomy for ABI placement as a stand-alone procedure.

It has also come to the attention of the authors that a strategy of tumor resection in one setting with ABI implantation at a second stage is sometimes considered. There are two disadvantages to this strategy. First, ABI implantation may be more difficult on second-stage surgery due to the usual issues related to re-operation, such as scarring. Second, and more germane to this discussion, the advantages of craniotomy risk-assignment to tumor resection are entirely lost.

17.3.1 Pediatric ABI Surgery

The use of ABI in the pediatric population also raises additional ethical issues. Due to an inherently emotionally charged situation, parents of young children who cannot benefit from cochlear implantation may be particularly credulous in terms of unrealistic expectations, and it is exactly these pediatric patients that may be exposed to the highest risk with the most uncertain benefit.

17.3.2 The Learning Curve

There is no direct data regarding the surgeon's learning curve for ABI placement. The presence of a learning curve has been demonstrated with other technically challenging operations.[26,27,28] There is no reason to think that a learning curve does not also exist for other such procedures. Certainly, acoustic tumor resection experience would be expected to translate to ABI placement. ABI placement, however, requires full exposure of the lateral recess and the foramen of Luschka in situations in which the normal features of the brainstem are typically distorted by tumors. In addition, there is significant variability of the anatomy of the lateral recess in children with congenital deafness due to abnormalities of embryonic and fetal development.[29] Furthermore, ABI electrode array and cable handling can be cumbersome due to their construction and inherent torque.

The most common indication for ABI is NF2, which has an estimated prevalence of 1/60,000.[30] Only a portion of these patients ever become candidates for ABI. Other indications, such as congenital absence of the cochlear nerves or cochlear malformations of the cochlea, appear to be yet less common. The rarity of potential ABI recipients would be expected to limit progress along the learning curve.

Review of the literature does suggest that there are differences in ABI outcomes among centers. For instance, the only centers that report any patients with significant open-set speech comprehension are those with the highest volumes. This is true both for patients with NF2 and for those without.

17.4 Who Should Be Implanting ABIs?

17.4.1 NF2 Patients

As discussed previously, in the group of patients with NF2 undergoing craniotomy for tumor removal, ABIs can be placed with little marginal risk since the major risk of the operation can be attributed to the need for tumor resection. For that reason, it is reasonable and wholly appropriate for centers with significant NF2 volume to develop programs and to engage in ABI placement.

We would recommend that training of ABI surgeons should involve observation of surgeons at existing higher volume centers. While some training should be in person in order to allow for real-time interaction, video demonstration is also useful. The development of high-definition intraoperative video along with the ability to disseminate such video on the internet has significantly elevated the resources available to prospective ABI surgeons.

Likewise, successful ABI centers require a high level of audiological expertise. ABI programs should not be initiated without a very high level of audiological commitment, such as might only be available at a large cochlear implant center. ABI programming is significantly more complicated that cochlear implant programming and must be recognized as such. The availability of video conferencing and internet communication may further facilitate the development of requisite programming skills.

It is important for prospective ABI centers to be realistic about patient volume. Even with a large number of NF2 patients, the percentage of patients with NF2 who are good ABI candidates at any one time is small. It is probably not realistic to expect sufficient volume if fewer than several dozen NF2 patients are being seen annually. The development of new therapies, such as bevacizumab, as well as an understanding that some NF2 patients benefit from cochlear implantation, has also served to delay ABI placement in many patients and to obviate the benefit of ABI placement entirely in some.[31]

The first few prospective patients of any ABI program should not be counseled to expect good audiological benefit. At least initially, ABI patients should undergo surgery for the primary purpose of tumor resection, and this should be stressed. A poor audiological outcome would be expected more acceptable to a patient in whom surgery was done for the primary purpose of tumor resection than to a patient undergoing craniotomy primarily for the ABI.

17.4.2 Adult Non-NF2 Patients

Due to the rarity of non-NF2 pathology that causes postlingual deafness in adults it is unlikely that any center will be able to specialize in this area. Thus, we would find it problematic if these operations were to be carried out by anyone other than experienced NF2 ABI surgeons in centers that provide the necessary audiological and programming expertise. In addition, these operations should probably only be undertaken at all if the expectations of audiological results are higher than with NF2.

17.4.3 Pediatric Patients

For a number of reasons, the standards must be "higher" when considering ABI surgery in pediatric patients. These reasons are both practical and ethical.

In pediatric, congenitally deaf patients, the entire craniotomy is being done for the sole purpose of ABI implantation. All of the risk of surgery is assigned to the ABI; ABI placement is not simply an incremental risk. Because of this, it is critical to both minimize risk and maximize benefit. Arguably, the best source of new pediatric ABI surgeons is adult ABI centers. Certainly, the surgeon taking responsibility for ABI implantation should be intimately familiar with and experienced in cerebellopontine angle surgery. In addition to experience, preparation for the nuances of brainstem surgical anatomy and device implantation is critical. Training should consist of multiple site visits, familiarization with the ABI receiver, cable, and electrode array, as well as, perhaps, simulation.

The lead ABI surgeon may, however, be the only one member of the necessary pediatric ABI team. If the lead ABI surgeon is a neurosurgeon, an experienced and interested neurotologist will be needed for patient selection and medical auditory management. In addition, if the lead ABI surgeon does not have a pediatric-focused practice, which could be expected to be the case due to rarity of lateral skull base pathology in pediatric neurosurgery practice, then a pediatric neurosurgeon must be involved as well.

It should also be recognized that ABI implantation is only the first step in optimizing ABI outcome. Proper device programming, audiological assessment, and speech pathology input are also critical. Enthusiastic participation of an entire such team, presumably constituted by specialists from a large pediatric cochlear implant program, is required in order to have any hope of achieving benefit that would make the surgery worthwhile in the first place. It should also be understood that an ABI program must also be considered a long-term proposition. Attention must be focused on these patients for 5, 10, or more years. A pediatric ABI program should not be initiated unless it is clear that there is institutional support for a long-term endeavor.

Pediatric ABI implantation also carries ethical concerns. It should be made clear to families that pediatric implantation is an off-label use. More importantly, it should be made clear to families that long-term benefit from ABI in this population remains uncertain. Parents of young, deaf children who either cannot undergo cochlear implantation or who failed to achieve benefit from cochlear implantation may make decisions on an emotional basis without understanding the risks or potential benefit. It is important for surgeons and teams both to be realistic about the state of the field as well as about expected results in their own hands rather than in the hands of a different surgeon who has done perhaps many dozens of cases.

17.5 The Role of Cochlear Implant Manufacturers

All ABIs are based upon cochlear implant platforms and are produced by the major cochlear implant companies. Fewer than 1,000 ABIs have been implanted worldwide, and, as such, ABIs represent a tiny fraction of the output of these companies.

Table 17.1 Components necessary for the development of ABI programs

NF2 ABI program	Adult non-NF2 ABI program	Pediatric ABI program
Sufficient quantity of NF2 patients	To be done only by established NF2 ABI centers due to very low volume of patients	Significant experience in adult ABI placement and programming or extensive preparation
Surgeons experienced in cerebellopontine angle surgery		Pediatric neurosurgical expertise
Cochlear implant program with commitment to ABI programming		Pediatric cochlear implant program with commitment to ABI programming and speech pathology
		Long-term dedication to patients through childhood and into adulthood

Although financial data is not made public, it is not possible that cochlear implant companies generate significant profit from ABIs. Cochlear implant manufacturers obtain two potential benefits from their ABIs. First is the prestige and public relation benefit of creating and providing ABIs, which can be marketed to the public as helping the most unfortunate deaf patients. Second is the ability to support their important cochlear implant customers in their own efforts to develop sophisticated and prestigious full-service hearing rehabilitation programs. For this second reason, it is in the interests of these corporations to accede to requests to provide ABIs. It is likely that these corporations impede the opening of new ABI centers at their own financial peril: Refusing to support cochlear implant customers who wish to implant a first ABI is probably a poor business decision in many cases. We have seen first-hand that the home offices of implant manufacturers face significant pressure from sales forces in the field to support their cochlear implant customers, even if the viability of various ABI programs is suspect from the start.

For similar reasons, cochlear implant centers cannot be counted upon to restrain the proliferation of ABI programs. Despite the fact that there would likely be no direct financial benefit from the procedure itself, placement of even a single ABI can be exploited by centers for both competitive and marketing benefit. In the end, it is up to any surgeon who will be directly responsible for assuming the risk of ABI implantation to ensure that patients' interests remain first and foremost when the question of opening a new ABI program is broached.

17.6 Conclusions

The decision to implant an ABI in any given patient is always based upon a risk–benefit analysis. The risk–benefit determination of ABI placement in nontumor patients is always less favorable than that in patients undergoing concurrent tumor resection. Centers with a high volume of NF2 patients and the expectation of sufficient volume of ABI patients should be supported in their effort to initiate ABI programs. On the other hand, there is a higher standard for potential pediatric ABI programs. These should only be facilitated if a strict set of criteria are met, including experience with NF2 ABIs, pediatric neurosurgical expertise, and a commitment to long-term audiological and speech pathology follow-up. Our proposed criteria for the development of ABI centers are summarized in ▸ Table 17.1. It is up to the ABI surgeons who will be assuming the risk and responsibility of ABI implantation to ensure that patients' interests are the highest priority.

References

[1] Hitselberger WE, House WF, Edgerton BJ, Whitaker S. Cochlear nucleus implants. Otolaryngol Head Neck Surg. 1984; 92(1):52–54

[2] Brackmann DE, Hitselberger WE, Nelson RA, et al. Auditory brainstem implant: I. Issues in surgical implantation. Otolaryngol Head Neck Surg. 1993; 108(6):624–633

[3] Otto SR, Brackman DE, Hitselberger WE, Shannon RV. Brainstem electronic implants for bilateral anacusis following surgical removal of cerebello pontine angle lesions. Otolaryngol Clin North Am. 2001; 34(2):485–499

[4] Ebinger K, Otto S, Arcaroli J, Staller S, Arndt P. Multichannel auditory brainstem implant: US clinical trial results. J Laryngol Otol Suppl. 2000 (27):50–53

[5] Otto SR, Brackmann DE, Hitselberger WE, Shannon RV, Kuchta J. Multichannel auditory brainstem implant: update on performance in 61 patients. J Neurosurg. 2002; 96(6):1063–1071

[6] Colletti V, Shannon RV. Open set speech perception with auditory brainstem implant? Laryngoscope. 2005; 115(11):1974–1978

[7] Matthies C, Brill S, Kaga K, et al. Auditory brainstem implantation improves speech recognition in neurofibromatosis type II patients. ORL J Otorhinolaryngol Relat Spec. 2013; 75(5):282–295

[8] Behr R, Colletti V, Matthies C, et al. New outcomes with auditory brainstem implants in NF2 patients. Otol Neurotol. 2014; 35(10):1844–1851

[9] Sollmann WP, Laszig R, Marangos N. Surgical experiences in 58 cases using the Nucleus 22 multichannel auditory brainstem implant. J Laryngol Otol Suppl. 2000(27):23–26

[10] Lenarz T, Moshrefi M, Matthies C, et al. Auditory brainstem implant: part I. Auditory performance and its evolution over time. Otol Neurotol. 2001; 22 (6):823–833

[11] Vincent C, Zini C, Gandolfi A, et al. Results of the MXM Digisonic auditory brainstem implant clinical trials in Europe. Otol Neurotol. 2002; 23(1): 56–60

[12] Nevison B, Laszig R, Sollmann WP, et al. Results from a European clinical investigation of the Nucleus multichannel auditory brainstem implant. Ear Hear. 2002; 23(3):170–183

[13] Kanowitz SJ, Shapiro WH, Golfinos JG, Cohen NL, Roland JT, Jr. Auditory brainstem implantation in patients with neurofibromatosis type 2. Laryngoscope. 2004; 114(12):2135–2146

[14] Grayeli AB, Kalamarides M, Bouccara D, Ambert-Dahan E, Sterkers O. Auditory brainstem implant in neurofibromatosis type 2 and non-neurofibromatosis type 2 patients. Otol Neurotol. 2008; 29(8):1140–1146

[15] Bento RF, Neto RVB, Tsuji RK, Gomes MQT, Goffi-Gomez MVS. Auditory brainstem implant: surgical technique and early audiological results in patients with neurofibromatosis type 2. Rev Bras Otorrinolaringol (Engl Ed). 2008; 74(5):647–651

[16] Maini S, Cohen MA, Hollow R, Briggs R. Update on long-term results with auditory brainstem implants in NF2 patients. Cochlear Implants Int. 2009; 10 Suppl 1:33–37

[17] Sanna M, Di Lella F, Guida M, Merkus P. Auditory brainstem implants in NF2 patients: results and review of the literature. Otol Neurotol. 2012; 33 (2):154–164

[18] Colletti L, Shannon R, Colletti V. Auditory brainstem implants for neurofibromatosis type 2. Curr Opin Otolaryngol Head Neck Surg. 2012; 20(5): 353–357

[19] Siegbahn M, Lundin K, Olsson GB, et al. Auditory brainstem implants (ABIs)—20 years of clinical experience in Uppsala, Sweden. Acta Otolaryngol. 2014; 134(10):1052–1061

[20] Colletti V, Shannon R, Carner M, Veronese S, Colletti L. Outcomes in nontumor adults fitted with the auditory brainstem implant: 10 years' experience. Otol Neurotol. 2009; 30(5):614–618

[21] Colletti V, Carner M, Miorelli V, Guida M, Colletti L, Fiorino F. Auditory brainstem implant (ABI): new frontiers in adults and children. Otolaryngol Head Neck Surg. 2005; 133(1):126–138

[22] Colletti V. Auditory outcomes in tumor vs. nontumor patients fitted with auditory brainstem implants. Adv Otorhinolaryngol. 2006; 64:167–185

[23] Wang NY, Eisenberg LS, Johnson KC, et al. CDaCI Investigative Team. Tracking development of speech recognition: longitudinal data from hierarchical assessments in the Childhood Development after Cochlear Implantation Study. Otol Neurotol. 2008; 29(2):240–245

[24] Buchman CA, Teagle HF, Roush PA, et al. Cochlear implantation in children with labyrinthine anomalies and cochlear nerve deficiency: implications for auditory brainstem implantation. Laryngoscope. 2011; 121(9):1979–1988

[25] Colletti V, Shannon RV, Carner M, Veronese S, Colletti L. Complications in auditory brainstem implant surgery in adults and children. Otol Neurotol. 2010; 31(4):558–564

[26] Samdani AF, Ranade A, Saldanha V, Yondorf MZ. Learning curve for placement of thoracic pedicle screws in the deformed spine. Neurosurgery. 2010; 66(2):290–294, discussion 294–295

[27] Snyderman CH, Fernandez-Miranda J, Gardner PA. Training in neurorhinology: the impact of case volume on the learning curve. Otolaryngol Clin North Am. 2011; 44(5):1223–1228

[28] Khan N, Abboudi H, Khan MS, Dasgupta P, Ahmed K. Measuring the surgical "learning curve": methods, variables and competency. BJU Int. 2014; 113(3):504–508

[29] Colletti G, Mandalà M, Colletti L, Colletti V. Surgical visual reference for auditory brainstem implantation in children with cochlear nerve deficiency. Otolaryngol Head Neck Surg. 2015; 153(6):1071–1073

[30] Evans DG, Howard E, Giblin C, et al. Birth incidence and prevalence of tumor-prone syndromes: estimates from a UK family genetic register service. Am J Med Genet A. 2010; 152A(2):327–332

[31] Plotkin SR, Merker VL, Halpin C, et al. Bevacizumab for progressive vestibular schwannoma in neurofibromatosis type 2: a retrospective review of 31 patients. Otol Neurotol. 2012; 33(6):1046–1052

18 Auditory Midbrain Implant

Thomas Lenarz, Amir Samii, Karl-Heinz Dyballa, and Hubert H. Lim

Abstract

The auditory midbrain implant (AMI) is a novel central auditory implant for hearing restoration in patients with neural deafness due to damage of the auditory nerve by bilateral vestibular schwannomas (mainly NF2). These patients cannot benefit from a cochlear implant nor from an auditory brainstem implant due to damage of the cochlear nucleus at the brainstem either by the tumor itself or its treatment.

The penetrating multichannel electrode arrays are inserted into the central nucleus perpendicular to the frequency layer. The tonotopic stimulation encodes different frequencies which can be used for speech discrimination. Five patients with a single shank and five patients with a double shank electrode have been implanted so far. The patients experience limited speech recognition scores comparable to those with auditory brainstem implants.

Overall the AMI provides an alternative treatment for hearing rehabilitation in NF2-patients.

Keywords: auditory midbrain, NF2, penetrating electrode

18.1 Introduction

Patients with neural deafness cannot benefit from a cochlear implant (CI) due to damaged auditory nerves, such as those with neurofibromatosis type II (NF2) who have had removal of tumors involving the cochlear nerve. There are also deaf individuals with cochleas that cannot be implanted with a CI due to anatomical distortions/ossification or damage of the cochleas. In these types of patients, electrical stimulation of structures of the auditory pathway central to the auditory nerve can be used for hearing restoration. Two types of central auditory prostheses have been realized for clinical application: the auditory brainstem implant (ABI) and the auditory midbrain implant (AMI; ▶ Fig. 18.1).[1,2,3]

The ABI has been in clinical use since 1979 in different versions including surface and penetrating electrodes.[5] Hearing performance with the ABI has remained substantially inferior to those achieved with cochlear implants and show a large variability in outcomes, spanning from no auditory sensations to some degree of open-set speech understanding.[6,7,8,9] Several possible reasons for the poor outcomes include the limited access or stimulation of the tonotopic organization of the cochlear nucleus, even with the penetrating electrode arrays used in a previous clinical study, and the preprocessing of auditory information from the cochlea to the brainstem that has been bypassed with the ABI. Current stimulation strategies for the ABI are derived from CIs and may not be able to sufficiently restore the auditory information at the brainstem level. Particularly in NF2 deaf patients, it has been proposed that poor ABI outcomes may be due to the damage caused at the brainstem level, associated with the tumor and/or tumor removal process, especially since hearing outcomes in nontumor patients have shown greater performance than those of tumor patients.[6,7,13]

Considering these limitations, as well as to attempt to overcome some of these limitations, the AMI has been developed.[4,14,15,16] The main concept of the AMI is the use of penetrating single-shank or double-shank electrode array with ring contacts that can stimulate the different frequency layers of the inferior colliculus, beyond the damaged tumor region in the brainstem area (▶ Fig. 18.2). This frequency layer stimulation could potentially improve speech discrimination by more precisely stimulating the tonotopic organization of the inferior colliculus in its central nucleus. In order to address the three-dimensional organization and the different neuronal presentation within one frequency layer, a double-shank electrode array was recently developed and brought into clinical studies with patients implanted in 2017 to 2019. This double-shank electrode array stems from research in animals and outcomes from a previous clinical study using the single-shank electrode array version in five deaf NF2 patients. The rationale, technology development and validation,

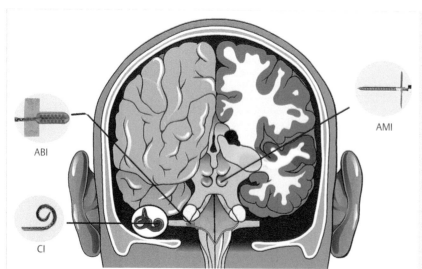

Fig. 18.1 Location of central auditory implants. Auditory brainstem implant (ABI) and auditory midbrain implant (AMI) compared to cochlear implant (CI). Different auditory neural prosthetics used in patients for hearing restoration. CI is implanted into the cochlea and used for auditory nerve stimulation. ABI is used for stimulation of the cochlear nucleus. AMI is used for penetrating stimulation of the auditory midbrain (i.e., the inferior colliculus). The examples shown in this figure were developed by Cochlear Limited (Australia). (Figure was taken from Lenarz et al, 2006 and reprinted with permission from Lippincott Williams & Wilkins.[4])

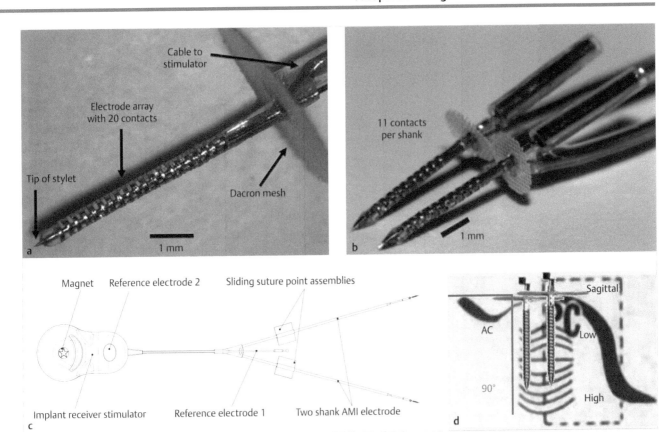

Fig. 18.2 (a) Single-shank and (b) double-shank auditory midbrain implant (AMI) electrode arrays. (c) Schematic of double-shank electrode array. (d) Schematic of double shank inserted into inferior colliculus. Fig. (a) shows the first generation of the AMI array that was implanted into five deaf patients in 2006 to 2008 consisting of 20 ring sites (200 µm spacing, 200 µm thickness, 400 µm diameter) along a silicone carrier. The Dacron mesh prevents over-insertion of the array into the inferior colliculus and tethers it to the brain. Fig. (b) shows new two-shank AMI array that was recently implanted into five deaf patients (2017–2019) in a second clinical trial. Each shank consists of 11 ring sites along a silicone carrier (300 µm site spacing except for one site positioned closer to the Dacron mesh for tinnitus treatment). Fig. (c) shows a schematic of the two-shank array. Fig. (c) shows schematic of inserted double-shank array into inferior colliculus along tonotope structure from low to high pitch. Images in (a) and (b) were taken from Samii et al[16] and Lim et al[3], respectively, and reprinted with permission from Wolters Kluwer and Elsevier. Schematic in Fig. (c) was taken with permission from Cochlear Limited (Australia). Image (d) was taken from Geniec and Morest[18] and reprinted with permission from Taylor & Francis.

and animal and human research supporting both human studies is described in detail in previous reviews.[3,17]

The penetrating electrode arrays are attached to a CI receiver-stimulator developed by Cochlear Limited (Australia). The electrode arrays have a tapered tip (▶ Fig. 18.2). For insertion purposes, each electrode shank is stabilized by a stylet with a sharp tip in a central canal of the shank. The stylet enables insertion of the shank into the brain and then can be pulled out after insertion, allowing the electrode array to become more flexible in order to adjust to the brain structure and creating less force on the brain tissue. The implant has a reference electrode with a separate wire which is ball-shaped placed into the temporalis muscle area in addition to the receiver-stimulator casing, similar to typical CIs developed by Cochlear Limited.

18.2 Preoperative Diagnostics and Selection Criteria for Patients

The AMI is indicated in patients with bilateral neural deafness due to damage of the auditory nerve, mainly in NF2 patients

with bilateral vestibular schwannomas (▶ Fig. 18.3). In those NF2 patients, the tumor itself or subsequent treatment such as microsurgical tumor removal and/or radiotherapy can create damage at the brainstem level, including the nearby area of the cochlear nucleus and/or the lateral recess of the fourth ventricle. The AMI can bypass the damaged brainstem areas by targeting the central nucleus of the inferior colliculus. Targeting of the inferior colliculus is possible through preoperative imaging of the midbrain structures and fusion of magnetic resonance imaging (MRI) and computed tomography (CT) images (▶ Fig. 18.4). These images can help identify key anatomical landmarks for the inferior colliculus, which includes the division line between the inferior colliculus and the superior colliculus, the midbrain midline, the tentorium, and the third ventricle. Audiological tests must document the neural deafness on both sides. The audiological profile is characterized by a severe to profound sensorineural hearing loss with pure speech discrimination in comparison to the pure tone threshold, missing auditory brainstem responses, and a negative (transtympanic) promontory test. These patients would not benefit from acoustic amplification.

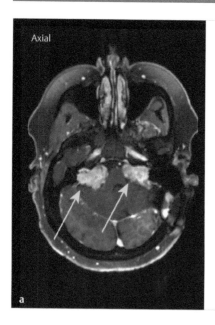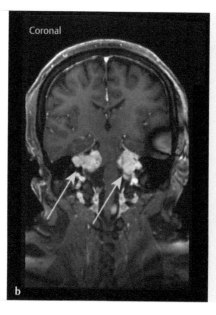

Fig. 18.3 Bilateral vestibular schwannomas in neurofibromatosis type 2 (NF2) patient. Vestibular schwannoma marked with *arrows* in axial (a) and coronal (b) views.

AMI should be especially considered in patients with distorted or damaged brainstem due to previous treatment or by the tumor itself. The anatomic situation shall be well documented using high-resolution imaging including MRI of the temporal bone and the brain as well as a CT scan of the temporal bone and the skull.

18.3 Surgical Technique

AMI implantation can be performed either with or without tumor removal depending on the individual case. Surgery is possible either in the semi-sitting or supine position. The preferred position is semi-sitting for retrosigmoid (suboccipital) approach with medial extension up to the midline (▶ Fig. 18.5). Navigation is advised in order to safely identify target structures, and determine the angles of electrode insertion. Bone anchored fiducials are placed in the skull around the craniotomy and a CT scan is taken. Surgery is done with the head fixed in the Mayfield clamp and using monitoring for facial nerve and long tracts and, depending on tumor extension, also other cranial nerves. After the exposure of the skull, a retrosigmoid craniotomy with extension to the midline is performed. After incision of the dura and opening the cistern for cerebellar relaxation a brain spatula is placed to hold the cerebellum, and tumor removal (e.g., vestibular schwannoma in the cerebellopontine angle) is initiated.

The next step is the exposure of the auditory midbrain through an infratentorial supracerebellar approach. In the semi-sitting position after removing the brain spatula from the cerebellopontine angle, the cerebellum shows a significant shift to the caudal direction due to gravity. This provides a sufficient surgical corridor to access the midbrain without any further retraction. The bridging veins from the tentorium can be typically preserved (▶ Fig. 18.6). The surface of the inferior colliculus is exposed (▶ Fig. 18.7). The inferior and superior colliculi,

the brachium, and the trochlear nerve are exposed with proper dissection of vascular structures that should be preserved (▶ Fig. 18.8).

The penetrating electrode arrays shall be placed into the central nucleus of the inferior colliculus with perpendicular penetration across the frequency layers shown to exist in previous anatomical and imaging studies in humans.[18,19,20] From the previous electrophysiological experiments and cadaver studies the optimum entry point on the surface of the inferior colliculus can be determined using anatomical landmarks (▶ Fig. 18.9). The landmarks include the midline between the two inferior colliculi, the horizontal division line between the superior and inferior colliculi, the brachium to the lateral side, and the exit point of the trochlear nerve as the inferior point of reference. The electrode shanks of the double-shank array are then inserted into the inferior colliculus in a rostral-lateral toward inferior-medial direction with an insertion angle of 40 degrees toward the midline. Special navigation tools have been developed to determine this angle (▶ Fig. 18.10). Placement of millimeter paper is useful to identify the two entry points, the rostral one being more lateral and the caudal one being more medial. The pia mater is first perforated with a special surgical tool (▶ Fig. 18.11). After placement of the receiver-stimulator in the drilled-out bony bed superior to the craniotomy, the electrode arrays are pre-positioned with their leads bifurcated intracranially. First, the rostral shank is inserted (▶ Fig. 18.12 and ▶ Fig. 18.13), followed by the caudal shank. The stylet is removed. The Dacron mesh defines the insertion depth (▶ Fig. 18.14). Electrode cables are protected in the bone canal between the bony bed and the craniotomy. The reference electrode is placed under the temporalis muscle. Intraoperative electrophysiology is performed to determine the electrode impedances and measure the so-called neural responses with the telemetry system of the implant. In addition, the electrically evoked middle latency responses (E-MLRs) are recorded

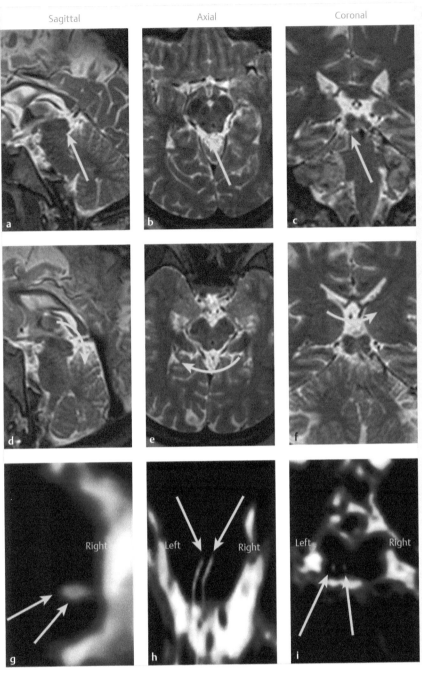

| Sagittal | Axial | Coronal |

Fig. 18.4 Imaging of the inferior colliculus with reconstruction of electrode positions. Figs. (a) to (i) show magnetic resonance imaging (MRI) images ([g] to [i] preoperative MRI fused with postoperative computed tomography [CT] images of one of the patients implanted with the double-shank auditory midbrain implant [AMI]) of the midbrain in different views, column by column, according to the headings. (a), (b), and (c) show a raw image dataset. *Arrows* point to the target region, which is the left inferior colliculus in this patient. (d), (e), and (f) are an aligned dataset that is used for the navigation which leads to the top peaks of the inferior colliculus and superior colliculus being aligned vertically in the sagittal view, both inferior colliculi being aligned horizontally in the axial view, and all four colliculi being viewed directly orthogonally to their top surfaces in the coronal view. (g), (h), and (i) show the two shanks inserted in the fused CT-MRI images. *Arrows* point to the shanks in the central portion of the inferior colliculus with appropriate angles to be aligned along the tonotopic axis.

(▶ Fig. 18.15). Watertight closure of the dura is (▶ Fig. 18.16) performed and the craniotomy is closed by cranioplastic approach with artificial bone cement wound closure.

18.3.1 Location of the Electrode Arrays

Postoperative CT scans are taken and the position of the electrodes within the inferior colliculus are reconstructed with superposition into the preoperative MRI scans (▶ Fig. 18.4). These data are still being analyzed to create three-dimensional anatomical reconstructions of the midbrain and shank positions, and will be published in a future publication.

18.4 Postoperative Fitting and Hearing Performance

About 1 month after surgery, fitting is performed with determination of the thresholds and comfortable loudness levels for each electrode site. Electrodes with nonauditory sensations are switched off. Remaining electrodes are ordered following pitch scaling or ranking (▶ Fig. 18.17). Loudness balancing across electrodes is necessary to present the different frequency bands of the acoustic signal in equal loudness. Daily intensive training on hearing with fine adjustments of the fittings is performed for up to a 2-year period that is

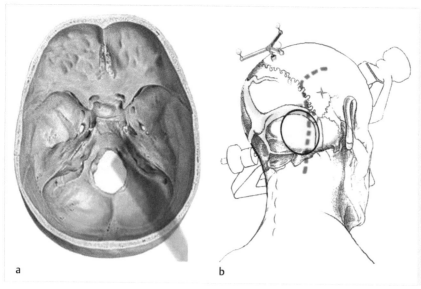

Fig. 18.5 Lateral suboccipital infratentorial supracerebellar approach. **(a)** Schematic drawing showing the area of exposure provided by the lateral suboccipital craniotomy including the ipsilateral cerebellopontine angle and the dorsolateral aspect of the mesencephalon. **(b)** Schematic drawing showing the skin incision (*red dotted line*), appropriate location for the receiver-stimulator of the auditory midbrain implant (AMI) in the temporoparietal area (*red star*), and the location of the lateral suboccipital craniotomy (*yellow circle*) exposing the inferior margin of the transverse sinus and the medial margin of the sigmoid sinus. (Image was taken from Samii et al[16] and reprinted with permission from Wolters Kluwer).

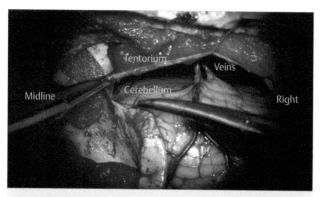

Fig. 18.6 Infratentorial supracerebellar dissection with preservation of bridging veins.

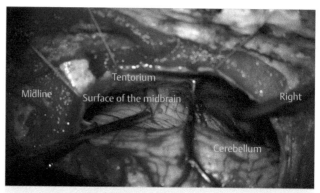

Fig. 18.7 Gentle dissection with exposure of the inferior colliculus.

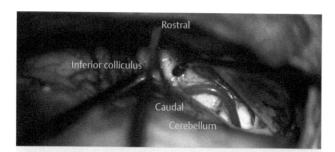

Fig. 18.8 Exposure of the surface of the inferior colliculus with preservation of all adjacent neurovascular structures.

required for the protocol of the ongoing clinical trial that is funded by the National Institutes of Health. The maximum rate of stimulation frequency has to be determined during these fittings. With a single-shank electrode array, rapid adaptation can occur with stimulation rates above 250 Hz. This can be partially overcome using a double-shank electrode where the stimulation sites are changed between the two shanks, and thus higher stimulation rates can be explored. Different types of stimulation strategies are being explored in these currently implanted AMI patients to build up speech and hearing performance. The clinical trial is still ongoing, and results will be presented at the close of the 2-year evaluation period for each patient.

18.5 Discussion

Hearing rehabilitation in patients with neural deafness is possible with central auditory implants. Besides the ABI, the AMI has been developed. So far two clinical studies with single-shank and double-shank electrode arrays have been performed. The results show that the patients experience hearing sensations and achieve some degree of closed- or open-set speech recognition, but further evaluation over time is required to make more definitive claims. The surgical procedure requires an appropriate exposure of the target structure and a precise definition of the insertion points on the surface of the inferior colliculus. This can be achieved using appropriately

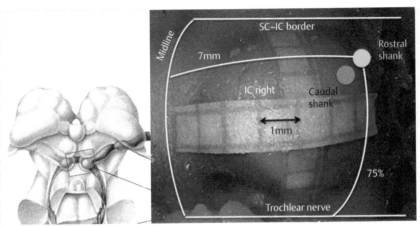

Fig. 18.9 Entry points of penetrating electrode arrays into the right inferior colliculus.

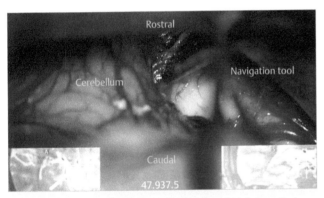

Fig. 18.10 Navigation tool on the surface of the right inferior colliculus indicating the angle toward the midline using a Fiagon navigation system.

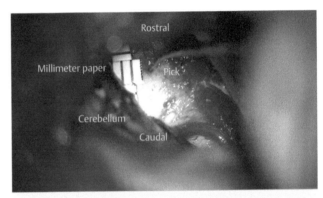

Fig. 18.11 Special surgical tool/pick to penetrate the pia mater in the right inferior colliculus.

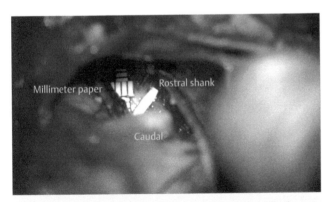

Fig. 18.12 Insertion of the rostral shank into the inferior colliculus.

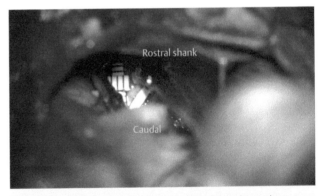

Fig. 18.13 Rostral shank completely inserted with stylet in place.

identified anatomical landmarks and proper brain navigation. These steps help to determine the locations and angles of insertion of each shank, although even with these landmarks, insertion into a small midbrain structure remains challenging. Encouragingly, the AMI from both studies has proven to be relatively safe and shows promise for restoring hearing relative to the ABI. Further evaluation of the implanted patients over the required 2-year period will reveal the extent of hearing improvements for the AMI in comparison to current ABI and CI devices, and whether it can serve as a successful hearing alternative in certain patient populations. These results are expected to be available by summer of 2021.

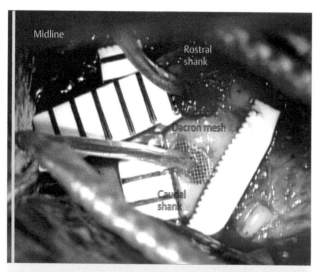

Fig. 18.14 Both shanks are inserted with stylets removed. The Dacron mesh helps to stabilize the electrode shanks in their position.

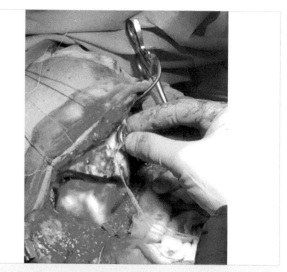

Fig. 18.16 Implant in bony bed. Dura closed.

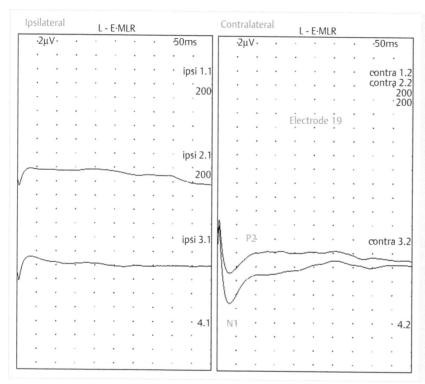

Fig. 18.15 Electrical middle latency responses (E-MLRs) intraoperatively recorded with electrical stimulation of the inferior colliculus.

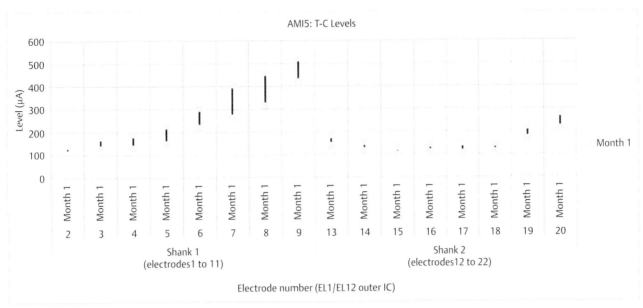

Fig. 18.17 Postoperative fitting with pitch scaling ordered electrodes. Depicted are threshold and comfortable current levels (endpoints of each vertical line) of one of the auditory midbrain implant (AMI) patients after first fitting.

References

[1] Schwartz MS, Otto SR, Shannon RV, Hitselberger WE, Brackmann DE. Auditory brainstem implants. Neurotherapeutics. 2008; 5(1):128–136

[2] Sennaroglu L, Ziyal I. Auditory brainstem implantation. Auris Nasus Larynx. 2012; 39(5):439–450

[3] Lim HH, Lenarz T. Auditory midbrain implant: research and development towards a second clinical trial. Hear Res. 2015; 322:212–223

[4] Lenarz T, Lim HH, Reuter G, Patrick JF, Lenarz M. The auditory midbrain implant: a new auditory prosthesis for neural deafness-concept and device description. Otol Neurotol. 2006; 27(6):838–843

[5] McCreery DB. Cochlear nucleus auditory prostheses. Hear Res. 2008; 242 (1–2):64–73

[6] Taslimi S, Zuccato JA, Mansouri A, et al. Novel statistical analyses to assess hearing outcomes after ABI implantation in NF2 patients: systematic review and individualized patient data analysis. World Neurosurg. 2019; 128: e669–e682

[7] Colletti V, Shannon R, Carner M, Veronese S, Colletti L. Outcomes in nontumor adults fitted with the auditory brainstem implant: 10 years' experience. Otol Neurotol. 2009; 30(5):614–618

[8] Colletti L, Shannon RV, Colletti V. The development of auditory perception in children after auditory brainstem implantation. Audiol Neurotol. 2014; 19 (6):386–394

[9] Matthies C, Brill S, Varallyay C, et al. Auditory brainstem implants in neurofibromatosis type 2: is open speech perception feasible? J Neurosurg. 2014; 120(2):546–558

[10] Meddis R, O'Mard LP, Lopez-Poveda EA. A computational algorithm for computing nonlinear auditory frequency selectivity. J Acoust Soc Am. 2001; 109 (6):2852–2861

[11] Shannon RV, Zeng FG, Kamath V, Wygonski J, Ekelid M. Speech recognition with primarily temporal cues. Science. 1995; 270(5234):303–304

[12] Sumner CJ, O'Mard LP, Lopez-Poveda EA, Meddis R. A nonlinear filter-bank model of the guinea-pig cochlear nerve: rate responses. J Acoust Soc Am. 2003; 113(6):3264–3274

[13] Colletti V, Shannon RV. Open set speech perception with auditory brainstem implant? Laryngoscope. 2005; 115(11):1974–1978

[14] Lenarz M, Lim HH, Lenarz T, et al. Auditory midbrain implant: histomorphologic effects of long-term implantation and electric stimulation of a new deep brain stimulation array. Otol Neurotol. 2007; 28(8):1045–1052

[15] Lim HH, Lenarz T, Joseph G, et al. Electrical stimulation of the midbrain for hearing restoration: insight into the functional organization of the human central auditory system. J Neurosci. 2007; 27(49):13541–13551

[16] Samii A, Lenarz M, Majdani O, Lim HH, Samii M, Lenarz T. Auditory midbrain implant: a combined approach for vestibular schwannoma surgery and device implantation. Otol Neurotol. 2007; 28(1):31–38

[17] Lim HH, Lenarz M, Lenarz T. Auditory midbrain implant: a review. Trends Amplif. 2009; 13(3):149–180

[18] Geniec P, Morest DK. The neuronal architecture of the human posterior colliculus:a study with the Golgi method. Acta Otolaryngol Suppl. 1971; 295:1–33

[19] De Martino F, Moerel M, van de Moortele PF, et al. Spatial organization of frequency preference and selectivity in the human inferior colliculus. Nat Commun. 2013; 4:1386

[20] Mansour Y, Altaher W, Kulesza RJ, Jr. Characterization of the human central nucleus of the inferior colliculus. Hear Res. 2019; 377:234–246

19 Future Development: Penetrating Multisite Microelectrodes as Cochlear Nucleus Implant

Martin Han and Douglas B. McCreery

Abstract

Auditory brainstem implants (ABIs) can restore useful hearing to patients with hearing loss who cannot benefit from cochlear implants. We provide an update on recent efforts to develop silicon-based, multisite, penetrating microelectrode arrays as a cochlear nucleus auditory prosthesis. We summarize technological advances with our devices in the feline model as steps toward validating the device for future clinical use.

Keywords: cochlear nucleus implant, penetrating microelectrode array, silicon-based multisite device, microstimulation, amplitude modulation

19.1 Introduction

19.1.1 Auditory Brainstem Prosthesis

While cochlear implants have become the most widely used neuroprostheses, patients without a functional auditory nerve or with a deformed or ossified cochlea cannot benefit from them. Studies have shown that electrode array implanted on the surface of the cochlear nucleus do convey auditory percepts that enable users to recognize important environmental sounds and aid with lipreading.[3] In some instances good recognition of speech ("open-set" speech recognition) has been reported for patients whose deafness was not due to neurofibromatosis type 2 (NF2), the most common indication for an auditory brainstem implantation.[4] In this context, an array of microelectrodes that penetrates into the ventral cochlear nucleus (VCN) may be applicable to non-NF2 as well as to NF2 patients. The non-NF2 group may include a subset of cochlear implant users who do not receive significant benefit from their cochlear implants.[4] A growing number of cochlear implant users who are middle-aged or older adults may lose their hearing by presbycusis including cochlear synaptopathy.[6] In a small clinical trial, an array of iridium oxide microwire electrodes with a single electrode site at the tip was implanted into the VCN of 10 patients following resection of auditory nerve tumors, but the effort had limited success.[11]

19.2 Multisite Arrays for Auditory Brainstem Prosthesis

Among the micromachining technology-based devices, the only silicon-based microelectrode array that has FDA approval is the Blackrock array (a version of the Utah intracortical array).[2] This device is approved for humans for less than 30 days and has only one microstimulating site on each shank that penetrates into the neural tissue. As a result, this device may not provide much additional benefit as an auditory prosthesis or implant. In contrast, it is possible that an array of penetrating multisite microelectrodes whose safety has been validated by adequate preclinical data may enable selective and localized access to the tonotopic gradients of the cochlear nucleus (CN), and thereby convey improved speech recognition to the users. ▶ Fig. 19.1 illustrates such an array of multisite penetrating electrodes intended for implantation into the feline VCN. Microelectrode arrays with multiple electrically independent stimulating sites on each penetrating shank have the potential for conveying electrical stimulation with high spatial selectivity

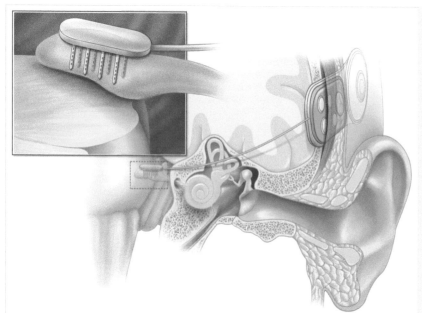

Fig. 19.1 Illustration of a three-dimensional penetrating multisite microelectrode array device configured for implantation into the ventral cochlear nucleus (VCN). *Right*: The device as it might be implanted into the human cochlear nucleus. *Left*: The device has eight silicon shanks, each with five activated iridium oxide microelectrodes distributed along the 2.5 mm from the tip of each shank. The geometric surface area of each microelectrode is approximately 2,000 μm^2. The array has been extensively validated in the feline cochlear nucleus. (From McCreery et al.)[9]

while minimizing the number of penetrating shanks and attendant risks of tissue injury. Having multiple electrode sites per shank ("multisite"), the device allows access to the topography of the cochlear nucleus. In the past, the Michigan/NeuroNexus probes have been widely used in animal studies,[1,10] mainly for recording neuronal activity. However, this device has not been approved by the FDA for human use, and their materials and designs are not generally known to satisfy the brainstem prosthesis requirements.

19.3 Device Development and In-Vivo Preclinical Evaluation

We developed our multisite silicon probes for neural stimulating and recording and validated their function and longevity through long-term implantation in the feline brainstem (▶ Fig. 19.2, left).[5] The photolithography-based micromachining technology allows the individual microstimulating sites to be three-dimensionally arranged as a cluster of multiple penetrating shanks. These probes are fabricated by the deep reactive ion etching process followed by and mechanical sharpening of their tip, yielding a mechanically sturdy shank with a sharpened tip that reduces insertion force and tissue displacement during implantation into the brain. The microelectrode sites are electroplated or sputter-coated with iridium oxide. We have implanted these multisite silicon-substrate microelectrodes into the cochlear nucleus of adult cats for up to 314 days and we have monitored the tonotopic specificity of the stimulation by recording in the central nucleus of the contralateral inferior colliculus (IC).[7,9] To our knowledge this is one of the longest durations of recordings and stimulation achieved by silicon-based multisite arrays. Histopathology evaluation of neurons and astrocytes using immunohistochemical stains indicated minimal alterations of tissue architecture after chronic implantation.

19.4 A Combinational Approach: Surface and Penetrating Electrodes

An important question is how the performance of a central auditory prosthesis may be enhanced by combining macrostimulation applied on the surface of the nucleus with simultaneous microstimulation within the cochlear nucleus. The premise is that the surface electrodes would convey most of the range of loudness percepts while the intranuclear microelectrodes would sharpen and focus pitch percepts. To delineate potential differences between the two devices, stimulating electrodes were implanted chronically on the surface of the animal's dorsal cochlear nucleus (DCN) and also within their VCN.[8,9] Recording microelectrodes were implanted into the central nucleus of the IC. The electrical stimuli were sinusoidally modulated stimulus pulse trains applied on the DCN and within the VCN. ▶ Fig. 19.2 shows contour plots of the time-depth distribution of the vector strength (VS) of the neuronal activity recorded in the cat's IC in response to charge-balanced electrical stimulation delivered through a microelectrode in the cat's contralateral posteroventral cochlear nucleus (PVCN) (▶ Fig. 19.2a) and to stimuli applied via a macroelectrode on the cat's DCN (▶ Fig. 19.2b), and then to simultaneous stimulation at both sites (▶ Fig. 19.2c). The plots' ordinate is along the axis of the recording microelectrode in the IC and approximately along the tonotopic gradient of the IC. ▶ Fig. 19.2a,b illustrate the much smaller spread induced by the microstimulation in the PVCN and the large spread by the stimulation on the surface of the DCN, respectively. ▶ Fig. 19.2c shows how the response to simultaneous microstimulation in the PVCN and the macrostimulation on the surface of the DCN retained the small focus of the near-maximum response while only slightly reducing the spread of the response induced by the surface stimulation. This illustrates how the intranuclear microstimulation focuses the maxima of the neuronal activity into a small part of the IC's tonotopic gradient while the surface stimulation retains the more broadly distributed activity.

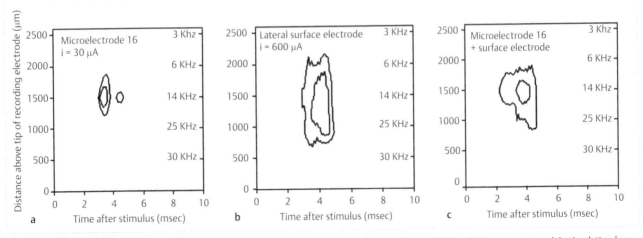

Fig. 19.2 Contour plots of the rate of action potentials elicited from a multiunit in a cat's inferior colliculus (IC) in response to: (**a**) stimulation by a microelectrode in the contralateral posteroventral cochlear nucleus (PVCN), (**b**) stimulation via a macroelectrode on the surface of the dorsal cochlear nucleus (DCN), and (**c**) when the microelectrode and the surface electrode were pulsed simultaneously. The inner and outer contour lines delineate, respectively, 75 and 50% of the unit's maximum discharge rate. The microelectrodes resulted in smaller foci than the surface electrodes (from McCreery et al[9]).

19.5 Temporal Encoding of Modulation

In the proposed clinical device, the functions of the surface and intranuclear microelectrodes could be best integrated if there is minimal variation in the neuronal responses across the range of modulation depth, modulation frequencies, and across the stimulation modes. To study this, VS and full-cycle rate of neuronal activity in the IC were measured for four stimulation modes: continuous and transient amplitude modulation of the stimulus pulse trains, each delivered via the macroelectrode on the surface of the DCN and then by the intranuclear penetrating microelectrodes.[9] Results showed that VS varied approximately 34% across modulation frequency and modulation depth within a stimulation mode, and up to 40% between modulation modes. However, the intra- and inter-mode variances differed for different stimulation rates, and at 500 Hz the inter-mode differences in VS and across the range of modulation frequencies and modulation depths were ±24% and the intra-modal differences were ±15%. The findings were generally similar for rate encoding of modulation depth, although the depth of transient amplitude modulation delivered by the surface electrode was weakly encoded as full-cycle rate. Modulation depth was encoded strongly when the maximum stimulus amplitude was held constant across a range of modulation depth. This "constant maximum" protocol allows enhancement of modulation depth while preserving overall dynamic range. Overall, our findings support the concept of a clinical ABI that employs surface stimulation and intranuclear microstimulation in an integrated manner.

19.6 Ramification for Clinical Translation

In the present study the one exception to the good concordance of the neuronal responses to the surface stimulation and to the intranuclear microstimulation was for the rate coding of the depth of transient modulation. However, the weak encoding of modulation depth as full-cycle neuronal firing rate may be of little consequence to the functioning of the proposed clinical device in which the role of the surface stimulation would be to convey most of the range of loudness. Therefore, our findings support the concept of a future clinical ABI that employs surface stimulation and intranuclear microstimulation in an integrated manner. The performance of ABIs may benefit from using pulse rates greater than those presently used in most ABIs, and by sound processing strategies that enhance the modulation depth of the electrical stimulus while preserving dynamic range.

19.7 Conclusions

The work completed to date has advanced the translation of our integrated ABI toward clinical use. In the cochlear nucleus ABI we envision, the primary role of the stimulation by relatively large macroelectrdoes residing on the surface of the cochlear nucleus would be to convey a wide range of loudness while the primary role of the multisite and microstimulation distributed across the tonotopic organization of the VCN would convey place pitch. While the overall size of the target patient population may be small compared to cochlear implants—a humanitarian use device designation with less than 8,000 patients per year—a penetrating array as discussed will provide great benefit to these individuals. In addition, a (first) success of multisite silicon device may remove a significant barrier to FDA approval, and additional benefits can be expected as the fabrication technology allows for modification to other sites along the auditory pathway (e.g., auditory nerve, auditory midbrain, and auditory cortex).

Acknowledgments

The authors thank the technical and animal care staffs at HMRI. Funding for the development of the silicon microelectrode array was provided by NIH grants R01DC013412 (DM) and R01DC014044 (MH).

References

[1] Basura GJ, Koehler SD, Shore SE. Multi-sensory integration in brainstem and auditory cortex. Brain Res. 2012; 1485:95–107

[2] Blackrock Microsystems. from http://www.blackrockmicro.com/

[3] Colletti V, Fiorino FG, Carner M, Miorelli V, Guida M, Colletti L. Auditory brainstem implant as a salvage treatment after unsuccessful cochlear implantation. Otol Neurotol. 2004; 25(4):485–496, discussion 496

[4] Colletti V, Shannon RV. Open set speech perception with auditory brainstem implant? Laryngoscope. 2005; 115(11):1974–1978

[5] Han M, Manoonkitiwongsa PS, Wang CX, McCreery DB. In vivo validation of custom-designed silicon-based microelectrode arrays for long-term neural recording and stimulation. IEEE Trans Biomed Eng. 2012; 59(2):346–354

[6] Liberman MC, Kujawa SG. Cochlear synaptopathy in acquired sensorineural hearing loss: manifestations and mechanisms. Hear Res. 2017; 349: 138–147–SI

[7] McCreery D, Han M, Pikov V, Yadav K, Pannu S. Encoding of the amplitude modulation of pulsatile electrical stimulation in the feline cochlear nucleus by neurons in the inferior colliculus; effects of stimulus pulse rate. J Neural Eng. 2013; 10(5):056010

[8] McCreery D, Han M, Pikov V. Neuronal activity evoked in the inferior colliculus of the cat by surface macroelectrodes and penetrating microelectrodes implanted in the cochlear nucleus. IEEE Trans Biomed Eng. 2010; 57(7): 1765–1773

[9] McCreery D, Yadev K, Han M. Responses of neurons in the feline inferior colliculus to modulated electrical stimuli applied on and within the ventral cochlear nucleus; Implications for an advanced auditory brainstem implant. Hear Res. 2018; 363:85–97

[10] Merriam ME, Dehmel S, Srivannavit O, Shore SE, Wise KD. A 3-d 160-site microelectrode array for cochlear nucleus mapping. IEEE Trans Biomed Eng. 2011; 58(2):397–403

[11] Otto SR, Shannon RV, Wilkinson EP, et al. Audiologic outcomes with the penetrating electrode auditory brainstem implant. Otol Neurotol. 2008; 29 (8):1147–1154

20 Future Developments: Conformable ABI Arrays and Light Stimulation of Auditory Brainstem Using Optogenetics

Osama Tarabichi, Elliott D. Kozin, M. Christian Brown, and Daniel J. Lee

Abstract

The auditory brainstem implant (ABI) is a neuroprosthetic device that provides hearing sensation to patients who are not candidates for cochlear implantation. The ABI provides meaningful sound detection that aids lipreading but overall outcomes are poor compared to the CI. ABI outcomes are highly variable and thought to be influenced by a number of factors related to patient characteristics, blind placement technique and ABI device design. The design of the ABI device has not changed significantly in about three decades and is thought to contribute to electric current spread and poor spatial specificity of stimulation. In this chapter we provide an update on ours and others work that is focused on improving ABI device design and exploring novel stimulation modalities. Specifically we will discuss (1) Conformable ABI array technology, (2) Novel electrode coatings and (3) Light-based neural stimulation modalities in the context of the ABI.

Keywords: hearing loss, deafness, auditory brainstem implant, cochlear nucleus, neurofibromatosis, optogenetics, inferior colliculus, conformable, opsin, optical stimulation, electrical stimulation, auditory cortex

20.1 Introduction

The auditory brainstem implant (ABI) is a neuroprosthetic device that provides hearing sensations to patients who are not candidates for cochlear implant (CI) surgery due to injury or absence of the cochlea or cochlear nerve.[1] The first surgery to place an ABI array on the cochlear nucleus (CN) was performed by William Hitselberger and William House in 1984.[2] A multi-channel (21-electrode) ABI manufactured by Cochlear Corporation was approved by the Food and Drug Administration (FDA) in 2000 for use in patients with neurofibromatosis type 2 (NF2), an inherited condition that causes the growth of large benign tumors of the vestibular nerve that invariably cause a significant degree of hearing loss.[3] In parallel, the MED-EL Corporation developed a multichannel (12-electrode) ABI for use outside the US that received the CE (conformité européenne) mark in 2003.

The ABI can provide meaningful sound detection that aids in lipreading but overall hearing outcomes are poor compared to those achieved by the CI. Only rarely do ABI users achieve open-set speech recognition compared to the majority of CI recipients.[4] The variability of ABI outcomes are likely influenced by a number of factors (difficulty of surgical approach, duration of deafness, neighboring nonauditory axons of passage).[5,6] Other contributors to the poor performance of the ABI include (1) damage to the CN caused by the tumor or its treatment (surgery or radiation), (2) suboptimal positioning of the array as a result of the "blind" placement during surgery, (3) inability of the ABI to replicate the advanced processing of the neurons of the CN, (4) poor spatial resolution of ABI stimulation caused by spread of the electric current, and (5) mechanical mismatch between electrodes and neural tissue due to stiff and noncompliant array.

The overall design of the ABI has not changed significantly over the past three decades. The primary aims of our research group at the Massachusetts Eye and Ear are to (1) examine clinical outcomes of the ABI in NF2 patients and nontumor children and adults who are deaf and are not candidates for the CI and (2) engineer and test new ABI electrode array technology that we hypothesize will reduce current spread and improve spectral resolution over existing designs.

In the following sections, we provide an update on our progress to develop (1) conformable ABI arrays that improve the mechanical mismatch seen with the current stiff array design, (2) novel coatings to improve electrical properties in smaller electrodes, and (3) "optical" or light-based stimulation modalities using optogenetics to modulate responses of the central auditory pathways.

20.2 Electrical Implant Modifications

20.2.1 Conformable Electrode Arrays for the ABI

As the field of neuroprosthetics has evolved, several engineering groups have sought to study ways to improve the electrode–neural interface. Neural implant electrode arrays in current clinical use, including the ABI, are manufactured on thick platinum and silastic substrates.[7,8] These materials are generally rigid and do not conform to the curved surface of neural tissues. We hypothesize that ABI electrodes mounted on a stiff backing will have suboptimal contact to the surface of the CN resulting in spread of current to neighboring structures. We also hypothesize that continuous micro- and macromotion of the pulsating brainstem may influence the durability of the electrode as well as increase scarring of the neural surface.[9] Our recent studies of perceptual thresholds as a function of electrode array position in children and adult ABI users highlight this phenomenon.[6] Some ABI users have a central cluster of usable channels with a peripheral rim of electrodes that produce side effects or do not confer any perception (▶ Fig. 20.1).

A conformable electrode array could theoretically solve this problem by improving contact with the brainstem surface. Conformability of implanted arrays made of a durable synthetic polymer called polyimide can be tuned by altering the thickness of the sheet (▶ Fig. 20.2).[10] Thinner polyimide sheets demonstrate greater conformability. Collaborating with Professor Stephanie Lacour at the École polytechnique fédérale de Lausanne (EPFL), we have shown in acute experimental preparations that

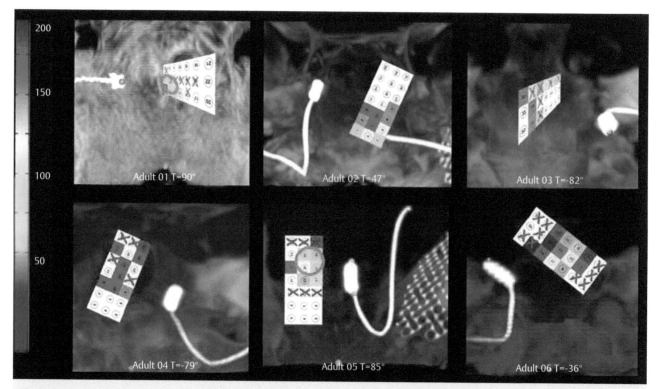

Fig. 20.1 Correlation of psychophysical responses of adult auditory brainstem implant (ABI) with three-dimensional (3D) reconstruction of array position in postoperative computed tomography (CT) images. Heat maps of perceptual thresholds are aligned to ABI array position (blue – low threshold, red – high threshold, white – no sound percept, red X – deactivated electrode due to side effects). We hypothesize that poor contact between the stiff and noncompliant array and curved brainstem surface may explain the small number of low threshold electrodes surrounded by high threshold or nonauditory electrodes. (Modified from and reproduced with permission from Barber et al.[6])

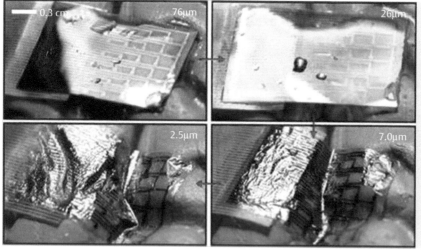

Fig. 20.2 Interaction of polyimide implants of various thicknesses to the surface of a simulated brain model. Thinner arrays (2.5 and 7.0 µm) demonstrate greater conformability to complex surface topography. (Reproduced with permission from Kim et al.[10])

conformable microelectrode polyimide arrays can elicit robust inferior colliculus (IC) responses in acute rodent models of the ABI.[11] Potential drawbacks of conformable technology are (1) increased fragility and (2) unfavorable surgical handling characteristics. These issues can be addressed by adding a spine or "handle" to the array to ease insertion (similar to existing designs) as well as including a rigid polymer coating that subsequently dissolves after surgery, allowing for conformation of the array to the curved brainstem.

Another important advantage of conformable materials is that their mechanical properties more closely match those of neural tissue.[9] Neural tissues are mechanically heterogeneous and exhibit Young's moduli (measure of the ability of tissue to be deformed elastically) in the kilopascal range.[12] In contrast, stiff electronics currently used clinically for central stimulation exhibit Young's moduli that are *orders* of magnitude higher. This mechanical mismatch is thought to contribute to inflammation at the electrode–brainstem interface and potentially

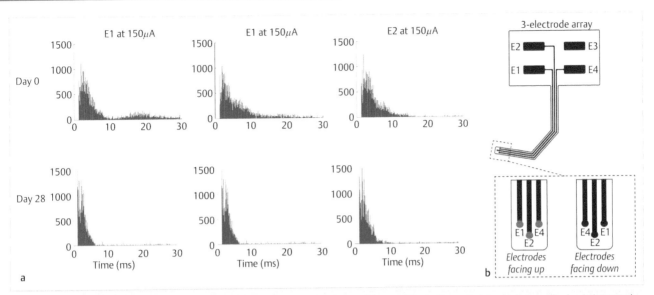

Fig. 20.3 Conformable arrays placed on dorsal cochlear nucleus (CN) can elicit multiunit spiking in the contralateral inferior colliculus (IC) 1 month after chronic implantation in mouse. **(a)** Day 0 and Day 28 peristimulus time histograms (PSTH) demonstrate IC spiking in response to monopolar electrical stimulation of CN (averaged over 412 trials). A 150 µA pulse was delivered at 28 Hz. **(b)** Three channel mouse ABI array design and electrode configuration (100 µm diameter contacts, coated with platinum elastomer mesocomposite).

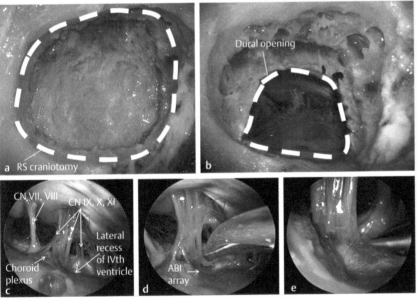

Fig. 20.4 Human cadaveric study of novel conformable auditory brainstem implant (ABI) array, right ear. **(a)** Microscopic view following retrosigmoid (RS) craniotomy. **(b)** Microscopic view of dural opening to access cerebellopontine angle (CPA). **(c–e)** 0-degree endoscopic view of right CPA. **(c)** Lateral recess of the fourth ventricle is identified by surrounding landmarks (choroid plexus, cranial nerve [CN] IX [glossopharyngeal nerve]). D/E: conformable polydimethylsiloxane (PDMS) arrays (thickness: 200 µm) placed under endoscopic control. In contrast, clinical ABI arrays are much thicker (700 µm) and much stiffer. CN VII, VIII: facial nerve and vestibulocochlear nerve; CN IX, X, XI: cranial nerves IX, X, and XI.

cause higher rates of electrode failure. One material used for conformable electrode arrays is polydimethylsiloxane (PDMS),[13] a silicone-based organic polymer that has been tested in rodent and primate models of spinal cord injury.[14,15] Multichannel electrode arrays made with PDMS have been used to stimulate motor spinal cord rootlets for the rehabilitation of lower limb paralysis in animal models with durable responses observed several months post implantation.[9,15] Empirical data from our laboratory suggest that these materials can reliably evoke activity in a rodent model of the ABI for up to 1 month post-op (▶ Fig. 20.3).[16] Minev et al[9] also showed that conformable spinal cord implants with elastic moduli more closely resembling those of neural tissue reduced the neuroinflammatory response

and extent of spinal cord deformation. In a pilot study, our group has recently demonstrated that conformable arrays can be scaled up to the size of a clinical device and implanted in cadaveric human specimens. We plan to use this model to determine optimal device dimensions and quantify differences in mechanical properties between novel conformable ABI arrays and those in clinical use (▶ Fig. 20.4).

20.2.2 Novel Electrode Coatings and Electrode Array Density

The contemporary ABI array approved for use has 12- (MED-EL, non-FDA approved) or 21-electrode contacts (Cochlear Corp,

FDA approved) that ranges in diameter from 550 to 700 μm, respectively.[17] Reducing electrode size has historically been limited by higher impedances associated with smaller contact diameters. To overcome this, a number of novel electrode coatings have been proposed to reduce impedance and increase safely injectable current levels with smaller contact sizes. This approach can improve the electrical properties of platinum electrodes by (1) optimizing the effective area of contact by creating a rough surface and (2) utilizing coatings that have excellent charge injection capacity. Conducting polymers such as poly(3,4-ethylenedioxythiophene) (PEDOT) and polypyrrole (PPy) can achieve this, and we have exploited these properties in an acute preparation of a rat ABI model.[18] Most conducting polymers, however, are stiff and can alter the mechanical properties of the array. Recent studies have examined the use of a platinum elastomer mesocomposite that is more compatible with conformable implant technologies.[19] Studies of durability of these electrode coatings *in vivo* are lacking and will be the focus of our chronic studies.

Whether increasing the number of electrodes will improve performance of the ABI is unresolved but channel interaction from electrical current spread is well described. Kuchta et al studied perceptual performance in ABI users with different numbers of active channels and found that the best performing patients had more than three active electrodes but those with five or more active electrodes had no additional benefit in sound perception abilities.[20]

20.3 Light-Based Stimulation Modalities

20.3.1 Infrared Neural Stimulation

Infrared neural stimulation (INS) is a term used to describe the activation of unmodified neural tissue by radiant energy emitted from a pulsed infrared laser source.[21] INS has been studied in various applications in both the peripheral and central nervous system.[22,23,24,25] For example, INS of the sciatic nerve can evoke more spatially restricted neural activity when compared to electrical stimulation.[22] In the peripheral auditory system, Richter and colleagues have demonstrated that INS of the cochlea has been shown to evoke multiunit firing in the auditory midbrain (IC).[26] INS has not yet been shown to generate far-field responses (optically evoked auditory brainstem response

or ABR) in a deafened ear. In the context of the ABI, our group has demonstrated that INS of auditory brainstem does generate neural responses of the auditory system in deafened rats but the mechanism may be related to an optophonic effect.[27] Delivery of INS via flexible optical fiber generates an intense broadband acoustic click due to the stress-relaxation wave created by pulsed radiant energy and so continued study of this modality must include deafened animal models to rule out the possibility of acoustic artifact.[27] Consistent with these observations by our lab, Thompson et al reported that INS of the cochlea does not evoke auditory activity in a deafened guinea pig.[28] These results suggest that evoked neural activity from INS in subjects with residual hearing is likely generated by an opto-acoustic effect and transduced by inner hair cells rather than a primary neural response. More recently, Bin et al reported that in a deafened rat model of the ABI, auditory responses from CN stimulation could be evoked if carbon nanoparticles are applied to the CN to enhance the thermal effect of INS.[29] Spike rates achieved by INS in hearing and deafened animals in this report differ significantly, signifying the need for further studies to discern the effect of an optoacoustic phenomenon from actual neural stimulation. While the concept of improving spatial resolution using light without the need to genetically alter CN neurons is intriguing, it is important to keep in mind some notable limitations of INS. The effects of repetitive thermal application from chronic INS on underlying tissue have not been well characterized.[23] Auditory implant usage requires continuous acoustic input from the environment and the cumulative thermal energy generated by an infrared laser at high rates of stimulation may have a detrimental effect on neural tissue in the long term. Contemporary implant and battery technology also cannot support the size and energy requirements needed to power a portable infrared device.[30]

20.3.2 Optogenetic Stimulation

Optogenetics is a powerful tool that has been extensively used by neuroscientists to probe neural circuits with millisecond precision[31] (▶ Fig. 20.5) and relies on genetic transduction of neurons to enable expression of light-sensitive ion channels called "opsins."[32] Optogenetics was developed in 2005 when Boyden et al reported the successful transduction of hippocampal neurons with channelrhodopsin-2 (ChR2), an opsin expressed by the bacterium *Chlamydomonas reinhardtii*, using a lentiviral vector.[33] Neurons that express ChR2 are rendered

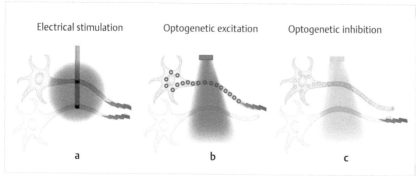

Electrical stimulation   Optogenetic excitation   Optogenetic inhibition

a   b   c

Fig. 20.5 Schematic comparing electrical stimulation with optogenetic control of neurons. (a) Electrodes in close proximity generate overlapping electrical fields that limit spectral resolution. (b and c) Optogenetics enables modulation of neuron activity with millisecond precision and with greater specificity than electricity. Only those neurons that (1) express opsins and (2) are exposed to light of a specific wavelength and radiant energy level will depolarize (b) or hyperpolarize (c). (Reproduced with permission from Deisseroth, K., Optogenetics. Nature Methods, 2010.)

photosensitive to blue light. In contrast to electricity, light can be focused to extremely narrow beams and can theoretically enable micrometer scale spatial selectivity.[34] Another advantage that is particularly useful in the complex cellular environment of the CN is that opsin gene delivery strategies can be modified to allow for the selective transduction and opsin expression of specific cell populations. Optogenetic stimulation also offers a more physiologic method of neural stimulation by recruiting smaller diameter nerve fibers first in contrast to electrical stimulation that preferentially stimulates large bore nerve fibers.[35] The spectrum of naturally occurring and synthetic opsins has increased dramatically since optogenetics was first developed a little over a decade ago.[36] Excitatory and inhibitory opsins that respond to a wide range of photon wavelengths are now available for research purposes.[32] Optogenetics has been extensively used in basic and translational research settings to achieve targeted control of neural circuits[37,38] and promises unprecedented selectivity of stimulation for ABI candidates. In this section we will provide an overview of the potential and challenges to incorporate optogenetics in future auditory implants such as the ABI.

Opsin Delivery

In animal models of optogenetics, opsin expression is usually achieved by viral vector delivery or through transgenic strategies such as the cre-lox recombinase system.[39] Safe, efficient, and selective introduction of opsins into neurons of interest presents the most prominent hurdle to clinical translation. The most promising avenue toward achieving safe expression of opsins in the CN is the use of virally mediated gene delivery. Adeno-associated virus (AAV) constructs have been shown to be safe and efficacious in alleviating genetic defects in clinical trials for hemophilia B and inherited blindness.[40,41] Darrow et al and Hight et al from our group showed that direct pressure micro-injections of AAV constructs into CN carrying opsins ChR2 or Chronos allow for robust expression in multiple cell types.[42,43] Preliminary results from our group also demonstrate that systemic injections of AAV into mouse temporal or tail vein are associated with robust opsin expression in the auditory brainstem.[44] Another notable hurdle toward translating optogenetics is the limited ability of current vector strategies to selectively target auditory neural networks. In optogenetics, promoter sequences carried by viral vectors allow for the targeting of specific neural subtypes. Opsin expression in mouse models of an optogenetic ABI is widespread throughout many cell types and involves many neural networks in the brainstem and cortex. The size of many promoter sequences far surpasses the carrying capacity of contemporary viral vectors, limiting the number of promoters that can be used to effectively target specific neuronal populations.[45] In a pilot study we studied the physiological responses and histological expression in transgenic lines designed to drive opsin expression using different promoters: Bhlhb5, VGLUT-2, Atoh-1, parvalbumin, and Nestin.[46] Preliminary data characterizing expression patterns and multiunit responses in the IC demonstrate variability among these transgenic lines. Our findings suggest that advancements in vector engineering coupled with improvements in our understanding of the genetics and physiology of the CN are needed to achieve more selective activation of neurons in

an optogenetic ABI. The theoretical ability of optogenetics to transfect different cell types with opsins that respond to different wavelengths can also lead to the development of more complex stimulation paradigms that may allow for further improvements in auditory performance with future optical implants.

Optogenetic Control of the CN

Shimano et al were the first to report *in vivo* optogenetic modulation of dorsal CN responses (see ▶ Fig. 20.6).[47] Later work by Darrow et al[43] using direct CN injections of AAV with a ChR2-EGFP fusion protein into wildtype mice and 4-week incubation period showed IC multiunit responses and optically evoked ABRs (oABR) in response to light stimulation of the CN.[43] In preliminary work we demonstrated that systemic AAV construct injections drove opsin expression to levels that allowed for physiologic responses to pulsed light stimulation.[44] One drawback to these methods is the high failure rate of systemic injections in producing physiologically significant levels of opsin expression.

The choice of opsin is important when developing an optical auditory implant. ChR2 is the most commonly used opsin in neuroscience and is ideal for slow-firing central nervous system neurons with its sluggish channel kinetics.[48] This property is suboptimal for hearing as the auditory pathways are unique in their ability to transmit high fidelity responses at fast rates of stimulation necessary to encode for the complexities of human speech. To address this issue Hight et al compared the temporal characteristics of the novel fast opsin Chronos in an optogenetic mouse ABI model to those of ChR2. We demonstrated that multiunit IC activity could be driven at much faster rates of stimulation in Chronos expressing mice compared to ChR2.[42]

Optical Devices

Another significant technical challenge that must be addressed is the development of durable and low power biocompatible devices that can safely deliver light to the CN. To date, light has been primarily delivered by either optical fiber-based devices or light-emitting diode (LED) based arrays. Optical fibers are extremely useful in laboratory settings but are not likely to be a feasible basis for an optical ABI due to several limitations. Optical fiber-based devices are restricted in the number of channels that they can carry as each additional channel will require the wiring of an additional fiber. This issue is partially resolved by the development of multipoint-emitting optical fibers,[49] although that technology is generally reserved for applications of penetrating neuroprosthetics and is not amenable to surface stimulation of the CN. Optical fibers also need to be tethered to a laser source, which limits their portability, as fully implantable laser sources have not been developed. Thus, future optogenetic based ABI technology will likely include micro-LEDs with electrical contacts in a hybrid configuration for both optical and electrical stimulation. Advancements in bioelectronics allow for fabrication of LED panels as small as 40 μm in diameter.[50] LEDs are driven by current sources removing the need for large, expensive, and power-hungry laser sources. Limitations of LED's include significant thermal energy when powered. It is well established that chronic heating of neural tissue with a 1 °C thermal gradient can induce detrimental

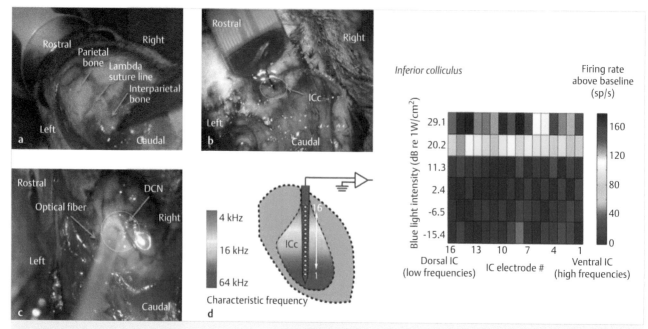

Fig. 20.6 Optogenetic control of the left auditory brainstem in mouse. **(a)** Skin and muscle are retracted laterally to expose lambda and coronal suture lines of the skull. **(b)** Placement of 16 channel penetrating recording probe into contralateral (*right ear*) inferior colliculus (IC). **(c)** *Left ear* posterior craniotomy and partial cerebellar aspiration expose surface of dorsal cochlear nucleus (CN). A 400 μm diameter flexible optical fiber mounted on a micromanipulator is introduced through the craniotomy and placed on dorsal CN surface. **(d)** Schematic of IC recording electrode array placed perpendicular to isofrequency lamina of central nucleus of the inferior colliculus (ICc). (Reproduced with permission from Hight et al.[42]) Right panel: heat map showing multiunit activity of IC neurons. Broad activation patterns in inferior colliculuc (IC) across the entire frequency range is consistent with the stimulation of a large number of CN neurons by a large bore optical fiber stimulating a large number of CN neurons. (Reproduced with permission from Darrow et al. [43])

physiological changes in neural activity.[51] Finite element models of thermal energy released by micro-LED arrays can define a safe stimulation paradigm for optogenetic stimulation.[52] However, these studies need to be coupled with chronic *in vivo* optogenetic experiments in animal models to prove safety. The attenuation and scatter of light as it passes through the brainstem tissue also needs to be characterized, as many of the targets of the ABI are deep from the surface.1

20.4 Conclusion

The fundamental design of the ABI has not changed significantly over the past several decades. Overall performance among ABI users continue to lag behind CI users and the reasons for this are complex. Continued study of improved electrical implant array designs and novel stimulation paradigms may help improve spectral resolution and reduce side effects associated with the ABI.

References

[1] Schwartz MS, Otto SR, Shannon RV, Hitselberger WE, Brackmann DE. Auditory brainstem implants. Neurotherapeutics. 2008; 5(1):128–136

[2] Hitselberger WE, House WF, Edgerton BJ, Whitaker S. Cochlear nucleus implants. Otolaryngol Head Neck Surg. 1984; 92(1):52–54

[3] Baser ME, R Evans DG, Gutmann DH. Neurofibromatosis 2. Curr Opin Neurol. 2003; 16(1):27–33

[4] Colletti V, Shannon RV. Open set speech perception with auditory brainstem implant? Laryngoscope. 2005; 115(11):1974–1978

[5] Matthies C, Thomas S, Moshrefi M, et al. Auditory brainstem implants: current neurosurgical experiences and perspective. J Laryngol Otol Suppl. 2000(27):32–36

[6] Barber SR, Kozin ED, Remenschneider AK, et al. Auditory brainstem implant aray position varies widely among adult and pediatric patients and is associated with perception. Ear Hear. 2017; 38(6):e343–e351

[7] Lacour SP, Courtine G, Guck J. Materials and technologies for soft implantable neuroprostheses. Nat Rev Mater. 2016; 1:16063

[8] Vincent C. Auditory brainstem implants: how do they work? Anat Rec (Hoboken, N.J.: 2007). 2012; 295(11):1981–1986

[9] Minev IR, Musienko P, Hirsch A, et al. Biomaterials: electronic dura mater for long-term multimodal neural interfaces. Science. 2015; 347(6218):159–163

[10] Kim DH, Viventi J, Amsden JJ, et al. Dissolvable films of silk fibroin for ultrathin conformal bio-integrated electronics. Nat Mater. 2010; 9(6):511–517

[11] Guex AA, Hight AE, Narasimhan S, Vachicouras N, Lee DJ, Lacour SP, Brown MC. (2019) Auditory brainstem stimulation with a conformable microfabricated array elicits responses with tonotopically organized components. Hear Res. 377:339-352.

[12] Harrison DE, Cailliet R, Harrison DD, Troyanovich SJ, Harrison SO. A review of biomechanics of the central nervous system—part II: spinal cord strains from postural loads. J Manipulative Physiol Ther. 1999; 22(5):322–332

[13] Guo L, Meacham KW, Hochman S, DeWeerth SP. A PDMS-based conical-well microelectrode array for surface stimulation and recording of neural tissues. IEEE Trans Biomed Eng. 2010; 57(10):2485–2494

[14] Borton D, Bonizzato M, Beauparlant J, et al. Corticospinal neuroprostheses to restore locomotion after spinal cord injury. Neurosci Res. 2014; 78:21–29

[15] Capogrosso M, Milekovic T, Borton D, et al. A brain-spine interface alleviating gait deficits after spinal cord injury in primates. Nature. 2016; 539(7628):284–288

[16] Tarabichi OVN, Kanumuri VV, Lacour SP, Brown MC, Lee DJ. Evaluation of a Flexible Auditory Brainstem Implant in Mice. American Academy of Otolaryngology-Head and Neck Surgery Annual Meeting; Chicago, IL, USA. September 2017

[17] Rosahl SK, Rosahl S. No easy target: anatomic constraints of electrodes interfacing the human cochlear nucleus. Neurosurgery. 2013; 72(1) Suppl Operative:58–64, discussion 65

[18] Guex AA, Vachicouras N, Hight AE, Brown MC, Lee DJ, Lacour SP. Conducting polymer electrodes for auditory brainstem implants. J Mater Chem B Mater Biol Med. 2015; 3(25):5021–5027

[19] Minev IR, Wenger N, Courtine G, Lacour SP. Research update: platinum-elastomer mesocomposite as neural electrode coating. APL Mater. 2015; 3(1): 014701

[20] Kuchta J, Otto SR, Shannon RV, Hitselberger WE, Brackmann DE. The multi-channel auditory brainstem implant: how many electrodes make sense? J Neurosurg. 2004; 100(1):16–23

[21] Wells J, Kao C, Mariappan K, et al. Optical stimulation of neural tissue in vivo. Opt Lett. 2005; 30(5):504–506

[22] Wells J, Kao C, Jansen ED, Konrad P, Mahadevan-Jansen A. Application of infrared light for in vivo neural stimulation. J Biomed Opt. 2005; 10(6): 064003

[23] Richter CP, Tan X. Photons and neurons. Hear Res. 2014; 311:72–88

[24] Cayce JM, Friedman RM, Chen G, Jansen ED, Mahadevan-Jansen A, Roe AW. Infrared neural stimulation of primary visual cortex in non-human primates. Neuroimage. 2014; 84:181–190

[25] Cayce JM, Wells JD, Malphrus JD, et al. Infrared neural stimulation of human spinal nerve roots in vivo. Neurophotonics. 2015; 2(1):015007

[26] Izzo AD, Suh E, Pathria J, Walsh JT, Whitlon DS, Richter CP. Selectivity of neural stimulation in the auditory system: a comparison of optic and electric stimuli. J Biomed Opt. 2007; 12(2):021008

[27] Verma RU, Guex AA, Hancock KE, et al. Auditory responses to electric and infrared neural stimulation of the rat cochlear nucleus. Hear Res. 2014; 310: 69–75

[28] Thompson AC, Fallon JB, Wise AK, Wade SA, Shepherd RK, Stoddart PR. Infrared neural stimulation fails to evoke neural activity in the deaf guinea pig cochlea. Hear Res. 2015; 324:46–53

[29] Bin J, Nan X, Xing W, et al. Auditory responses to short-wavelength infrared neural stimulation of the rat cochlear nucleus. Conference proceedings: ... Annual International Conference of the IEEE Engineering in Medicine and Biology Society. IEEE Engineering in Medicine and Biology Society. Annual Conference. Jul 2017;2017:1942–1945

[30] Richter CP, Rajguru SM, Matic AI, et al. Spread of cochlear excitation during stimulation with pulsed infrared radiation: inferior colliculus measurements. J Neural Eng. 2011; 8(5):056006

[31] Boyden ES, Zhang F, Bamberg E, Nagel G, Deisseroth K. Millisecond-timescale, genetically targeted optical control of neural activity. Nat Neurosci. 2005; 8 (9):1263–1268

[32] Guru A, Post RJ, Ho YY, Warden MR. Making sense of optogenetics. Int J Neuropsychopharmacol. 2015; 18(11):pyv079

[33] Boyden ES. A history of optogenetics: the development of tools for controlling brain circuits with light. F1000 Biol Rep. 2011; 3:11

[34] Bernstein JG, Han X, Henninger MA, et al. Prosthetic systems for therapeutic optical activation and silencing of genetically-targeted neurons. Proc SPIE Int Soc Opt Eng. 2008; 6854:68540H

[35] Llewellyn ME, Thompson KR, Deisseroth K, Delp SL. Orderly recruitment of motor units under optical control in vivo. Nat Med. 2010; 16(10):1161–1165

[36] Deisseroth K. Optogenetics: 10 years of microbial opsins in neuroscience. Nat Neurosci. 2015; 18(9):1213–1225

[37] Tye KM, Mirzabekov JJ, Warden MR, et al. Dopamine neurons modulate neural encoding and expression of depression-related behaviour. Nature. 2013; 493 (7433):537–541

[38] Ordaz JD, Wu W, Xu XM. Optogenetics and its application in neural degeneration and regeneration. Neural Regen Res. 2017; 12(8):1197–1209

[39] Madisen L, Mao T, Koch H, et al. A toolbox of Cre-dependent optogenetic transgenic mice for light-induced activation and silencing. Nat Neurosci. 2012; 15(5):793–802

[40] Maguire AM, Simonelli F, Pierce EA, et al. Safety and efficacy of gene transfer for Leber's congenital amaurosis. N Engl J Med. 2008; 358(21):2240–2248

[41] Nathwani AC, Tuddenham EG, Rangarajan S, et al. Adenovirus-associated virus vector-mediated gene transfer in hemophilia B. N Engl J Med. 2011; 365 (25):2357–2365

[42] Hight AE, Kozin ED, Darrow K, et al. Superior temporal resolution of Chronos versus channelrhodopsin-2 in an optogenetic model of the auditory brainstem implant. Hear Res. 2015; 322:235–241

[43] Darrow KN, Slama MC, Kozin ED, et al. Optogenetic stimulation of the cochlear nucleus using channelrhodopsin-2 evokes activity in the central auditory pathways. Brain Res. 2015; 1599:44–56

[44] Sinha SKA, Hight AE, Kozin ED, et al. Systemic Delivery of Opsins to Cochlear Nucleus Neurons Using Adeno-Associated Virus. Association for Research in Otolaryngology-midwinter meeting 2014. 2014:Poster Presentation. 2014, San Diego, CA

[45] Wu Z, Yang H, Colosi P. Effect of genome size on AAV vector packaging. Mol Ther. 2010; 18(1):80–86

[46] Hight AE, Narasimhan S, Meng X, Hirschbiegel C, Edge AS, Brown MC, Lee DJ. Optogenetic Stimulation of Mouse Cochlear Nucleus Using Transgenic Lines for Cell-Specific Expression of Opsins. Association for Research in Otolaryngology-midwinter meeting. 2014, San Diego, CA

[47] Shimano T, Fyk-Kolodziej B, Mirza N, et al. Assessment of the AAV-mediated expression of channelrhodopsin-2 and halorhodopsin in brainstem neurons mediating auditory signaling. Brain Res. 2013; 1511:138–152

[48] Nagel G, Szellas T, Huhn W, et al. Channelrhodopsin-2, a directly light-gated cation-selective membrane channel. Proc Natl Acad Sci U S A. 2003; 100(24): 13940–13945

[49] Pisanello F, Sileo L, Oldenburg IA, et al. Multipoint-emitting optical fibers for spatially addressable in vivo optogenetics. Neuron. 2014; 82(6):1245–1254

[50] McAlinden N, Massoubre D, Richardson E, et al. Thermal and optical characterization of micro-LED probes for in vivo optogenetic neural stimulation. Opt Lett. 2013; 38(6):992–994

[51] Elwassif MM, Kong Q, Vazquez M, Bikson M. Bio-heat transfer model of deep brain stimulation-induced temperature changes. J Neural Eng. 2006; 3(4): 306–315

[52] Guex AA, Lacour S. Selective electrical and optical neuromodulation of the central nervous system with conformable microfabricated implants. Graduate Thesis-École polytechnique fédérale de Lausanne. 2017

Index

Note: Page numbers set **bold** or *italic* indicate headings or figures, respectively.